Conducting
Clinical Trials

Conducting Clinical Trials

Frank L. Iber, M.D.

Hines Veterans Administration Medical Center
and Loyola University Stritch School of Medicine
Mayfield, Illinois
Formerly University of Maryland School of Medicine
Baltimore, Maryland

W. Anthony Riley, M.D.

Baltimore Medical System, Inc.
Baltimore, Maryland

and

Patricia J. Murray, B.A.

Boston, Massachusetts

Plenum Medical Book Company
New York and London

Library of Congress Cataloging in Publication Data

Iber, Frank L., 1928–
    Conducting clinical trials.

    Bibliography: p.
    Includes index.
    1. Drugs—Testing. 2. Clinical trials. I. Riley, W. Anthony (Wallace Anthony) II. Murray, Patricia J. III. Title. [DNLM: 1. Clinical Trials. QV 771 I12c]
RM301.I24   1987   615.5   87-15273
ISBN 0-306-42626-9

First Printing—September 1987
Second Printing—May 1989

© 1987 Plenum Publishing Corporation
233 Spring Street, New York, N.Y. 10013

Plenum Medical Book Company is an imprint of Plenum Publishing Corporation

Printed in the United States of America

To Alan G. Woodman,
whose vision of the clinical trials process
brought us together

Preface

A few years ago, two of us joined our senior colleague at Pharma-Kinetics Laboratories, a newly public contract research firm just undertaking a major expansion into the clinical trials market. The company's unique concept of clinical research held great promise and had successfully endured many of the fits and starts characteristic of entrepreneurial organizations. With a staff of highly enthusiastic, albeit inexperienced, field personnel located in 30-odd cities around the country, we found ourselves off and running with several critical research programs for major pharmaceutical manufacturers. Our excitement with the innovation was tempered with the reality of staffing and bearing responsibility for more than 30 field offices and 300 new staff persons, more than half of whom had no previous experience in the pharmaceutical industry.

In the ensuing few years, we explored by trial and error many workable and unworkable patterns of training, delegation, data collection, and auditing. The ideas expressed in this book benefited greatly from that experience and from the willingness of our co-workers and clients to share insights and problems. During those years, we also sought guidance from the works available on the clinical trials field. Although we found numerous references on research ethics, little guidance was available on the practical aspects of conducting a clinical trial. Our decision to collaborate on this work was largely the result of our inability to find such a work when it was so badly needed by our many new investigators and staff members. Although, in retrospect, we expanded too rapidly, trained too poorly, and intervened too slowly, we hope the lessons of our own experience will make the road to successful research a little easier for future research physicians and personnel.

This book represents a blend of the very different outlooks from which each of us considers the research process. Frank Iber has had extensive experience conducting research in an academic setting and has served as a member and chairman of several institutional review boards. His seasoned perspective has served this work well in tempering his colleagues' occasionally misplaced enthusiasm for the intellectually correct though highly unworkable solution. Tony Riley has brought to our collective experience a relentless insistence that all of the policies, practices, and reward systems we have developed reflect some very fundamental principles of competent health care delivery. His experience in medical practice management has provided the expertise with which to develop a process for incorporating personal ethics and values into an effective organizational design. P. J. Murray has had the opportunity to observe the clinical trials field from both the institutional and industrial perspectives, first as the administrator for an institutional review board, and subsequently as a field clinical monitoring associate for a major pharmaceutical firm. Her fearless idealism, unfettered by awe of physicians and grounded firmly in both the ethics and the economics of the research discipline, added greatly to this work. We did not always agree, either in the workplace or in recording our views, but completed this book with a rich respect for one another and a tolerance for our divergent opinions.

This book is intended for the new clinical investigator and his staff in need of practical advice on how to overcome the problems of recruitment, data management, and preserving the quality of a clinical trial. It also should be useful for the new entrant into the pharmaceutical industry who must evaluate the performance of clinical investigators and understand the workings of the institutional committees that have a prominent place in research regulation. The goal of this book is to provide the new investigator with a solid grounding in basic research procedures that will enable him to successfully execute his first clinical trial.

Actual examples from our own experience are presented in this book for amplification of key points. One of our colleagues in the pharmaceutical industry who read an early draft was skeptical of some of the more negative experiences presented—notably, an example of a sponsor's clinical research associate who encouraged data falsification. Still another colleague expressed great surprise in learning that we had characterized our experience with an FDA audit as quite positive. Although the research field is so complex that it cannot easily be represented in a selection of anecdotes, we can assure our readers that we have done our best to choose actual examples that reflect the variety of situations a clinical investigator may expect to face. Although names and identifying details have been changed to protect the confidentiality of those involved, we have attempted to preserve the essential elements of each case.

No preface would be complete without acknowledging the behind-the-scenes efforts of those who helped make the project a reality. Special thanks are due to Victoria Hanbury, whose tireless search for the perfect phrase produced a much more readable work than we otherwise could have achieved. We also owe a substantial debt to Mary Brooks-Ellis, who typed and organized our numerous drafts. She successfully overcame what seemed at times an insurmountable problem of coordinating the work styles of three very busy and geographically distant people. Many other of our industry and academic colleagues have read and reread portions of this book and have offered excellent suggestions and additions that have enhanced the book's utility and clarity. We extend to all of them our sincere thanks.

Chicago, Illinois   Frank L. Iber, M.D.
Baltimore, Maryland   W. Anthony Riley, M.D.
Boston, Massachusetts   Patricia J. Murray, B.A.

Contents

I. Introduction

II. Entering the Field of Clinical Trials

III. The Institutional Review Mechanism

IV. The Recruitment Process

V. Critical Decision Points in a Clinical Trial

VI. Data Management

VII.   Drug Accountability

VIII.   Enhancing Credibility

IX.   Appendixes

Introduction

This section traces the development of the many scientific advances and evolving concepts of research ethics that continue to influence contemporary research practices. It also includes an overview of the current regulatory approval process.

CHAPTER 1

Introduction

Science, Animal Testing, and Statistics • *Research Ethics and Regulation* • *Investigators, Subjects, and Sponsors* • *The Drug Approval Process* • *Prognosis for the Future*

Most of the scientific methods relating to human drug testing are undergoing orderly change. Animal testing of toxicity, evaluation of human therapeutic effects, statistical analysis, monitoring of improvement in disease, and design of human studies have changed in progressive steps that appeared slow and appropriate to those who lived through these changes but are dramatic when the changes are looked at in brief review. All of these changes result in better standards of laboratory and human testing such that what was commonplace and accepted even ten years ago is no longer up to the standard of today. Regulations, on the other hand, have usually changed abruptly in response to one or more seminal issues arising from abuse of the public. This introductory chapter will trace the development of the ethical and regulatory concepts that have influenced and controlled current research practices to provide a framework that the new investigator or research administrator may find useful in interpreting this work.

SCIENCE, ANIMAL TESTING, AND STATISTICS

Before 1930 new medicines and new formulations emerged from a limited number of university and industry laboratories testing for specific effects in animals or, occasionally, in man. There were very few drugs to be tested and most new entities arose from empirical data generated throughout the world. The pharmaceutical industry's production of new chemical substances to test as possible drugs increased from a few new ones each year before 1920 to several hundred each year in the 1930s and 1940s. Now computer design of many thousands of new molecules is undertaken. Each year new animal models to test possible drug effects appear that enable predictions to be made about the therapeutic value of a potential drug. Toxicological, oncogenic, and teratogenic effects of drugs can also be identified from animal cell test systems. As these new bodies of information have become established, the standards of the industry and regulation have usually changed to conform to the new technology.

Testing of drugs in humans has also evolved. Short-term changes in organ function such as the kidney or the heart can now be assessed with about the same precision as in animal experiments. Noninvasive monitoring using isotopes and scintillation cameras and computer storage of data have permitted more detailed evaluation of drug effects on the heart, GI tract, and brain, allowing much more precise assessments of what has taken place. Experimental design has shifted from an imprecise clinical evaluation, including patient perception of benefit, to the direct quantification of improved function of the whole person or the organ under study. The double-blind, placebo-controlled study design that became the standard of the industry in the late 1950s still remains important. However, many alternative designs are also contributing in a major fashion to assessment of drug effects. Sequential analysis has lessened the number of participants necessary in controlled trials; rank-sum techniques permit quantification in many studies that formerly could not be so treated.

Such progress imposes new responsibilities and unprecedented economic commitments. From 1962 to 1972, it is estimated that the industry's cost to produce a new drug application (NDA) needed to secure marketing approval of a new product increased by a factor of 5.[1] Analyses that take into account the attrition rate of new drugs at various stages of the development process reveal that approximately $100 million are spent over a period of 12 years to produce a new product that actually reaches the point of marketing approval.[2] In addition, greater public interest in the drug-testing process has enhanced appreciation of its important role in establishing the safety and effectiveness of new medicines. However, many well-motivated patients still harbor great suspicions of the drug-development process that make them reluctant to take medication described as producing toxicity of any kind, whatever the anticipated benefits. Teaching prospective research subjects to feel comfortable with the responsibility of making informed choices among competing therapies will demand all of the professional expertise and resources a clinician can bring to bear.

In reaching its current state of maturity, the research field faces a difficult challenge. Investigators and sponsors must not only meet ex-

acting scientific and regulatory standards, which demand highly sophisticated testing and record-keeping procedures, but also persuade
an ambivalent public to accept its crucial role in the risk–benefit assessment process.

RESEARCH ETHICS AND REGULATION

The ethics of human experimentation were codified following
World War II in *The Nuremberg Code,* which addressed the extreme
abuse of prisoners in Nazi Germany in medical experiments. The
World Medical Association subsequently expanded on these principles
in its 1964 *Declaration of Helsinki: Recommendations Guiding Medical Doctors in Biomedical Research Involving Human Subjects* (revised
in 1975). These landmark documents in the field of medical ethics, on
which all current regulations and practices are based, formalized such
concepts as voluntary and informed consent, risk–benefit assessment,
and the conflict of interest inherent in a physician's dual role as practitioner and investigator. These documents have been reprinted widely
and can easily be found in most textbooks on medical ethics. Aside
from these two broad ethical codes and similar guidelines issued by
professional organizations such as the American Medical Association,
the field of clinical research received little outside attention until the
1960s.

The Food and Drug Administration came into being initially to test
the quality of food sold in interstate commerce, following reports of
widespread abuse. Expansion in the FDA's mission and responsibilities usually has been in reaction to popular clamor resulting from
some abuse of the public trust. The thalidomide tragedy occurring
mostly in Europe in which children were born without hands and feet
because their mothers took the drug during pregnancy resulted in extensive review and revision of drug-testing regulations under the Kefauver commission.

In the 1960s, a study of rejection of transplanted cells from one
human to another conducted at the Jewish Chronic Disease Hospital in
Brooklyn drew considerable public attention. Live cancer cells were
injected into 22 patients who had been hospitalized with various
chronic illnesses. During the disciplinary proceedings, in which the
investigators were censured for their actions, they revealed that they
had not informed subjects that the injected material contained liver
cancer cells because they wished to avoid both emotional responses
from the patients and refusals of participation.[3] Henry K. Beecher published a classic study in the *New England Journal of Medicine* in 1966

citing published research papers involving possible unethical practices.[4] These were widely publicized and amplified in the lay press.

In 1966 the concept of peer review, long preferred by physicians
and scientists as a method of regulating their professional activities,
was formally extended to clinical research. In that year, the Public
Health Service issued a policy requiring that all of an institution's
research grant requests involving human subjects be reviewed by one
peer review committee with official standing within the facility. Ten
years earlier, the National Institutes of Health (NIH) had instituted such
a requirement at its own Bethesda facility. However, the precedent was
not widely applied until the 1966 requirement became effective. Although these initial policies and those of the Department of Health and
Human Services (DHHS) today officially apply only to research under
federal sponsorship or involving regulated products, most institutions
have established multidisciplinary institutional review boards (IRBs)
to guide physicians on the conduct of all protocols regardless of their
funding source. These IRBs have become the primary vehicle by which
the federal government administers regulations governing the protection of human subjects.

Since several federal agencies have the authority to regulate some
aspects of clinical research activities, it is worthwhile to review their
unique mandates and how they are reflected in current legislations.
The DHHS, which essentially replaced the Department of Health, Education, and Welfare (DHEW) in 1980, is the parent agency of the United
States Public Health Service (USPHS), which contains the NIH and
FDA. The FDA's role in overseeing clinical trials encompasses prescription drugs, over-the-counter (OTC) products, biologics, and medical devices. Research on food products, cosmetics, and certain health-
promoting but not disease-curing devices (e.g., sunlamps) is excluded.
The FDA Bureau of Drugs maintains a staff of scientists and statisti-
cians who review applications for marketing and periodic safety reports on commercially available drugs. Agency personnel also conduct
laboratory research that may aid in the evaluation of new submissions.
The agency's authority in the health research area encompasses pharmaceuticals, biologics, and devices moved in interstate commerce for
either investigational or commercial purposes. As a funding agency,
the NIH issues ethical and scientific policies applicable to biomedical
and behavioral research, both projects conducted at its own facility in
Bethesda and those extramural projects to which it provides grant support. The Drug Enforcement Administration, an arm of the Department
of Justice, has statutory authority to oversee the storage and dispensation of controlled substances used for investigational purposes.

Of these agencies, the NIH and the FDA are specifically charged with supervising the ethical aspects of research involving human subjects. The NIH maintains an Office for the Protection from Research Risks (OPRR), whose administrators have been heavily involved in the development of regulations governing IRBs and research involving vulnerable groups such as children and prisoners. In the past, the research community had strongly advocated that the OPRR and FDA adopt a uniform set of regulations applicable to clinical investigations under either agency's jurisdiction. This desire for uniformity led the two agencies to collaborate successfully in producing revisions to the regulations governing IRBs. The 1981 regulations, issued separately by OPRR and FDA, are nearly identical in form and reflect a common philosophy regarding the IRB's role in the protection of human subjects. These regulations represent the first collaborative effort by the NIH and FDA to produce a uniform set of requirements for IRB and consent functions and extend the FDA requirement for IRB review to research on outpatient populations. They also include a requirement that even research not expected to involve any risk to human subjects must be approved by a qualified IRB. The regulations do include a provision for no- or minimal-risk studies to be reviewed by an expedited committee procedure and give even greater autonomy to committees.

Much of the pressure for regulatory reform can be attributed to the National Commission for the Protection of Human Subjects of Biomedical and Behavioral Research. This commission met extensively over a four-year period to develop ethical guidelines for research involving human subjects that could be applied to projects receiving federal funding. Its influence was felt most heavily in the 1981 revisions to the regulations governing the protection of human subjects. The current IRB regulations reflect many of the practices that the IRBs of major teaching institutions have developed over the years and at their inception in 1981 involved few procedural changes for experienced committees. The implementation of these regulations is discussed in greater detail in Section III, which describes the IRB process. Several private institutes, such as the Kennedy Institute of Ethics, the Hastings Center for Ethics, Medicine, and the Life Sciences, and the Institute for Medical Humanities, also provide an ongoing forum that makes important contributions to the discipline. The President's Commission for the Study of Ethical Problems in Medicine and Biomedical and Behavioral Research, which met from 1980 to 1983, also has been a major contributor.

Although federal endorsement of the IRB process reflects the government's growing concern with the ethics of research activities, the NIH and FDA have clearly indicated that the IRB is not expected to take on a policing function. Rather, IRB review is meant to provide a forum for clinical investigators to receive assistance in making the difficult ethical choices involved in any project involving human subjects. While the IRB has the authority to prohibit research from being conducted if it does not satisfy minimum conditions for ethical acceptability, or if there is evidence that it is being conducted in a manner that does not follow the protocol, the IRB strives to collaborate with the investigator to design a project that meets appropriate scientific and ethical standards. The greatest portion of the IRB's review activities occur while a project is in proposed form, and with annual reviews. At present, IRBs are not required to supervise the actual conduct of a research protocol once it has been approved, or to verify independently that the conditions of approval are, in fact, being adhered to. Neither are IRBs expected to conduct detailed scientific reviews of research proposals or clinical data to verify that they are accurate and complete. While IRBs do enjoy considerable latitude to undertake such activities if so mandated by their parent institutions, the FDA continues to emphasize that the responsibility for the integrity of the study lies completely with the investigator and sponsor. This point is clearly reflected in the many other regulations NIH and FDA have issued in the health research area.

The OPRR has issued several sets of regulations that may be of interest to research teams, namely, those governing research on fetuses, children, prisoners, and patients institutionalized as mentally disabled (proposed regulations). Although investigators conducting FDA-regulated research are not currently required to comply with these regulations, the OPRR's policies do reflect the views of the research community and are widely accepted as ethical guidelines. The FDA has independently published proposed regulations on the obligations of clinical investigators and sponsors that have been in existence for several years and so have been adopted by much of the pharmaceutical community despite their tentative status. The FDA regulations governing the IND/NDA process for drug approvals (21 CFR Part 312 and 21 CFR Part 314, respectively) and postmarketing toxicity surveillance (21 CFR Part 314.8) exist in final form. Both the NIH and the FDA have independent mechanisms for overseeing the IRB process. OPRR has developed an extensive general assurance mechanism to assure that IRBs reviewing federally funded research are, in fact, organized as the agency requires. The FDA maintains an agencywide bioresearch monitoring program in which it periodically inspects IRBs reviewing research on new drugs, biologics, and devices.

INVESTIGATORS, SUBJECTS, AND SPONSORS

It is currently estimated that at least 500 new physicians take part in clinical trials each year as principal investigators (PIs) and that an equal number participate as members of teams investigating new products or devices. Only a minority of these physicians have specific training in the area of clinical trials. Most gain experience as they proceed, depending heavily on representatives of industry, their IRBs, and independent study for guidance. This highly unstructured learning process involves considerable trial and error, which can expose research subjects to some unnecessary risks. In fact, it can be estimated that the data of approximately 10 to 30% of the patients taking part in outpatient drug testing are excluded from eventual regulatory submissions because the selection, compliance, or documentation of their participation was found lacking.[5] Since many patients choose to take part in clinical research partly to further medical knowledge about new treatment modalities, investigators who fail to contribute evaluable data compromise their commitment to their subjects. Furthermore, if deficiencies at individual sites render a whole study unusable, the entire study population has been subjected to the risks of investigational therapy without societal benefit. In an environment of limited research resources, errors can delay the introduction of worthwhile new medications and engender public distrust of the drug-development process. The magnitude of these potential resource and ethical issues demands that the new investigator or administrator gain familiarity with current standards before undertaking a new research endeavor.

In addition to demanding regulatory requirements, the investigator faces new challenges with a changing population of research subjects. The public, heavily influenced by the mass media, is better informed about the therapeutic advances that were made possible through scientific discovery. Yet the public remains suspicious because of the many tragedies that have resulted when the pharmaceutical industry has not lived up to the ethical and scientific standards it has established. Now that competitors of the traditional health care system have begun to offer patients advantages (e.g., cost-free care) that formerly were unique to the research setting, the investigative team faces greater pressure to offer prospective research subjects benefits that are not being delivered by practitioners, health maintenance organizations, medical teaching institutions, or free-standing clinics. The increasing importance of the concept of voluntary informed consent also poses a challenge for the contemporary investigator. He now must teach prospective subjects to distinguish between the more passive role they may have chosen to adopt as patients and the decision-making responsibility for the risk–

benefit assessment they must accept as research subjects. Many new investigators, unaccustomed to restricting their authority in routine clinical interventions, find it difficult to train reluctant subjects in the responsibility for evaluating complex scientific information and deciding whether or not to participate in a research study. While the medical profession as a whole is acknowledging the necessity of making patients active partners in their own health care, the research community emphasizes more strongly that investigators must *not* take on this decision-making authority in experimental situations. The fears of ethical abuses and mistrust of the discipline as a whole can be abated only by more open discussions of the uncertainties in the scientific process.

The pharmaceutical sponsor has the following responsibilities, which are essential to a successful clinical program: (1) selecting the strategic business objective and compound that is suitable for R&D investment, (2) assembling the research team qualified to develop and execute a testing program for the new product, (3) supervising the conduct of the study to confirm that current regulatory and scientific standards are being met, (4) monitoring adverse experience data to determine whether any unexpected or significant side effects are being observed with clinical use, (5) promptly reporting the outcome of the study or any significant findings to the medical community and regulatory agencies, and (6) conducting postmarketing surveillance of a newly approved agent to follow any potential adverse experiences associated with long-term or widespread use. The manner in which these responsibilities are executed will determine the ultimate success or failure of the study.

The sponsor completely assumes the financial and strategic risks associated with drug development. Excluding overhead expenses, the cost to study 500 patients in a multisite investigation may be as high as $5 million, with a poorly executed clinical trial delaying introduction of a new medication for two to three years. The manufacturer must also accept liability for any adverse effects of the protocol or study drug. Product liability suits and regulatory pressure have provided the impetus for firms to acquire the scientific and regulatory expertise needed to fulfill the above responsibilities more effectively.

THE DRUG APPROVAL PROCESS

Regulations governing the purity and safety of drugs appeared in 1938, when the large number of ineffective and unsafe medications appearing on the market raised public consciousness about the destructive potential of insufficiently tested and improperly labeled medications. In the 1960s, the FDA's authority was broadened to include efficacy testing of new drugs. The Kefauver–Harris amendments to the Food, Drug, and Cosmetic (FD&C) Act stipulated that "adequate and well-controlled clinical trials" would be required to support an application to market a new drug. These amendments, therefore, allowed the agency to evaluate the scientific validity of any research data submitted as evidence of a new drug's safety and effectiveness. They also gave the agency greater authority to remove drugs from the market if they were found to be unsafe and extended this authority to removal of drugs found ineffective. This authority has significantly shaped the way the agency views its regulatory mandate today and has gradually increased standards of effectiveness.

The American system of drug regulation is characterized by a lengthy regulatory process that is discussed quite often in the lay press. This system reflects a strong scientific preference for limiting testing of unproven products to a well-defined population studied under controlled conditions, an ethical viewpoint that is manifest in all regulations promulgated on the field of research. In contrast, some European nations permit the release of drugs on the market at a much earlier stage of the testing process, thereby depending on postmarketing surveillance studies to reveal any significant toxicities that may occur with widespread use.

The Kefauver–Harris amendments initiated the development of new drug-testing standards that now encompass all phases of the R&D process and establish specific conditions under which human testing may begin. Before a new medication may be administered to human subjects, extensive studies must be undertaken in at least two animal species (usually rodents, dogs, and, rarely, primates). These studies must provide toxicity data on short- and long-term dosing, including the LD50, or dose of the study medication that succeeded in producing death in 50% of the animal test population. These animal studies suggest the dosage required for efficacy in animal models of the illness. Although animal studies can successfully predict toxicities likely to occur with human use, they have little value in suggesting possible hypersensitivities or idiosyncratic reactions that might be observed in clinical testing or with widespread use. The experienced pharmacologist John Arnold has estimated that even with extensive animal data, about one-third of more than 300 compounds his research group tested showed properties that could not easily be predicted from animal data.[6] Since the life-threatening toxicities can be predicted, however, death among the first few hundred test subjects is extremely rare.

Once animal and preliminary manufacturing data are available, a sponsor makes a submission to the FDA to initiate clinical testing in the form of an investigational new drug (IND) exemption. An IND represents a notice that the sponsor wishes an exemption from the restriction on interstate shipment of drugs not approved for commercial distribution. It requires that the sponsor provide data on the chemical structure, manufacturing, animal studies, and plans for clinical study of the new agent. Upon receiving an IND notice, the FDA has 30 days to request additional information on the proposed research activities. Once that deadline passes, the research activities may proceed. A "new drug" subject to clinical investigation is defined very strictly for regulatory purposes. A drug is considered a new entity if it comprises a combination of commercially available drugs not currently available in a combined dosage form in those proportions; or if the drug is being used to treat a new disease for which it is not currently approved; or if the drug is being administered in a new dosage, dosage form, or dosing schedule; or, finally, if the drug is being manufactured with a different combination of fillers or inert ingredients.[7]

Within six months of an IND's submission to the FDA, the new entity is given a rating that will establish its priority for review within the agency. This rating takes into account the results of early pharmacologic studies and any research experience with the drug abroad. Drugs are classified numerically on a scale from 1 to 6 as to whether they represent new molecular entities, new salts or other derivatives of available drugs, or duplicates of drugs already on the market. The drugs also receive a letter rating that "represents the FDA's opinion about whether they represent a major (A), a modest (or moderate) (B), or little or no appreciable (C) therapeutic advance over currently available drugs; other letters are used to designate, for example, whether a drug would be useful in children or whether it is marketed abroad."[8] This rating may be updated as new safety and efficacy findings emerge.

Clinical testing of new drugs occurs in four phases. Phase I investigations involve the earliest administrations of the drug to man. These are ordinarily open-label or single-blind studies conducted in healthy male volunteers and serve to establish appropriate dosage schedules, pharmacology, dose tolerance, and a preliminary side-effect profile of the drug. Increasingly, special populations (such as the elderly) for whom a medication is most likely to be prescribed in clinical practice are being asked to participate in pharmacology studies early in testing to identify any safety differences unique to those populations.

Following Phase I studies, the sponsor initiates Phase II studies, which represent the earliest trials in a limited population (50–200 subjects) with the disease for which the drug will primarily be marketed. These constitute some of the "adequate and well-controlled clinical trials" and may be designed to determine the effective dose for larger trials. Studies are considered "adequate and well-controlled" if they include the following: (1) a clear statement of objectives and methods for final data analysis; (2) a design that permits comparison of the test group with a control to quantitatively determine the study drug's effectiveness and safety; (3) procedures for selecting subjects that include methods for verifying that they have the condition being studied; (4) a method of treatment assignment selected to minimize bias and assure comparability of subjects with respect to age, sex, severity and duration of disease, and uses of concomitant therapy; (5) sufficient blinding procedures to minimize bias on the part of the subjects and investigative team; (6) outcome measures that are well defined and reliable; (7) an analysis chosen to determine outcome that is appropriate to the design. All of the above principles must be both incorporated into the study design and documented in the protocol itself.[9] For many classes of drugs, the FDA has guidelines for protocol design, and its staff will informally review and advise on protocols that are in the formative stage.

Once Phase II studies have been completed, the FDA holds a formal conference with the sponsor of a 1A or 1B drug to review findings and discuss plans for additional studies. All further clinical trials are labeled Phase III investigations. They represent the expanded controlled and uncontrolled clinical trials designed to gather additional data supporting effectiveness in major indications and specific data on adverse experiences. At the conclusion of Phase III trials, the sponsor files a new drug application, or NDA, which provides complete data on the drug's pharmacology, animal toxicology, clinical study results, and manufacturing and labeling information.

This NDA application is reviewed by a team of FDA personnel, consisting of a physician, a pharmacologist, a chemist, a pharmacokineticist, and, where appropriate, a biometrician or microbiologist.[10] Significant NDAs are forwarded to advisory committees of outside experts in the fields in which the drug will be used. These committees recommend whether or not the NDA should be approved and specify labeling requirements and postmarketing surveillance testing that should be included as conditions of approval. Postmarketing studies are being required more frequently to assure identification of possible toxicities associated with long-term use or rare adverse experiences that did not emerge in the IND phase. These postmarketing studies, combined with additional clinical trials in secondary indications and comparative studies against available competitive products, constitute the Phase IV investigations of the drug. Phase IV investigations begin anytime after the NDA has been filed.

The philosophy guiding the four-phase testing process is that the standard testing sequence provides an effective means of determining safety and effectiveness with the smallest possible population. For example, a clinical trial comparing a test product with a competitor's agent requires a larger population to achieve statistical significance than a trial comparing the test agent with placebo. Thus, marketing studies comparing similar medications are not considered ethically justified until Phase II studies establishing the new agent's basic safety profile have been completed.

PROGNOSIS FOR THE FUTURE

The process of drug testing is rapidly evolving in a fashion that produces research which is of better quality but, unfortunately, more expensive to conduct. Increasingly, all aspects of bioavailability and improvements to dosage forms are being evaluated in the population targeted for use of the drug. Establishing bioavailability in the desired patient population rather than in young, healthy males provides important clinical data that will benefit both the investigative team and private practitioners who subsequently prescribe the drug. Increasingly, sustained-release forms of drugs to permit once-daily or once-weekly dosages are under development. Skin absorption patches or oral sustained-release methods are growing in availability. The methods of measuring drug efficacy are becoming more sophisticated and more directly related to the disease. The availability of state-of-the-art diagnostic tests, such as isotopic function tests (e.g., gated thallium scans of the heart), and emptying tests of the esophagus, stomach, and bladder, is allowing more detailed and precise cataloguing of side effects. It has been the authors' experience that the design of a clinical trial becomes obsolete in approximately three years at the present rate of progress.

The practitioner interested in conducting clinical trials will also face new pressures in the form of greater competition for the research dollar. For-profit contract research firms have gained sufficient expertise in the recruiting sphere to outdo their academic counterparts in performing large-scale clinical trials, particularly outpatient studies. Health maintenance organizations, municipal clinics, and other provider organizations are increasingly open to the economic and educational possibilities afforded by involvement in the clinical trials process.

As far as the prospective test subject is concerned, some difficult choices must be faced. With prepaid health care plans removing many of the financial incentives for participating in clinical trials, the public at large must increasingly accept its social responsibility to advance medical knowledge by participating in research activities. Without the public's willingness to share equally in the risks associated with the development of new medicines and technologies, scientific knowledge will not be able to advance at a rate compatible with its technical potential. As changing industry and professional views of the importance of research subjects and scientific inquiry are increasingly reflected in contemporary research practices, the public should become more willing to respond to the research community's calls for its participation. Some progress in encouraging public cooperation in the testing process can already be seen. A recent demographic study of volunteers for ulcer-healing studies revealed that the majority were employed suburbanites who had insurance to support their care yet chose to participate.[11]

The FDA also faces many pressures that will provide the impetus for more stringent regulatory practices as well as some seemingly conflicting goals to lower costs. Many consumer advocates and congressional committees interested in the health care industry have put forth the view that the agency allows too many unsafe and ineffective drugs to reach the market. Meanwhile, the pharmaceutical industry cites considerable academic research suggesting that the agency is deserving of criticism for its excessive delay in approving new products. The FDA also has been the subject of criticism in a number of executive branch studies that revealed a variety of administrative deficiencies.[12] These pressures, combined with the agency's skepticism about the caliber of some of the clinical work performed to support the approval of new drugs, will undoubtedly result in greater scrutiny of investigators who conduct clinical trials.

The cost of the R&D process has increased substantially, forcing smaller firms to rely on acquisitions from foreign drug manufacturers, notably Japanese firms, to provide products suitable for clinical R&D. Generic firms are already entering the clinical trials field. In addition, the increased acceptance of clinical data generated outside of North America is also to be anticipated as worldwide research practices evolve to meet U.S. standards.

The drug industry should continue to benefit from the many legislative changes that have been instituted within the past few years. The Waxman-Hatch Act, which became law in 1984, offers the generic industry an abbreviated review procedure for generic versions of patented prescription drugs. Major pharmaceutical manufacturers also benefit from this legislation in that it offers them extended patent rights to compensate for the lengthy FDA drug-approval process. At this writing, legislation is also being considered that will allow manufacturers to export drugs not yet approved by the FDA to 15 foreign countries, provided that they license the products before exporting them. In spite of these many possible legislative advantages, the industry faces sky-rocketing R&D costs that demand substantial cost-cutting measures. Service industries, such as contract research, that may allow a firm to staff its research divisions with fewer administrative personnel should become an increasingly attractive option as overhead expenditures are examined more critically.

All this considered, although the investigator who is just joining the field of clinical research is participating in a much more demanding regulatory environment than in the past, he also has a wealth of history on which to draw. The ethical abuses that have been publicized in the past two decades have given rise to a great many worthwhile works on the ethical considerations and regulatory requirements governing the research process. A few of these have been listed in the references and offer excellent background for an investigator wishing to become better acquainted with the literature. The investigator striving to prepare his team for a challenging professional future must be willing to contribute to, and take advantage of, any of these professional resources that might help get the job done.

Part of an investigator's preparation for the future must include a willingness to evaluate critically his current research practices with respect to rapidly evolving standards and regulations. Adherence to these standards becomes even more important as the bias for large-scale research programs demands greater organization and clinical record-keeping skills. This book should provide a framework for considering each of the fundamental aspects of conducting a clinical trial, namely, its planning and budgeting, important clinical decision points, data management, and the auditing process. In each of the sections an effort has been made to distinguish between suggested methods of admin-istrative record keeping and those practices that have become accepted as standard, are required by regulation, or are optional. Clearly the investigator and his staff must evaluate the suitability of the many alternatives presented for the setting and the particular research being conducted. However, the reader is encouraged to keep in mind that one important purpose of research record keeping is to engender confi-dence in the quality of the process that produced the clinical data. While a suggestion need not be implemented simply because it has been presented as useful in one type of investigation, neither should it be discarded simply because the additional record keeping is expected to prove cumbersome. In evaluating these alternatives, the reader is encouraged to consider how well the team's proposed documentation practices would stand up to outside scrutiny in our present demanding environment. Such forethought is often the critical ingredient in developing successful research techniques.

REFERENCES

1. Weimer, D.L., Safe—and available—drugs, in: *Instead of Regulation: Alternatives to Federal Regulatory Agencies* (R.W. Poole, ed.), Lexington Books, Lexington, 1982, p. 261.
2. Tucker, D., *The World Health Market*, Euromonitor Publications, Ltd., Guildford, 1984, p. 62.
3. Hershey, N., and Miller, R.D., *Human Experimentation and the Law*, Aspen Systems Corporation, Germantown, 1976, pp. 6–7.
4. Beecher, H.K., Ethics and clinical research, *N. Engl. J. Med.* **274:**1354–1360, 1966.
5. Shapiro, M.F., and Charrow, R.P., Scientific misconduct in investigational drug trials, *N. Engl. J. Med.* **312:**731–736, 1985.
6. Barber, B., *Informed Consent in Medical Therapy and Research*, Rutgers University Press, New Brunswick, 1980, p. 157.
7. Code of Federal Regulations, Title 21, Part 310.3.
8. Finkel, M.J., The FDA's classification system for new drugs: An evaluation of therapeutic gain, *N. Engl. J. Med.* **302:**181–183, 1980, p. 181.
9. Code of Federal Regulations, Title 21, Part 314.126.
10. Finkel, M.J., The FDA's classification system for new drugs: An evaluation of therapeutic gain, *N. Engl. J. Med.* **302:**181–183, 1980, p. 182.
11. Lyon, J., and Riley, W.A., *Demographics of 400 volunteer subjects with peptic ulcer disease.* Manuscript in preparation.
12. Weimer, D.L., Safe—and available—drugs, in: *Instead of Regulation: Alternatives to Federal Regulatory Agencies* (R.W. Poole, ed.), Lexington Books, Lexington, 1982, pp. 252–253.

FURTHER READING

Bezold, C. (ed.), *Pharmaceuticals in the Year 2000: The Changing Context for Drug R&D*, Institute for Alternative Futures, Alexandria, 1983.
Shapiro, S.H., and Louis, T.A. (eds.), *Clinical Trials: Issues and Approaches*, Marcel Dekker, Inc., New York, 1983.
Tygstrup, N., Lachin, J.M., and Juhl, E. (eds.), *The Randomized Clinical Trial and Therapeutic Decisions*, Marcel Dekker, Inc., New York, 1982.

Entering the Field of Clinical Trials

There are many differences between the research care setting and that of the routine office practice. This section describes the detailed planning and preparation that must be accomplished before deciding to conduct regulated clinical trials and suggests how a new investigator might evaluate a pharmaceutical sponsor with whom he is considering taking on these activities.

CHAPTER 2

Deciding to Enter the Research Field

Considerations in Deciding to Conduct Clinical Research • *Personal/ Professional Motivations* • *Financial Considerations* • *Impact on Staff, Colleagues, and Facility* • *Clinical Issues*

CONSIDERATIONS IN DECIDING TO CONDUCT CLINICAL RESEARCH

The physician who sets clear objectives for his participation in a clinical trial has a greater likelihood of reaping the desired rewards of such an undertaking. There are many worthwhile reasons for entering the research field, but there is also a price for doing so. The purpose of this chapter is to outline these potential rewards and drawbacks so the prospective investigator will be better prepared to assess the scope of the responsibility he is considering. While research may seem to offer a ready solution to short-term economic or professional needs, hastily initiated protocols rarely produce the desired results for either the investigator or the sponsor. Conversely, investigators who take the opportunity to prepare their colleagues and employees for the changes that can be expected will enjoy much more cooperation when the new responsibilities and tasks must be faced. The motivation of the PI is such a critical ingredient to the success of a clinical trial that he should make the effort to define his expectations and consider their price before entering into a commitment from which he cannot withdraw easily or inexpensively. The investigator must be willing to weigh the benefits he has identified against the many personal or professional sacrifices that will be required. These considerations must be addressed at two critical points in the planning process: (1) when the possibility of entering the research field is being considered, and (2) when a specific protocol is being reviewed so the staff does not find itself saddled with a burdensome protocol not suited to the facility. If the general objectives of the endeavor have been clearly established, deciding whether a particular research protocol is an appropriate undertaking should require little effort.

These cautionary words are not meant to discourage the new investigator or practice group anxious to diversify their professional activities or revenue base—quite the contrary, well-executed clinical trials produce many attractive rewards. However, clinical research is an activity that demands considerable intellectual energy and commitment, particularly in this era of increasing regulation. Clinical R&D has become quite a costly undertaking for pharmaceutical manufacturers and, while they may be generous in their remuneration, they do expect investigators to adhere to ambitious performance objectives. The investigator who is committed to meet those goals and has the support of his colleagues and staff is much more likely to find enjoyment in the challenge and diversity of the research experience.

PERSONAL/PROFESSIONAL MOTIVATIONS

The investigator may consider entering the research field as a means of diversifying his medical work for the sake of self- or career development. The excitement of delving into new areas and discussing the latest scientific developments with colleagues provides powerful intrinsic rewards to some investigators. Participation in multicenter programs usually includes opportunities to enjoy travel and collegiality at investigators' meetings. The investigator may also desire the prestige and the special professional expertise patients and peers often attribute to the research physician. The prospect of these rewards must be considered in light of the reality that the work of clinical research is at times a mundane, repetitive chore that must be attended to every day of the year. Its fruition, even just reaching the point of discussing preliminary findings, is a long time coming and only briefly savored.

The opportunity to procure clinically useful sophisticated equipment or to recruit technical staff that otherwise would not have been affordable is also attractive. Sponsors do not expect that equipment supplied for research purposes will be used exclusively for the study. They may also choose to donate study equipment to the institution or group at the project's conclusion. Further, research techniques often become the state-of-the-art clinical practice. The competitive advantages of being on the leading edge are obvious.

EXAMPLE 1. High Tech

An automated recording apparatus for taking blood pressure and pulse is widely used in intensive care units. This technology was used to obtain highly uniform blood pressure readings in an outpatient study of a new antihypertensive agent. This equipment provided an efficient means of collecting highly uniform blood pressure data. Funds provided from the study enabled the investigative team to purchase five sets of this apparatus.

EXAMPLE 2. Better Way

The end point of a study on gastric acidity was measured by visually titrating to an indicator change with phenol red. The suggestion that an automated titrimeter using an automatically determined end point be used was accepted. A superior apparatus was purchased for this and was used in many subsequent studies.

Clinical trials may provide a vehicle for an investigator to expand his clinical practice, particularly when the research will require extensive patient recruitment efforts. Patients who are caught up in the excitement of participating in a clinical trial often recommend the study to friends or relatives whose medical care they may not have discussed under other circumstances. Advertising can yield considerable numbers of subjects stimulated to seek treatment for a condition they had previously ignored. The effects of a large, well-publicized clinical trial on patient flow in private practice can be substantial. Many investigators are even offered opportunities to participate in local media activities to discuss new research developments.

FINANCIAL CONSIDERATIONS

Pharmaceutical research does offer a source of revenue. The physician's time, facility, staff, or equipment that is not currently being utilized optimally can be directed to this remunerative activity very easily. Since some research work is administrative in nature, it can be performed during the brief spans of time that often occur between clinical commitments. However, this reallocation cannot be accomplished without paying an opportunity cost. The investigator faced with imminent recruitment deadlines and frequent sponsor visits, or excited about the sheer novelty of the experience, will feel pressure to shift his priorities in favor of the research activity. Although this commitment may not often conflict with the physician's other professional activities, more lucrative opportunities occasionally will need to be sacrificed in favor of the research project.

Clinical research is also beginning to require greater financial planning. Sponsors are becoming increasingly strict in requiring that investigators return funds to the company if the requirements of the study have not been fulfilled satisfactorily. Such a request is not ordinarily made unless several thousands of dollars are involved. However, it can pose significant hardship if the investigator is not prepared for this possibility. Potential investigators should be aware that sponsors ordinarily issue grant installments prospectively at selected enrollment checkpoints so a team will not find itself without the funds to continue recruitment. As the study nears conclusion, some percentage of the funds due will be withheld, both to provide an incentive for prompt data submission and to permit a final determination of patient evaluability. Thus, the investigator could be asked to return funds that he has already used for other purposes, or he might not receive an anticipated final payment due to disqualification of some subjects' records. Maintaining a detailed accounting of research funds may be an inconvenience but is a necessity if the investigator wishes to avoid unpleasant contingencies.

Clinical trials are conducted most economically if the investigator has a highly motivated staff member who can supervise or conduct the day-to-day activities and optimize the use of the physician's time in a review capacity. A physician should not undertake a research protocol with the idea that it will prove cost-effective for him to complete the majority of case records and administrative forms himself. The advantages to research budgeting come from being able to bill the sponsor at established fee scales for activities that may be performed competently by a technician or nurse. Although the investigator must be available should any questions or problems arise, it may not be necessary for him to see a patient at each visit. Research funds allocated for clinical activities may allow an investigator to add part-time personnel who can assist him in his practice as well as conduct basic research procedures.

IMPACT ON STAFF, COLLEAGUES, AND FACILITY

STAFF ISSUES. The potential drawbacks to participating in clinical trials are also experienced at the organizational and staff levels. While the suboptimally utilized facility may be used for research purposes, the use of this resource for research tasks requires considerable effort, particularly if the staff is not compensated for the real or perceived increase in activity. The authors frequently have observed very willing, enthusiastic investigators whose efforts to conduct a clinical trial were undermined by a reluctant, poorly oriented, and poorly supervised staff. The staff may neither feel the same need for greater diversity of work that the investigator does nor see the benefits or rewards of participating in the project. While some economic and professional justification can quell resistance to the increase in workload, the investigator nevertheless must be prepared to motivate and supervise his employees more actively than before. Suggestions for securing employees' full cooperation in a project are included in a later chapter.

The investigator who plans to hire staff members for a particular project has an obligation to assure that they are fully aware of the project-specific duration of the job, that they are given adequate notice when a project is nearing completion, and that the employment understanding includes some provision for an orderly termination if a project is abruptly and unexpectedly discontinued. These are the responsibilities of any employer and are emphasized here because of the potentially serious morale and ethical dilemmas the staff may face when their jobs are so closely linked to the success or failure of a particular project.

IMPACT ON COLLEAGUES. The investigator must also consider the impact of the research on his colleagues. The thoughtful prospective investigator will discuss the proposed activities at length with his colleagues to work out the potential conflicts that are certain to arise in the critical areas listed below.

Cross-Coverage. How do his colleagues feel about caring for research patients while cross-covering? Is the covering physician willing to learn enough about the protocol to take on emergency administrative procedures, e.g., notifying the sponsor of significant adverse experiences, in the investigator's absence? Will the PI be available to clarify any of the procedures or protocol requirements if issues arise during coverage hours? How will the colleague react when the research patient, with expectations of immediate access to the investigator, demands this same treatment from the covering physician? Will he be willing to cooperate so that the study is not jeopardized?

Recruitment. When the recruitment pressure heightens, how will the PI react toward his colleagues who appear to be insensitive to his requests for patient referrals, or who do not wish to take part in screening and recruiting patients for the study? Will his colleagues understand that recruitment objectives may require that the investigator make the facility available to prospective subjects at the subjects' convenience?

Compensation. How will the colleagues be compensated for their limited roles in the study? Will the research revenue be treated as part of the group's income, or as the PI's income exclusively?

The administration and accounting of research revenue are issues that are often underemphasized. Whatever the investigator's professional environment, the use of research funds is undergoing greater scrutiny to explore possible cost shifting and rates of return associated with research activities. Separate accounting records should be maintained for each protocol so one's colleagues or institution will feel satisfied that the activities are, indeed, self-supporting endeavors.

FACILITY ISSUES. The investigator must also consider the impact of the research activity on the facility. Is the facility adequate for the increased patient flow that will result, including the space and time for the patient's family to wait or participate in the informed consent process if they so choose? Can space be set aside or cabinets purchased for adequate and secure medication storage? Will space be available for record storage as well? Is there sufficient space away from high traffic areas in which regulatory auditors and sponsors can work during their visits? Does the facility contain the necessary equipment and space for the special types of emergencies that may arise? Is the group prepared to submit administrative and clinical records for outside regulatory scrutiny?

EXAMPLE 3. Too Much of a Good Thing

Recruitment of patients with gallstones who were willing to participate in a placebo-controlled study of an agent designed to dissolve the gallstones was undertaken by radio. After a single announcement was aired, 100 to 150 telephone inquiries were received. These telephone calls disrupted the office and prevented regular patients from reaching doctors or making appointments. A staff member was assigned to take names and telephone numbers and contact the prospective subjects within the following two weeks. The phone lines could then be kept open for more urgent communication and orderly scheduling of potential study subjects.

CLINICAL ISSUES

The investigator and his staff should find that the rigors of the research process sharpen their clinical skills and enhance their interest in their private patients as well. While research is a valuable stimulus for developing one's powers of observation and techniques for communicating with patients, the physician should also make certain that this "spillover" of research technique does not adversely affect his practice habits. The investigator may find he has a desire to conduct more tests than would ordinarily be required to make a diagnosis with sufficient certainty to initiate treatment. He may also be inclined to adopt new prescribing habits, even though the approaches and regimens he is using have not yet been proven effective for use in the general population. This is particularly true if the investigator is conducting post-marketing studies to examine similar medication regimens of available products. If the necessary care is taken to observe these tendencies, however, the nonresearch patient can certainly be expected to benefit from the attentions of a more interested and involved research physician. It is also very likely that the research physician will be motivated to seek and detect adverse events from drug therapy prescribed for his nonresearch patients.

The research physician is also in a position to offer numerous care advantages to his patients. Indigent or underinsured patients can be provided with better follow-up, plus more intensive health monitoring and screening, when medical costs are subsidized by a research protocol.

These advantages clearly reveal that the investigator must be prepared to practice differently with the research patient. The investigator-physician has a dual role that is a source of constant conflict and stress to both the patient and the physician. Both experience a loss in the degree of freedom to individualize a therapeutic regimen. The management of potential side effects is also difficult because the patient may have some concerns about whether or not to take note of and report minor symptoms. His trust in the physician may be undermined if he is uncertain whose interests the investigator may have uppermost in mind when making clinical decisions in a research setting. The physician will feel similar stresses, which, if not properly resolved, can become serious obstacles to the successful conduct of a clinical trial. For example, his frustration with noncompliant behavior may become more pronounced when such behavior compromises the validity of the study. He could also find himself unable to discontinue the necessarily close relationship with research subjects once they have returned to the private practice sphere (see Example 4 below). The physician must be prepared daily to confront possible conflicts between his interests as an investigator and his immediate duties as a clinician. When substantial academic and financial rewards are riding on the success of a research project, these conflicts may be difficult to face.

EXAMPLE 4. In Need of Referral

During a 16-week study of an antiarthritic drug, the investigators met regularly with the 20 subjects and provided them with a great deal of counsel about their general health, immunizations, intercurrent illnesses unrelated to the drug, and their disease. One subject completed the study and continued to call for these services. Initially they were delivered, but with a great deal of frustration that evolved into hostility. The investigator did not fully appreciate, however, that while he had been an enthusiastic general health provider while the patient was in the study, his attitude had subsequently shifted to one of lack of interest after the study was completed. The nature of the change in the relationship from a research care to a private practice setting and its significance had not been shared with the patient. This problem is discussed more fully in the chapter entitled "The Referral Process."

Participation in clinical research will impose burdens on the investigator's staff, colleagues, and facility. However, it can also add considerable excitement and novelty to the professional routine. The physician who secures his colleagues' cooperation in expanding into the area of research medicine will find that establishing a relationship with pharmaceutical sponsors can offer numerous rewards and opportunities. Involving the staff in the research activities can provide a cost-effective means of increasing practice volume and diversity of income sources. Choices of suitable research projects must be made carefully, however, if the physician wishes to minimize the disruptions to his practice that result from this expanded activity. The prospective investigator who establishes clear objectives for his involvement in the research process will not find himself burdened with a responsibility for which the team has not been properly prepared.

Physicians

During the conduct of drug or device research, two distinct types of physicians are usually interacting with the patient. One group is primarily responsible for the conduct of the research and consists of the principal investigator (PI) and his associates as well as the several physicians in the sponsoring company. Another group of physicians provides the patient's ordinary health care in a practice mode and usually has little or no knowledge of the research protocol and its proper execution. The protocol physicians derive benefit from the completion of the protocol and, therefore, are considered to some degree in a conflict of interest with pure advocacy of what is beneficial for the patient (see Spiro, 1986).

The relationship between the research-team and nonstudy physicians can greatly influence the ease with which a research protocol can be filled and carried out. This chapter will explore the many roles physicians can be expected to play in caring for a research subject. Included are suggestions for addressing many concerns or criticisms that initially may be raised by physicians unfamiliar with the clinical trials process. Other professional issues of concern to be considered by physicians involved in research are discussed in Chapter 2 and Chapter 15.

TYPICAL ROLES OF STUDY-EMPLOYED PHYSICIANS

The principal investigator (PI) is the responsible scientist (usually a licensed physician) listed on the FDA Form 1572/3, accepted by the

TABLE 1. *Physicians Employed by or Receiving Funds from Research Sponsors*

Title	Responsibility	Relationship with patient	Comments
Principal investigator	Responsible for all aspects of study—following protocol, evaluating reactions, training, supervising all personnel; reviews all safety checks	Available to patient at all times	Major contact, resolves all problems
Medical monitor	Can approve minor protocol, deviations, advise on safety, ask company scientists about drug effects	Remote from patient at sponsor's headquarters	Central source of all adverse reaction data
Specialist	Gives consultation for specific problem; may be collaborating investigator	Sees patient for limited diagnostic evaluation, either for routine testing or emergency consultation	Selected by PI to perform routine protocol services
Staff physician	Substitutes for or assists PI; may be collaborating investigator	Available to patient	
Emergency consultant	Addresses a specific urgent question in consultation	Sees patient for acute complaint in area outside of research team's specialty in the event that regular physicians and specialists are unavailable	Renders opinion on possible side effects the agent or study
Recruiting physician	Refers patient to study for a fee	Identifies and may screen patient	

sponsor as the responsible scientist, and accepted by the local IRB as the responsible person. Although major portions of this responsibility may be shared and delegated, the legal, professional, and ethical responsibilities reside with the PI. Table 1 lists titles and relationships of various study physicians to one another and to the PI.

All of the physicians at the local study level (i.e., collaborating investigators, consultants, and specialists) are selected by the PI and should work effectively together. The PI and his associates are expected to be highly knowledgeable about the research protocol and the potential side effects of the agent or device under study. Consultants and specialists are informed about the drug and protocol to the degree needed to fulfill their role. The sponsor's medical monitor is usually apprised of all possible reactions and has the authority to permit deviations from the protocol in enrollment and in uncritical details of operation. While the medical monitor must concur in the continuation of a subject when a possibly significant adverse event occurs, the PI is free to discontinue a drug at any time without the medical monitor's permission.

EXAMPLE 1. Approved Deviation

An admitted alcoholic known to us to have been compliant with a treatment program for seven months presented for an ulcer study for which we were the investigators. The patient met all other inclusion criteria with the exception of the previous history of alcoholism. Since he was an otherwise ideal candidate for the study, we contacted the medical monitor by phone and the patient was allowed to participate. The patient satisfactorily completed the study and was enrolled in an additional study of long-term prophylaxis of ulcer.

It should always be recognized that the patients' safety and their health have a much higher priority than the completion of the protocol. However, with concerned, informed physicians on the spot, it is often possible to meet both the needs of the patient and the protocol. Discussions between the PI and the medical monitor are nearly always needed to find a solution.

EXAMPLE 2. A Relaxing Solution

A patient satisfactorily progressing in a yearlong new-drug study for the control of hypertension had an opportunity to take a Caribbean cruise after about six months on the protocol. Since this vacation would disrupt the visit schedule, the patient considered dropping from the study. We presented this problem to the medical monitor with our recommendation that this patient be permitted to continue. A sufficient supply of study medication was made available so the patient could both enjoy her cruise and continue in the study.

TABLE 2. Patients' Physicians Encountered in the Research Setting

Title	Ideal action for PI	Relation to patient	Comments
Regular doctor	Inform of study, provide consent form and letter outlining any protocol-required restrictions	Takes care of all basic medical needs, usually sees patient two to four times annually	Best provider with whom to share ECGs and useful lab results
Specialist	Inform of study, provide consent form and letter outlining any protocol-required restrictions	Sees and treats patient for the same condition being investigated in the study or an area being monitored for safety	Should have clear understanding of his role with the patient and research team during the study
Finding physician	Thank for the referral and discuss what is mutually expected	May be either of the above or another practitioner involved with a patient who referred him for study	Should state his expectations in return for the referral
Emergency care physician	Telephone and write about the protocol; gain cooperation to care for the patient within the restrictions of the protocol if appropriate	Physician engaged by patient during the study to manage an emergency complaint	May provide valuable information on possible adverse events

ROLES OF NONSTUDY PHYSICIANS INVOLVED WITH A RESEARCH SUBJECT

The roles of the patients' regular doctors, consultants, and emergency room physicians for those engaged in a research study are presented in Table 2. Many patients entering a study have regular physicians or a specialist doctor for the area of study (e.g., a rheumatologist for arthritis or a gastroenterologist for ulcer). Each of these physicians has a responsibility for the care of the patient that is predominantly motivated by the patient's health needs. Lesser concerns are the desire of the physician to keep his professional options open by avoiding the restrictions of the protocol, his wish to continue the patient in his practice, and his trained caution to avoid the new until it is established. More often than not, these doctors are reluctant to refer patients for study and discourage patients from entering studies, usually because protocol participation would restrict their freedom of choice. Only when a totally new therapy is available, and the patient is not responding to his current treatment, do they seek out and endorse the study. Patients under their care may themselves have responded to announcements of screening in conjunction with the study and are thus self-referred. Some of these patients seek the counsel of their physician; others ask that their physician not be told of their participation.

The PI must judiciously weigh the consequences of not telling a regular physician about the study, basing his decision upon the patient's wishes, the nature of the protocol, and possible harm to the patient. Thus, a study of a new diuretic, requiring discontinuation of all other medications under competent medical supervision for three days, with close monitoring of the patient, has little possibility of harm. Both the patient and the PI need a clear understanding in this situation that the regular physician has not been informed and that all emergency care during the experimental period should be known to the PI to arrange communication. On the other hand, a mildly hypertensive patient entering a study requiring a four-week period on placebo medication before a new antihypertensive drug or placebo is utilized for the next year has a high likelihood of needing services from his regular physician. The physician will be understandably irate about the deception associated with the study, and may, in an effort to help the patient, prescribe an agent that would interact with the treatment, or otherwise unknowingly produce harm. Such patients must consent to notification of their physician or not be enrolled (see Figures 1 and 2).

Nearly all studies generate data of value to physicians managing the patient. Any such material should be transferred to the patient's regular doctor or, if appropriate, to the new one managing his condition. Sample letters addressing some of these situations are shown in Figures 3 through 6. Chapter 15 addresses referral of patients to non-study physicians.

A frequent situation arises when a patient seeks emergency care for new symptoms that may be related to the experimental drug. In this circumstance, the PI or his physician associate should talk with the emergency care physician by phone to inform him of the details of the study and what is known of the side effects of the agent. The patient's copy of the written informed consent is valuable to provide some information about the study. Unless the situation requires an antidote (e.g.,

Re: Mary Jones, Birthdate May 16, 1946

Dear Dr. Samuels:

Mary Jones was endoscoped July 23, 1985, and found to have an ulcer in the duodenum and decided to enter a study of a new cimetidinelike agent on that date. This study continues for 8 weeks and she will receive either the new agent or a placebo. She can take as many Gelusil tablets from a supply we have given her as needed to control abdominal pain, and we have also provided a bottle of Tylenol, 300-mg tablets, should any other aches and pains need treatment. She will be endoscoped again at 4, 6, and 8 weeks and if she is healed, no further treatment or endoscopy will be required.

During this period she may not take other agents to treat ulcers and should not take analgesics for other causes. If the pain cannot be controlled by the Gelusil she can be discontinued from the study, an endoscopy performed by our physician, and then alternative treatment arranged.

We are enclosing copies of her initial screening chemistries and endoscopy reports for your records. If you wish further information about her study please call me at 123-4567.

Sincerely,

Ann C. Harrison, M.D.
Principal Investigator

FIGURE 1. Letter to a physician providing regular care for patient Jones.

patient's child ate the entire bottle of experimental medication), the code need not be broken (see Chapter 14 on adverse experiences). In all such emergency situations, the drug should be discontinued, with appropriate medical care administered, substituting, if necessary, a known effective medication. A decision as to whether the drug may be started again can then be made later when the situation has become much clearer. Contact with the emergency room physician administering care will permit the PI to learn the details of the possible reaction so an eventual decision can be made as to whether or not to restart the drug. Problems sometimes arise in which the relationship between these outside physicians and the study physicians is perceived as adversarial. These are among the most challenging situations in drug research with patients.

WHO "OWNS" THE PATIENT?

This issue generates much misunderstanding between doctors. There is an assumed contractual relationship between each patient and

Re: Rasputin Long, Birthdate May 17, 1946

Dear Dr. Fishman:
    Mr. Long responded to our posted notice seeking patients with mild
hypertension and upon our examination qualified. He was willing to
discontinue his methyl-DOPA treatment for 1 year and to try our new agent or
placebo under conditions of careful monitoring. He stopped his medication on
July 23, 1985, and in the subsequent 2 weeks has changed his blood pressure
very little, with the usual values in his twice-weekly visits being 146/96 after 5
minutes of relaxation. It is our plan to continue this washout with no drug for
an additional 2 weeks and then start him on a new agent similar to minoxodil
(or placebo). The dose will be adjusted to bring his diastolic blood pressure to
85 mm Hg or less for a full week and that dose continued for 10 additional
months. Should this drug (or placebo) fail to control his BP to less than
diastolic 85 mm Hg in two successive measurements at least 2 days apart, or
should either his systolic or diastolic pass the limits of 155/102 mm Hg, he
will be discontinued from the new therapy and restored to his methyl-DOPA. We
will adjust this sufficiently to obtain control, and then plan to return him to
your care.
    The initial ECG, chemistries, urine examination, and ophthalmological
consultations that we obtained are enclosed for your records. If we can supply
further information about this study please call me at 123-4567.

                         Sincerely,

                         Maurice Se, M.D.

FIGURE 2. Letter to a physician providing regular hypertensive treatment to a patient
who is about to be enrolled in a one-year, placebo-controlled trial.

his physician that is seldom clearly articulated and almost never written. For the doctor's part, the assumption is that the patient will have
fidelity to him and only him unless he approves referral or alternative
arrangements for treatment. In actual practice, whom a patient consults, how much of the advice given is followed, and for how long
constitute the patient's choices. The patient is getting less than his
money's worth from any physician if he is not forthright about other
treatments that are being used and other health providers employed.
Nonetheless, all doctors are familiar with patients' less than full dis-
closures about over-the-counter medications, illicit drugs, and use of
chiropractic, mental health counselors, or extreme fad diets, or even
simultaneous physicians.
    The clear responsibility of the investigative team is to do all that is
possible to preserve good physician relationships for the patient, to
enhance subsequent ones, and to advise on measures that may improve
his health. Only a limited number (about one-quarter) of study patients

Re: Renalda Semovitz, Birthdate May 18, 1936

Dear Dr. Stephens:
    During the course of a 10-week, placebo-controlled trial of SEMOLINA, a
new vegetable-origin nonsteroidal antiarthritis agent in rheumatoid arthritis,
the following studies were obtained on Ms. Semovitz. Goniometry of the right
and left knee, respectively, 55–160, 80–180 initial, and 35–180, 35–180 final.
Her global activities index rose from 16 to 45 (see enclosed scale), indicating a
marked response. Her consumption of Tylenol dropped from a mean of 26 300-
mg tablets to zero during the 10th week. Needless to say, she markedly
improved, but we do not know whether she received placebo or active
SEMOLINA and this cannot be identified until all 750 subjects complete the
study nationwide. I am enclosing some chemical, X ray, and immunological
tests conducted on Ms. Semovitz for your records. At the termination of the
study on September 31, 1985, she did not require pain medication and felt very
good. She will be returning to your care for recommendations in a few weeks.
Should you need further information I can be reached at 123-4567.

                                    Sincerely,

                                    Pat Rally, M.D.
                                    Principal Investigator

FIGURE 3. Letter to a rheumatologist regarding a patient who had completed a study.

Re: Anna Banana, Birthdate June 15, 1942

Dear Dr. Emory:
    I appreciate the sincerity of your call regarding Anna Banana, who is
currently enrolled in our study (placebo-controlled) of a novel molecule in the
long-term treatment of hay fever. Ms. Banana answered our advertisement in
the newspaper, was thoroughly examined, and qualified for this study, starting
on April 1, 1985, in time for the full allergy season. I thought it would be of
interest to you to know something of the study we are undertaking and I have
enclosed a copy of the informed consent. The initial laboratory tests on Ms.
Banana are also enclosed for your subsequent management of her condition.
This study will continue until October 1, 1985, to encompass an entire hay
fever season. At the time of this writing, Ms. Banana rates her symptoms as
the least she has ever had, but she stayed away from work 3 days during the
spring.
    If I can assist you in the care of Ms. Banana with further information
about this study, please call me again.

                                    Sincerely,

                                    D. Strawberry, M.D.

FIGURE 4. Letter to a concerned physician about entry of *his* patient into study without
his consent.

Re: Antonio Civellini, Birthdate May 13, 1946

Dear Dr. Wallace:

Mr. Civellini has just completed a 12-week trial of a sustained-release appetite suppressant in treating his long-standing problem of overweight. This agent is a peptide related to cholecystokinin and only caused diarrhea in animals, and in previous trials no substantive side effects were noted. Although Mr. C lost 19 lbs. during this trial, we do not know whether he was on placebo or the active agent. During the 10th week of the trial, his previously normal liver test, the AST, rose from 13 (before the trial) to 37 (not abnormal), and just after the trial ended (after 12 weeks of medication) the level was 88. A repeat determination 1 week later was 86, indicating that the elevation is real and persisted. He had no symptoms of liver illness and a complete battery of liver tests done on December 19, 1985, is enclosed. His physical examination on December 28 frankly was nearly normal, but it was impossible to assess liver size because he remains fairly fat. However, there was no tenderness.

It is my opinion that this minor elevation of the AST is coincidental to the drug trial, but we would be interested in his subsequent follow-up and values. If, in your judgment, further testing is advisable (e.g., sonography, liver biopsy) I can arrange to have it done at no cost to Mr. Civellini, but I did not feel further evaluation is needed, particularly if the abnormality disappears. I will be calling you in a few weeks as to how he has done.

Sincerely,

Candice Thin, M.D.
Principal Investigator

FIGURE 5. Abnormal laboratory tests communicated back to the private physician.

Re: Mary Jones, Birthdate July 1, 1924

Dear Dr. Filmore:

Mary Jones, age 62 and living in Apt. 314 at 100 Charles Street, Baltimore, is a patient in your office and currently enrolled in our experimental study of a new oral drug for glaucoma. She had mild emphysema and asked me about vaccination for influenza and pneumonia after hearing about these at the Senior Center. I believe both influenza and pneumovax would be helpful for her condition and have recommended that she schedule a visit with you to obtain an update on her immunizations as you find necessary.

She is a very compliant patient. I am enclosing her most recent tonometry and visual acuity measurements indicating that her intraocular pressure is well controlled and her vision is improving. Her study will continue for 2 additional years ending in December 1989.

Sincerely,

Elaine Day, M.D.

FIGURE 6. Referral to a personal physician for indicated services, not part of protocol.

will have ideal relationships with their physicians. In those cases, the PI and his staff can enhance the current relationship by encouraging communication. The better the relationship between the patient and the physician, the more important it is for the investigative staff to enter into that relationship to strengthen it and avoid strain or disruption.

Hospitalized patients recruited for study fall into a different category. The responsible physician, as defined by the hospital's bylaws (which differ from one hospital to another), must be fully knowledgeable about the experimental treatment and the protocol. The challenge of securing the private physician's cooperation is considerably less than in outpatient practice and outpatient studies because more clinical research is undertaken in the hospital. A relationship usually exists already between the PI and the patient's physician, with the PI and staff interacting with him more frequently.

ETHICAL AND MARKETPLACE CONSIDERATIONS

Almost all physicians who provide some services to the patient (Table 1) are paid for them by a commercial sponsor and, thus, have a conflict of interest. They are paid for performing the protocol or recruiting. This payment may impede their judgment as the patient's advocate. On the other hand, physicians employed by the patient may counsel the patient not to enter a study because of concern that services provided at no cost will lead to loss of income from the regular visits made to them. In such situations, the private physician's judgment may be compromised.

It is essential in any research intervention that the well-being, comfort, and good health of the patient at all times dominate. In well-run studies, all staff members clearly recognize this and display an attitude of concern in all of their dealings with research patients. Furthermore, they are aware that the many advantages and kindnesses of being in a well-designed study should overcome the bother to subjects and easily overcome the additional risks. The best way to avoid concern about a team's potential conflict of interest is to be open in discussing all of the financial arrangements with both the IRB responsible for the study and the patient (see Spiro, 1986). In this way, nothing is uncovered that may arouse suspicion. Paid recruiters and PIs who are also the patients' doctors should indicate to their patients that they are paid for the time to explain the study, and the staff should indicate that they are employees of the commercial sponsor. It is entirely appropriate that they add that "because we are paid for this we have more time to spend on your problems and welfare."

SOME METHODS OF AVOIDING COMMON PROBLEMS

Whenever possible, and in nearly all circumstances, the private physician with any relationship with the patient should be informed about the patient's participation in the study. If the patient has an excellent relationship with his physician, he will not be willing to enroll without prior discussion of the study with his physician. When the patient is indifferent about communication with his doctor or is somewhat negative but does not insist the doctor be denied information, from the authors' experience it is recommended that the physician be told *after* the patient is enrolled to avoid a reflex action to discourage the patient from participation. If there are important health considerations that may lead to the patient's also consulting a regular physician, sharing the study information with the physician is of benefit and essential for good health care. For example, there are many studies in which a drug with predictable side effects may be employed, or a drug-free interval may be utilized for washout. Sharing this information and the dates with the physician is of great benefit in maintaining the patient in the protocol. An indication of concern for the patient's welfare in the communication with the personal physician will allay much of his concern. Referring appropriate services to his office must be done meticulously (see Figure 6).

The patient should be encouraged to keep the informed consent and appropriate emergency call numbers in several locations. Providing the patient with adhesive labels containing the day and night phone numbers of the study physicians, with advice to paste them in several locations, including on the telephone, is useful. All letters to doctors about patients should include phone numbers. To the extent that the study physicians are called about a problem and that they maintain contact with the regular physician, one can evaluate the quality of overall communication. The informed consent usually contains sufficient detail to allow a physician to consult with a patient on a study medication.

APPROPRIATE RESPONSES TO RECURRENT CONCERNS, COMMENTS, OR CRITICISMS

A physician learns that his patient has entered a study and is irate and calls the study number insisting that the team has "stolen" his patient. A calm reply indicating that the patient chose to come to the study and entered with informed consent is in order. An offer should be made to send to the physician a copy of the informed consent and study details as well as reports that are of value medically. The investigator responding to the complaint should not become defensive or argumentative. A letter documenting the details of the call should follow shortly (see Example 3 and Figure 4).

EXAMPLE 3. *Angry Private Physician*

A patient with rheumatoid arthritis entered a protocol after reading a newspaper advertisement. Her local doctor learned of this during a routine visit and irately called the PI insisting that his patient had been stolen, that the patient should immediately be discontinued from the study, and that he be informed of the nature of the medication. Calmly talking with the physician, explaining the nature of the recruitment and the study, and sending him some information led to a reversal of his position and his referring subsequent patients for the study. We acknowledged this support of the research by referring several new patients who had no practitioner to this man when their participation in the study concluded.

A patient in a study develops a new complaint that he does not think is related to the study and consults a doctor in an emergency room or one who has not previously heard of the study. Upon learning of the experimental medication, the physician contacts the PI or the on-call study physician to learn something of what the investigators might attribute to the study and whether or not there are interdictions in what they may undertake in treatment. Such callers should be aided in every possible way. If required by the situation, the PI may need to contact the medical monitor to see whether the situation is known to have occurred before. When appropriate, the PI may agree to pay for special tests needed in follow-up, explaining that well-documented outcome is needed for future reporting. Such an action will demonstrate the concern of the study group for the subject. A thank-you note to the doctor would then be in order.

The local medical society has received complaints about "advertising," "individuals practicing medicine without a license," or "unethical" practices and wishes more information for a review of this matter. Documentation of IRB review of the protocol and the study procedures, an explanation that any patients in question chose to undertake the study without notifying their physician, and a summary of the PI's own actions are usually all that is required. It goes without saying that all study doctors should be licensed in the region where they are working. The authors have been through medical society review several times and have found that as long as the PI is a fully licensed physician in the jurisdiction in which he is working and in good standing, with records indicating communication with many of the patients' doctors, there is not a major problem.

A physician calls with an urgent problem requiring a forbidden medication and the request is appropriate and urgent. The required medicine is forbidden because it changes the evaluable characteristics of the patient not because of a probable toxic reaction. The PI or representative of the PI can phone the medical monitor and get prior permission for this or, if this is not possible, can notify the medical monitor at the earliest possible time after the action. Since the patient's welfare must at all times dominate, this is the only reasonable action. On the other hand, if an alternative compatible treatment exists (e.g., cimetidine is totally contraindicated, while sucralfate is an acceptable alternative), it may be possible to preserve the letter of the protocol and totally fulfill the patient's needs.

A physician calls insisting on knowing what drug the patient is taking for the purpose of records and his management. A calm explanation that the blind cannot be broken and the patient still remain in the study is usually sufficient, but sometimes the insistence becomes overwhelming. At such times, the patient must make the choice of whether to remain in the study or not.

A physician refers a patient to a study and asks to be paid for his "case finding." In such circumstances, it is ethically reasonable to pay the physician for the time spent delivering services to the study patient that are used in the study, but not for case delivery unless this is a clear written policy defined with the responsible IRB. Although such problems are often less frequent if the physician is asked to outline in writing what he is charging for, occasionally the IRB may be called upon to adjudicate reasonable differences of opinion.

FURTHER READING

Glaser, W.A., Paying the Doctor: Systems of Remuneration and Their Effects, Johns Hopkins University Press, Baltimore, 1970.

Kammerer, W.S., and Gross, R.J., Medical Consultant: Role of the Internist on Surgical, Obstetric, and Psychiatric Services, Williams and Wilkins Company, Baltimore, 1983.

Levinksy, N.G., The doctor's master, N. Engl. J. Med. 311:1573–1575, 1984.

Pellegrino, E.D., and Thomasma, D.C., A Philosophical Basis of Medical Practice, Oxford University Press, London, 1981.

Relman, A.S., The new medical-industrial complex, N. Engl. J. Med. 303:963–970, 1980.

Spiro, H.M., Mammon and medicine: The rewards of clinical trials, J. Am. Med. Assoc. 255:1174–1175, 1986.

Wohl, S., The Medical Industrial Complex, Harmony Books, New York, 1984.

CHAPTER 4

Evaluating a Sponsor

Experience of the Company • Features of the Company • Company Personnel • General Policies • Protocol • Relationship with the Investigator • Patient Issues

Companies conducting testing of drugs in humans differ from one another in previous experience, market focus, and approach to investigators. These companies spend up to $100 million to develop an effective new drug that actually reaches the market (see page 4). To bring a generic drug onto the market costs up to $3 million. Only a minor fraction of these costs are expended on the actual clinical trials because extensive animal testing, regulatory interactions, patent reviews, and manufacturing standards also must be completed.

The clinical investigator as PI is but one link in this process and must depend heavily upon many others to perform their tasks adequately in order to carry out his. For instance, sloppy manufacturing control can deliver a very impure substance to the investigator, who administers the material to test subjects with possibly bad results. The research process carries with it uncertainty of clinical outcome. The sponsor's support in certain common unexpected turns, such as evaluation of side effects, determines the satisfaction of the investigator with the relationship. This chapter discusses important issues for patient-oriented practitioners who must evaluate pharmaceutical firms.

All companies, large or small, eventually have to show a profit. The pressures of stockholders, regulatory agencies, and recent performances on profitability lead to major variability in the approaches for achieving returns on R&D investment. Not too long ago, most drug investigation was a cottage industry, with the investigator having a very close one-on-one relationship with the responsible person in the company. Now the industry has evolved to the point that it is highly efficient, computerized, and to some degree impersonal. Although these changes may be advantageous for the investigator, they can also prove frustrating if he is not in agreement with the policies sponsors may

TABLE 3. *Useful Areas in Evaluating a Sponsor*

Experience in the past decade
Company issues
  Stated company goals
  Quality assurance program on drug testing in humans
  Indemnity policies
  Resources
  Encouragement to publish
Protocol issues
  State of the art
  Indications of need to know the truth about the agent under study
  Demonstrated knowledge of typical problems encountered in conducting
    human research
Interaction with the investigator
  Clear line of authority of personnel
  Quality and longevity of personnel
  Authority of the team's contact
Patient issues
  Responsiveness to safety issues
  Promptness in reporting results to FDA

---

develop. Table 3 lists some areas that a physician may wish to investigate before agreeing to work with a pharmaceutical firm. These are discussed in subsequent paragraphs.

EXPERIENCE OF THE COMPANY

Companies who have engaged in clinical research for any length of time have encountered problems and have learned to handle them. Less experienced companies often go no further on ethical, safety, and recruitment requirements than the written letter of the regulation. As a result, their policies may present problems in areas important to patient care, particularly the management of possible adverse reactions. The many areas described subsequently will allow a person to "test the water" of newer companies.

EXAMPLE 1. *You Get What You Pay For*

An identical protocol was submitted to an investigator by two sponsors, each testing its new antiulcer treatment in gastric ulcer. Although both companies are considered pioneer and have excellent reputations, one company was paying investigators 190% of the offer of the other

*company. The difference was that the more experienced company was
very desirous of paying an assistant to assure compliance with the medication, multiple visits, and careful diary entries. The company paying
the lesser amount was cutting every corner possible. The company paying the higher rate obtained prominent, highly respected investigators.
The company paying the lower rate obtained many performing their first
drug study. The inexperience of the company paying lower fees for this
sort of investigation almost certainly led to its decision.*

FEATURES OF THE COMPANY

All companies have a mission or stated goal. This says to the world
as well as to its own employees what the company stands for. Better
firms conducting drug research emphasize truth, knowledge, and safety. A commitment to use the best available tools, skills, and experience
to perform its research work better is found in the most satisfactory
sponsors.

The presence of a quality assurance program reviewing all aspects
of clinical testing and defining when a study is reviewed and who
conducts the review reveals a great deal about a company's priorities.

The quality and morale of sponsor personnel can also influence
both the final product of the research effort and the ease with which an
individual investigator can conduct his study. The sponsor's personnel
with whom the investigative team relate are noted in Table 4.

TABLE 4. Sponsor's Personnel

Title	Role	Level of interaction
Clinical research associate (CRA)	Field liaison with team	Frequent phone contact and visits
Medical monitor	Sponsor's medical decision-maker	Phone contacts, rare visits
Regulatory affairs and QA	Sponsor's regulatory decision-maker Audits forms and data collection	Variable
Corporate lawyer	Sponsor's legal advisor	
Biostatistics	Protocol guardian	

COMPANY PERSONNEL

The clinical research associate (CRA) is the field contact for the investigative team. This person always participates in orientation and is the first person who is called for supplies, questions about the CRFs, or operational details. This person observes some of the data collection, reviews some raw documents, instructs the staff in avoiding and correcting errors in CRFs, and is always present at the orientation and eventual closeout of the study. The initial recruitment of the investigator, the planning of budget, assisting with regulatory documents, and approval of payments may be carried out by the CRA, but in some companies other persons may be responsible for these functions.

A CRA is very knowledgeable about the protocol and usually is responsible for multiple investigators. He may share useful recruitment or record-keeping methods from one investigator with another. The CRA also may be able to provide information about future studies, or other investigators in the region who may be of assistance to the team.

The medical monitor is the final authority for all study-related medical matters. He participates in protocol development and contributes to and reviews the investigator's brochure. He monitors all new toxicity and reaction reports and serves as a readily available clearinghouse for this information. He usually coordinates publication at the end of the study.

The regulatory affairs section is responsible for submitting the IND and NDA and assuring compliance with all of the regulations. Many sponsors have separate quality assurance (QA) departments that are part of regulatory affairs. They conduct on-site reviews of investigators and other company departments to document that data have been collected properly and that the protocol has been followed.

Corporate lawyers are involved in the clinical trials process to the extent that they interpret FDA regulations on research and are often asked to determine whether a written informed consent form satisfies the regulations. They also interpret the indemnification policies. Biostatistics departments heavily influence protocol design and make decisions on evaluability of patients with minor or major protocol deviations.

GENERAL POLICIES

Resource issues are a reality in any endeavor but are a particular problem in research because of the unpredictability of the outcomes of the research process. In clinical research, the budgeting must be done up front, and it is highly desirable not to have to worry about money after a project is under way. A very low-budget, low-margin study allows for none of the uncertainties of the research process and may foster a corner-cutting, short-term mentality. This can be particularly dangerous if it affects the diligence with which adverse reactions are followed and evaluated.

The investigator should discuss the sponsor's position on liability coverage to ascertain the degree to which he will be protected in the event of a lawsuit by a research subject. It is customary for sponsors to offer indemnification to investigators who have enrolled and followed subjects as specified in the protocol. Whatever its policy, the sponsor's willingness to provide such information reveals a great deal about how well the sponsor has prepared itself for entry into the research field. The investigator also should ascertain whether he will be offered any assistance in publishing data.

PROTOCOL

Is the protocol state-of-the-art or does it use obsolete design or methods? The FDA develops guidelines for testing nearly all classes of drugs and most sponsors adhere to these.

EXAMPLE 2. Better Method

A protocol measured the quantity of organic-bound iodine to assess the activity of a desiccated thyroid preparation. The ability to suppress TSH (thyroid-stimulating hormone) in normal subjects seemed a much better evaluation. Largely on the basis of our recommendations and evaluation of a new desiccated thyroid, the standard method of evaluating these preparations was changed from organic-bound iodine to levels of T-3 and T-4 and the physiological evaluation in normal subjects of the ability to suppress TSH.

Is the protocol compatible with the realities of practice and the way the investigator is willing to treat his patients? Such factors as the definition of entry criteria, timing of multiple coordinated laboratory and consultative visits, and acceptable laboratory variations must be realistic. Further suggestions for evaluating new protocols are discussed in Chapters 5 and 8.

RELATIONSHIP WITH THE INVESTIGATOR

The quality of the CRA and the medical monitor can greatly influence the PI's performance. Their longevity in this type of work, background, and personal experience with this company are pertinent. The

CRA should be knowledgeable about FDA recommendations on record keeping and on many of the common dilemmas associated with the specific study. By discussing hypothetical situations on recruitment eligibility, proposed method of record keeping, and recruitment methods, the PI can quickly determine the extent of the CRA's experience.

The PI should determine the level of authority of the sponsor's staff with whom he has direct contact. In large companies, nearly everything must be separately approved by a special person. These decisions must be made as quickly as possible so that the team is not inconvenienced. An experienced sponsor will promptly respond to requests for wording changes in the informed consent document. A first-rate CRA can often obtain approval by phone while sitting in the investigator's office; an undersupported one may suggest that the PI himself call or mail requests to get the fastest response.

EXAMPLE 3. Good

A study involved several overnight gastric aspirations in order to compare a new acid-suppressing agent with cimetidine. Each patient had to have a nasogastric tube placed by fluoroscopy and 10 to 12 hours of study, emptying the stomach each 60 minutes. The pH and titratable acidity had to be carried out promptly. The CRA interviewed all patients, came to each fluoroscopic session, and remained all night through two studies and returned at about 5:00 a.m. after leaving about midnight in all others. He unobtrusively watched all phases of the data collection and was pleased. This is one of the best monitoring jobs we have ever seen.

EXAMPLE 4. Bad

A study of a topical liniment versus oral nonsteroidal antiinflammatory tablets was undertaken in a variety of outpatients with work-related or athletic muscular injuries of moderate nature. All patients used a liniment and all took tablets. Global relief of pain and restoration of activity were determined by daily diaries of medication and symptoms. The initial evaluation for injury and the initial and final interviews were conducted directly by the staff, but the in-between observations were undertaken by the patient, usually with two phone calls from the staff if they could be successfully completed. The sponsor monitored no phase of this activity other than via the case report forms. This was the least involvement with a project we have ever witnessed.

The PI must carefully consider the influence of the protocol on his usual level of care for the type of patient being studied and delineate precisely the authority delegated to him to make his usual decisions. Thus, a protocol in acute myocardial infarction must give the PI much more authority for hour-by-hour variations than a protocol treating acne. Discussions of minor laboratory abnormalities or a patient taking cold or headache medications in long-term studies usually will reveal the company's policy regarding the need for approval of minor violations. Sponsors vary widely in the latitude they provide investigators.

EXAMPLE 5. No! No!

A new analgesic was undergoing evaluation in postoperative patients who had to accept the possibility of a placebo with no escape until a full hour of evaluations were made. Recruitment was difficult because the patients had to have taken four or more doses of standard analgesic in the previous 24 hours. Recruitment picked up immediately after a CRA visited, watched our recruitment, and indicated that two analgesic doses in the previous 24 hours was sufficient, a full hour was not needed to escape, and several other modifications. In attempting to get these protocol changes confirmed in writing, we were told they could not be changed and that no one from the company had indicated that they could. The CRA had acted without authority, and his actions led to the disqualification of a large group of patients recruited under the relaxed criteria. This is an example of very poor performance by a CRA.

PATIENT ISSUES

The latitude permitted the PI in evaluating possible adverse reactions and the policy of reimbursement for costs of such evaluation reflects the sponsor's attitudes regarding patient safety. The sponsor's willingness to make a drug available for compassionate use (continuation of a therapeutically useful drug in Phase III evaluation for the benefit of the patient) also reflects its attitudes toward patient care.

The PI files safety reports on significant adverse reactions experienced with a drug. Most sponsors have a mechanism in place to collect these data and forward them on an FDA-1639 form immediately or at intervals required by the agency. Generic firms may require the investigator to complete and submit the FDA-1639 form to the FDA himself. In any event, the sponsor should not impose any restrictions regarding the investigator's ability to report results directly to the FDA if he wishes to do so.

Even new investigators will be approached by multiple companies interested in conducting clinical trials. Since companies differ so strikingly from one another, it is wise to review the strengths and weaknesses of each prospective sponsor to assure that the relationship will be workable and mutually rewarding.

FURTHER READING

Coulter, H.L., Drug industry and medicine, in: *Encyclopedia of Bioethics* (W.T. Reich, ed. in chief), Macmillan and Free Press, New York, 1978.
Matoren, G.M. (ed.), *The Clinical Research Process in the Pharmaceutical Industry*, Marcel Dekker, Inc., New York, 1985.

CHAPTER 5

Budget Planning and Development

*Planning the Budget • Evaluating the Protocol • Recruit-
ment • Payments or Reimbursements to Subjects • Converting
Plans into Cost Estimates • Administrative Support and Paper
Work • Personnel • Overhead • Contingency Fund-
ing • Cost Cutting and Savings • Money Management •
Submission and Negotiation of the Budget • Final Contracting*

A budget is awarded as a part of each contract to conduct drug or device research and to a large degree determines what can be accomplished as a part of the investigation. A budget can be developed only through careful planning of exactly how the study will be carried out.

PLANNING THE BUDGET

The initial step in planning requires the PI to obtain the protocol, at least in preliminary form. The protocol should be broken down into five large sections for planning; budgeting is required for each. These are recruitment and enrollment, conducting the study, paper work and administrative support, personnel costs, and overhead. Table 5 further subdivides these areas, addressing both planning the execution of the study and assigning costs for budget purposes.

Many times sponsors have planned approximately what they can pay to an investigator for each completed patient and will share this figure upon request. The internal budget range established by the sponsor usually allows a 10% deviation above or below the quoted price. Obtaining this figure and comparing it with a rough approximation of what is required to conduct the study may indicate that the PI's planning process is in error, for wide departures from the anticipated budget suggest that the strategies planned are different from those that others have used. It is not necessary to conduct the study exactly as the sponsor suggests on items of recruitment and other such details. How-

TABLE 5. *Planning a Study and Estimating Its Cost*

Activity	Planning steps	Cost estimates
Recruitment and enroll-ment	Identification of subjects	Finder's fees
	Screening	Advertising costs
	Estimate of % screened who are eligible and enroll	Costs of test and staff time required for screening
	Payments to subjects	
	Consultants' fees	
Conducting protocol	Is special site needed?	Cost of each item and test
	Must equipment be rented or purchased?	
	Clinic personnel	
	Estimate of staff needed for scheduling and actual visits	
Paper work and admin-istrative support	IRB submission and reports	$300 to $1000
	Keeping research records	$200 to $500
	Completing CRFs	$200 to $300
	Photocopies	$200 to $1000
	Typing	
	Correspondence with patients and physicians	
Personnel	Secretarial	
	Research assistant	Coverage at night
	Physicians	Coverage for vacations
	Consultants	
	Clinical staff	
Overhead	Rental, facility fees	Vary with institution
	Drug storage costs	
	Phone, postage, paper	
	Overhead for fund management	
	Rental of pager or tele-phone-answering service	
Contingency and alter-native plans	Repeating abnormal tests	At least 5% of test costs
	Evaluating possible adverse reactions	Minimum of $50/pt.
	Hospitalizations	Usually covered by sponsor
	Alternative recruitment plans	Separate budget

ever, it is wise to assure that the costs of any proposed methods fall within the acceptable range.

A quick review of the items in Table 5 should reveal that many activities can be precisely estimated as to cost, such as laboratory work and cost of consultants. Some may require consultation with other departments but can be determined precisely. The variables that cannot be precisely estimated are the cost of recruitment, the fraction of those who start who will continue long enough to provide evaluable data, and the study's overall duration. Since this work is labor-intensive, costs of receptionists, research assistants, and the PI's own time are all dependent upon the duration of the study. It is evident, therefore, that recruitment and retention of patients are the critical planning issues in establishing a budget.

In some cases, the nature of the patient's illness may justify transferring some of the costs related to the investigation for payment by the patient or his insurance. In other instances, the desire of the investigator to gain experience with a new agent, or his attempt to benefit his patient, may lead to the study's being undertaken with little or no funding. However, an inadequate budget often leads to poor research because the necessary things cannot be done. A full-cost budget should be developed for every investigation. Once it is developed, it may be possible to identify economies to the research that can be brought about by efficiency, use of pooling to lower costs of laboratory tests, use of less costly personnel to perform certain tasks, and assignment of appropriate costs to the patient's care. Preparing the budget is an ideal time to plan details of protocol performance as noted above, placing particular emphasis on planning recruitment and retention of subjects in the study.

Physicians new to drug and device investigations usually overestimate the ease of obtaining subjects, underestimate the time and bother of complying with regulatory affairs, underbudget for the unexpected, and overestimate their own efficiency. Their initial budgets, therefore, are often inadequate to perform the research, and they become irritated when the studies are partially completed but inadequately funded. Each study should be separately considered along the lines noted in Table 5, with recruitment and enrollment getting the greatest share of planning. A knowledgeable person can price out the other items in the table fairly accurately once recruitment statistics are available for estimating the time required to complete the study. Each of these budget areas is specifically discussed in the subsequent sections, with emphasis on the decisions needed for budget planning. In separate chapters or sections, a great deal more is presented on recruitment, enrollment, and compliance that can also be used in the detailed planning and execution of the study.

EVALUATING THE PROTOCOL

As the first step in developing a study budget, the PI must undertake a careful review of the protocol to assess how difficult it will be to recruit subjects with the inclusion criteria and study them on the schedule that is required. Even sponsors who are experienced in protocol development may underestimate the percentage of laboratory abnormalities, concomitant medication use, or scheduling conflicts likely to be encountered in the target population. Designing a protocol necessarily involves some give-and-take between biostatisticians, who strive to minimize the variability in all aspects of the study plan, and clinicians, who must assure that the criteria for selection and compliance are not so strict that the desired subjects will never be located. The investigator who reviews the potential project with clinical and operational considerations in mind will be better able to work with the sponsor to identify any areas for potential cost-cutting. While some protocols must be designed to meet specific FDA guidelines and hence can be altered very little, others may allow flexibility to expand inclusion criteria and visit schedules.

INCLUSION/EXCLUSION CRITERIA. Do the age, weight, and sex requirements of the protocol reflect the characteristics of the PI's own practice population with the disease? Even for the simplest study, an investigator should be able to identify in his records at least ten times the number of patients being studied in the protocol. Investigators who undertake a study with the expectation that they will have to recruit from sources other than the population immediately available to them rarely complete the study on schedule. Do the inclusion criteria describe a stage of the disease that the investigator encounters less frequently? For example, physicians in specialty clinics often agree to conduct seemingly simple protocols of early stage disease without taking into account that they see such patients rather infrequently in comparison to more severely ill populations. Would the proposed treatment be accepted within the community for treating the stage of disease? For example, a protocol requiring that patients be hospitalized for treatment of an infection may prove difficult to conduct if subjects are routinely treated on an outpatient basis for the affliction. Are the ranges of acceptable laboratory tests wide enough for the population being studied? Are the restrictions on concomitant medication use reasonable for the population under study? Does the sponsor expect that X rays or ECGs will be read by radiologists or cardiologists, or can these functions be performed by the research physicians?

STUDY PLAN. Is the visit schedule sufficiently flexible to allow for conflicts that may arise such as car trouble, forgotten appointments, and difficulties with baby-sitters? If not, are the potential benefits such that subjects will still wish to participate? Is it important to have the same medical and administrative personnel evaluate the subject throughout his course of study? If so, have adequate budget provisions been made to assure their continued availability? Since laboratory results must be available prior to dosing, does the protocol allow enough time between the baseline evaluation and dosing for the results to be returned? If the disease being treated requires presumptive therapy while awaiting laboratory results (e.g., some antiinfective studies), how will the team be remunerated for having enrolled subjects who later prove ineligible? Do the medication kits include a few extra days of medication in the event that a subject cannot return on schedule? If not, do the compliance limits account for the fact that patients who skip a visit may miss a day or two of medication until a new supply can be provided for them?

OUTCOME/SAFETY MEASUREMENTS. Most protocols specify some minimum period for which the patient must be on therapy in order to be considered an evaluable case. Is the time period chosen appropriate for the type of drug being studied? Would the investigator be willing to leave subjects on the study drug for this period of time even if they were showing no improvement? Is the maximum period of therapy appropriate for patients with more severe disease who may be included in the study? Are the frequency and timing of the study tests suitable for the population being studied? For example, if a study restricts enrollment to women over 50, do pregnancy tests need to be conducted at every visit? Are the laboratory evaluations frequent enough in view of the type of disease and anticipated side effects of the medication?

This detailed analysis of a protocol is required not only to identify hidden costs that may be involved in conducting the study but also to assure that the protocol will prove medically acceptable to the research team. Protocols that are much more inconvenient or involve more paper work than similar studies being conducted at the facility will not likely benefit from so many referrals or so much staff enthusiasm as the other research. While those factors should not necessarily deter the investigator from choosing to participate in the research, he should be prepared to budget for those inconveniences and offer other advantages unique to the more complex study. Often such advance planning can make the critical difference in whether a protocol enjoys the support of the research team and is considered an attractive option for prospective subjects.

RECRUITMENT

The planning and attainment of recruitment is the critical step of any drug investigation. The protocol must be read carefully as discussed above to abstract the precise inclusion criteria, the precise exclusion criteria, and some formulation of the bother and hassle factor for the participant. Should the observations needed on the patient require a great number of trips to the office, the inclusion criteria may be altered to include living within a 20-minute ride or possessing a personal vehicle in order to enhance the number of patients retained in the study. Once all of this has been determined, thought must be given as to just where subjects are located who meet all of these criteria and, having identified their location, what inducements relative to this study would successfully motivate them to participate. A very successful biostatistician once suggested that the planning investigator should make the best possible estimate of the number of patients he can recruit and then divide that number by *at least* 4 and as much as 10, reflecting the many problems that can arise between initial and sometimes unrealistic planning and performance.

The new investigator should test the recruitment strategy to some degree by actual surveys of colleagues, clinics, hospital admissions, laboratory logs, or an HMO to determine exactly how many eligibles are present in the sample. An experienced recruitment colleague can review the inclusion, exclusion, and hassle criteria and estimate knowledgeably the fraction of eligible patients that can be recruited, and separately estimate the fraction who will complete the study. Such surveys, though laborious, positively impress sponsors and provide useful decision-making and budgeting information for the PI before committing his staff and his services to a study.

Several basic decisions regarding recruitment must be made in budget planning. Patients in hospitals can be utilized only with the permission of the responsible physician as well as that of the patient. A recruitment strategy involving a department all of whose members participate is vastly superior to one involving individual negotiation with each patient and his doctor. Identifying patients before a close doctor–patient relationship is developed (such as in screening areas and new patient areas, or by advertising directed at the patients) produces better results than depending upon physician referrals. The direct appeal to the patient who has the qualifying condition is usually more successful than negotiating through several other parties.

Completion of recruitment in the shortest possible time results in savings in personnel costs, rent, and consumption of the PI's services. Often these efficiencies will lead to the sponsor's paying a premium price. Reimbursements to case-finders for their time, advertisement, or personnel to explain the study to those who inquire are all excellent economies. For example, if a PI is searching for patients with proven ulcer or urinary tract infection, arrangements could be made for administrative personnel to scan available records and receive a bonus for any pertinent cases of which the team is notified.

When a plan has been formulated and is ready, expected recruitment rates should be defined (e.g., one patient each week after the initial start-up month) and the criteria for failure established (e.g., fewer than two patients in the first two months of recruitment and fewer than three patients in any subsequent two-month period) so an alternative plan or decision to default on the contract can be instituted. If possible, an alternative plan and a budget for it should be formulated and included as a separate item in the budget submission.

EXAMPLE 1. *Alternative Strategy*

Recruitment of normal males for a bioavailability study was simply inadequate despite substantial unemployment. Two storefront offices were procured in totally different sections of town targeted for recent layoffs from industry, and local weekly newspapers were used heavily for announcements about the program. Great numbers of applicants appeared and were taken by van to the regular facility after screening. This program increased the costs of identifying suitable subjects by about 5% and allowed much more rapid completion of protocols.

The screening and enrollment process should minimize inconvenience to the interested patient and be designed to obtain needed results rapidly. Sometimes laboratories involved in the screening process or physicians conducting a key review may need to be paid a premium for their rapid response. Often taxi fares may need to be reimbursed to allow a subject to go to two or three sites in a short period of time. Occasionally, when a single nationwide laboratory system is utilized, services may be intolerably slow in some communities. In such cases the PI may need to obtain duplicate values in a local laboratory and enroll the patient on the basis of those values while awaiting findings of the reference core lab. Physicians are not always available when needed, and to lessen the wait and inconvenience for the client, paying another doctor to conduct a necessary physical examination may be advisable.

The costs of screening patients who do not qualify or do not participate once qualified to join the study must be included in the budget. Obviously, keeping these costs low will increase the financial value of the study. In all studies at least 1 in 10 fail to qualify or refuse to participate. In complex studies, only 1 in 50 or 1 in 100 screened patients may participate. The investigator must keep in mind all the "consumed" personnel costs in these calculations. If personnel costs are a large budget item, available means of economizing should be considered. For example, can a less skilled employee perform certain tasks? Often proper telephone screening alone will eliminate candidates with common disqualifying factors and save everyone time. Good telephone screening for a study that is limited to women who cannot become pregnant will eliminate most women of childbearing potential. Effective telephone techniques for a study that requires arthritis patients who take no other medication will usually eliminate many with severe pain at the initial review.

A research assistant is a good value in expediting screening and recruitment and in assisting with or conducting much of the paper work. Sometimes existing staff can carry out this function, but more often a new employee should be considered. The many functions delegated to such a person are discussed more fully in the next chapter on staff selection.

PAYMENTS OR REIMBURSEMENTS TO SUBJECTS

Virtually all investigative studies will inconvenience subjects and require unessential testing (from the vantage point of proper care for the subject's condition). It is, therefore, customary and proper to pay subjects for extra travel and out-of-pocket expenses associated with participation. These payments also provide some motivation for complex, bothersome tasks such as keeping detailed diaries, collecting 24-hour urines, and similar duties. The marketplace clearly dictates what one must pay, but it is traditional to reimburse travel and other costs of the visits at approximately the cost of gasoline, parking, minimum wage for travel time, or taxi fare. Usually a bonus is given for completion of the study that approximates $5 to $10 for each transaction. The bonus payment is increased for undesirable studies and diminished if it is a popular one. At all times, the sponsor's and IRB's policies on payment to subjects must be followed.

Thus, a patient undertaking two unnecessary endoscopies and six trips for the study, and keeping a daily symptom diary might be paid $10 for each trip at the time of the trip and be given $100 for completing the study. The bonus would not be given if the patient dropped out. A patient undertaking a study of acute diarrhea might be given $25 for the first trip, which includes the provision of a stool sample, and $10 for one follow-up visit (both paid at the time of the visits), with a $125 bonus for completing the study, with diary, test medication, etc., and final telephone interview on side effects. A patient appearing every other week for one year for routine visits might be given $10 for each visit and a $500 bonus for completion.

EXAMPLE 2. Money Talks

A study of an antiinflammatory drug for knee and hip arthritis required many return trips to quantitate ease of walking. Dropouts were high. Rearranging the payment so that each trip was rewarded with $10 in cash paid during the visit seemed to eliminate the problem.

Out-of-pocket expenses of the patients should be paid immediately (in cash if possible) and should be treated as study expenses.

CONVERTING PLANS INTO COST ESTIMATES

This process may require someone from the PI's office, hospital, or region knowledgeable with cost accounting to aid him, but it is not difficult. Each activity in the recruitment process requires an expenditure of someone's time and may involve a direct service for which the PI will be billed (advertising, laboratory tests, subject payments). The estimate of rate of recruitment, efficiency of converting screened eligible applicants into enrollees, and estimates of retention to completion in the study are all used to estimate costs. Although there is moderate to marked uncertainty in this business, it is not an overwhelmingly risky problem, for most of the personnel costs and physician costs will be those of the PI and his staff. Table 6 is an example worked through to plan a budget.

Some commonly overlooked costs occur because of local policy. Thus, drugs may have to be stored and dispensed in the pharmacy and a charge rendered for each patient or each transaction. A cost for the IRB review of sponsored research may be assessed. Charges for certain support services such as dietetics, social service, rental of the facilities, and record use may be separately assessed. In certain circumstances,

TABLE 6. Per Patient Budget for Study of Prevention of Ulcer in Patients on Nonsteroidal Antiinflammatory Agents

Regulatory requirements and paper work	
Peer review $400/10	$ 40
Completion and filing of records	$ 300
Recruitment costs	
Payments to physicians $300	$ 150
(only half obtained in this way)	
Secretarial screening of charts	$ 300
and phone calls—40 hrs.	
PI discussion with patients	$ 100
Screening physical and verification	$ 100
of old ulcer, records, phone	
SMA 12, urine, ECG, pregnancy test	$ 42
Failure to enter study after	$ 242
eligible (half enter)	
(i.e., screening costs)	
Study costs	
Safety check, eyes, lab, Hx and Px (2	$ 242
sets)	
Cost/visit—blood, office nurse × 11	$ 935
@ $85	
Patient payments—15 visits @ $10 + 600	$ 750
at end	
Endoscopy costs—3/pt. @ $310	$ 930
PI supervision—5 hrs. @ $150/hr.	$ 750
Contingency costs	
Reaction evaluation $50/patient	$ 50
Repeat labs, ECGs, 5% total	$ 45
Total	$4976
Profit 20%	$ 995.20
Subtotal grant	$5971.20
Overhead to hospital to dispense funds	
15%	$ 895.68
Total grant	$6866.88

the IRB may require a visit by the alcoholism counselor or a review by the anesthesiologist, and these services will be charged against the study budget. Some hospitals require that their laboratories be used for all sponsored studies, a factor that may change the budget estimates. Soliciting the advice of an experienced person reviewing a budget before submission, preferably one who works in the PI's own administrative structure, is of great value.

ADMINISTRATIVE SUPPORT AND PAPER WORK

No investigator should plan a study without planning for assistance in the many contacts with the patients and completion of the paper work. All studies require a great deal of communication as a part of the recruitment, screening, and enrollment processes and in keeping patients compliant during the study. The IRB submissions and the case report forms (CRFs) are time-consuming and, with training, much of this can be carried out by a research assistant. Preparing a typical submission to an IRB, with informed consent and appropriate documentation, usually requires two hours of the PI's time and another two hours of secretarial time. Follow-up and final reports require about one additional hour of secretarial time. More complex submissions, including those requiring radioisotope review or submissions to multiple hospitals, can be very time-consuming and, hence, more costly. The authors believe that the actual value of the preparation is seldom less than $300. Some committees charge for each review and these charges vary from $300 to $1000 per protocol.

Patients' research records and case report forms must be prepared and maintained separately from patient care charts. While their cost may be slight in time, some cost must be assigned to them. The authors' experience supervising skilled clerical workers indicates that the cost of preparation, filing, and distribution is usually about $200 per patient for a multiple-visit study. It is preferable for a person with secretarial skills to be specifically assigned to these tasks and planned for in the budget. Even if an investigator has a secretary, specific payments or bonuses for these special services encourage their being done well and saves the PI time and bother. Cutting costs or trying to save in this area is inappropriate, for it leads to poor documentation and extreme frustration for the PI and the sponsor.

PERSONNEL

In the previous section, costs were assigned on the basis that new employees were not hired to perform the work. Depending upon the complexities of the protocol and its major needs, staff with secretarial-receptionist skills, patient-motivation and contact skills, or nursing technical skills may be needed. Most studies fund the salary of only one full- or part-time person to assist the PI with the research protocol. Other employees working with the PI may perform services on the protocol for no specific payment but derive benefit from the one study employee who performs other duties in the unit. In any event, should a person be hired, a salary must be included in the budget. The estimated duration for recruitment, enrollment, and completion of the study becomes critical in this planning, for it is essential to have the assistant for the duration of the study. If a person has not been identified, the budget should permit the hiring of someone with some experience or provide a great deal of extra time for training. If the starting salary is $15,500 for a college graduate not experienced in research, two months of his time might well be required for training. If this is the case, a person paid $17,500 with two years of experience is a bargain. Providing a salary also requires payment of benefits, which approximate 13 to 20% of the salary, depending upon the administrative system through which that person is hired.

OVERHEAD

Almost all research sites charge the funded investigator for some of the services that are consumed. Rent or facility fees may be assessed for each use of a site or clinic. Phone charges, postage costs, paper, photocopying services, and maintenance of photocopiers, computers, or word processors are common charges. Nearly all money management will require payment (3 to 8%) and many institutions "tax" drug grants from 15 to 40% as the overhead costs. These must be carefully considered in budgeting.

CONTINGENCY FUNDING

In all studies it can be expected that 5 to 15% of tests that are performed will be abnormal, unsatisfactory, or simply confusing to interpret. These must be repeated. Sponsors desire evaluation of possible reactions by follow-up testing and visits, additional tests to clarify the nature of a reaction, or alternative explanations. At least $50 per subject should be included for these items. Alternative recruitment plans may be included but usually are paid for only if the alternative plans have to be used.

The pharmaceutical industry usually earns a return on sales of 15 to 20% each year, and it is not unreasonable to expect this amount of yield on an efficiently organized, well-planned study. This profit may be calculated after all reasonable costs have been included and is conditional upon the estimates of recruitment being reasonably accurate.

Clearly, a prolongation of recruitment could easily cost more than this amount to complete the study.

COST CUTTING AND SAVINGS

In budgeting, prices that will be in effect at the time the study will be done should be used. In performance it is often possible to obtain a 20 to 30% reduction on laboratory and consultant prices by agreeing to pay a single bill within ten days and in some instances allowing them to process study samples after their more urgent ones are completed. X rays and ECGs can be obtained more cheaply if the study physicians are willing to read them. Occasionally, a physician's assistant or a nurse practitioner can perform tasks usually done by a physician. Physicians should not be utilized in filling out questionnaires when a less costly person can undertake this function.

MONEY MANAGEMENT

All funds should be maintained in separate accounts from which an audit can be conducted. They should not be placed in private checking accounts, which may be construed as personal income by the Internal Revenue Service. The funds should be easily accessible to meet the needs of immediate payment for expenses to patients.

The sponsor should provide payment to keep up with disbursements. Vendors usually will accept a lower fee for their services if payment is prompt but will need a higher payment if it is to be delayed. Accordingly, the payment schedule needs to be carefully worked out by the PI and the sponsor and should accurately reflect the investigator's costs. A good budget will make this easy. Standard plans, wherein 25% of the total contract is paid up front, 25% when half the contract is fulfilled, 25% when all of the contract is fulfilled, and 25% when all paper work is done, usually fail to cover out-of-pocket expenses when patients and suppliers are paid promptly. Costs of employees' salaries and all of the ongoing expenses must be met and the payment schedule adjusted to match reimbursement schedules. These things are all negotiable but must be clarified before the contract is accepted.

Sponsors differ markedly from one to another in policies for paying for dropouts, patients who miss clinic visits but finish the study, and evaluations of possible adverse events. Clarification should be obtained from the company on all considerations involved in deciding whether to reimburse the PI for any cases falling into the above groups. The company's policies on paying for evaluations of possible reactions also should be stated. This information should be utilized in planning the budget.

EXAMPLE 3. Disagreement on Payment

A sponsor agreed to fund costs related to reactions separately. A patient developed rising AST and ALT during the sixth to tenth week of exposure to a new agent and was discontinued from the study. In evaluation of this problem after discontinuation, the patient was seen three times and $72 worth of blood and antibody tests were obtained showing a rising antibody level to Hepatitis B, thereby ruling out a reaction to the sponsor's medication. The sponsor refused to pay for the studies because the event was not drug-related. The sponsor prorated the stipend on the basis of the actual time in study, paying about half of the contracted value for this patient. The sponsor reversed this position when no information beyond the dates paid for was supplied on the CRF.

Table 6 illustrates a budget submitted for a protocol testing a single daily dose of a prostaglandin derivative versus placebo in patients with rheumatoid arthritis who require at least four tablets of nonsteroidal antiinflammatory agent daily, who are not taking H2 blocking agents, but who can take sucralfate or antacids. All patients must have had a verified ulcer in the past two years (X ray or endoscopy) in the stomach or duodenum. Patients will be seen monthly for compliance and safety check of blood, urine, and ECG, and will continue the study for one year. Any new stomach symptoms lead to endoscopy. If an ulcer is identified, that patient has completed the study. If there is no ulcer, endoscopy is repeated each month until three studies have been completed and the patient is dropped. Detailed ophthalmological exams are needed at the beginning and end. All female patients must have a pregnancy test at every visit. The contract is planned for ten patients to be completed in two years or less.

In planning the recruitment, two strategies are undertaken. A payment to physicians of $300 for each patient who enrolled is planned, but only half of the patients are expected to be obtained in this manner. Thus, the cost per patient is listed at $150. A secretary will screen charts in several offices and clinics for past history of ulcer and contact such patients. It is estimated that 80 hours will be required for each patient enrolled. This estimate was based upon the need to screen 30 charts for each one with an ulcer and the assumption that one patient would join the study for every 200 charts screened. Half the patients are to be recruited in this way. The PI will be used for discussion with patients, including the informed consent, calculating 40 minutes of time for each patient. The laboratory costs are as offered by the pathology department. It is estimated that half of the patients screened and found eligible will enter the study so that $242 per patient will be screening costs for those reluctant or unwilling to enter or those found ineligible. Once patients enter the study, they must have a safety screen of eyes and test on two occasions, even if they receive only a single dose of study medication, and this will cost $242. In the actual conduct of the study, there are 11 required visits that include physical examination, interaction with the staff, blood tests, and a pregnancy test for women, at a cost of $85 for each visit. Patient payments are calculated at 15 trips because separate trips are often required for visits to the ophthalmologist and to the laboratory. To motivate the patients to complete the study, keep the diary, return medications, and put up with the three unnecessary endoscopies, they will be paid $600 at the end of the study. Endoscopy costs, including facility charges, are $310 per procedure. PI supervision for each patient, including contact with the patient after recruitment, telephone conversations, and a brief examination at each of the visits, is calculated at five hours per patient. A contingency of $50 per patient is included for testing for possible reactions. Five percent of the cost, or $45, of all laboratory work, including ECGs, is included for repeats that may be necessary and payment for the patients to come back for the repeat tests.

The preparation of IRB submission and follow-up reports is estimated to cost $400, and this is divided over the ten patients. The completion of each record and preparation of the CRF, including copying, is calculated at $300 per patient. A profit of 20% is included and the cost to dispense the funds is 15% of the total grant. Some sponsors prefer not to approve a line item of profit and request that all prices be increased to reflect that 20% fee.

SUBMISSION AND NEGOTIATION OF THE BUDGET

The final budget figure can usually be reviewed by phone and subsequently submitted in writing. Most sponsors will indicate whether the cost is appropriate and, after consideration, may seek to negotiate. If the cost is too high, the sponsor may agree to pay certain charges directly (e.g., all endoscopies will be paid separately from the budget, all extra health checks, repeat tests, etc.). The sponsor may accept a less costly approach, for example, visual fields performed by a resident in ophthalmology, PE and Hx done by a nurse practitioner, or dispensing with the pregnancy tests. Each of these will result in a saving and may be eliminated from the investigator's budget. The PI may want to perform the study for the reasons discussed in Chapter 2 and may wish to undertake it at any cost. All of these factors must enter into the negotiation. Quality work, the need for little supervision by the sponsor, and rapid completion of the contract justify premium payments.

Several budget items presented in Table 6 are negotiable. The recruitment costs could probably be reduced by $100 per patient and patient payments reduced by $200. Lab and endoscopy costs could probably be accomplished for $300 less per patient and the PI supervision could be diminished by $150, for a total reduction in the actual subtotal of $750. With the overhead, this would be a reduction of more than $1000 per patient. If the sponsor should choose to pay a maximum of $5000 per patient, the study could be performed only if another project contained enough funds to subsidize the sponsor's study. Alternatively, perhaps the endoscopies could be performed at no cost in the context of a training program, the patients need not receive a final bonus, and all staff functions could be performed as part of salaries already paid. These several maneuvers would make the study possible at less than $5000 per patient.

FINAL CONTRACTING

The final contract must be a written document. The policies of the sponsor for adverse event reimbursement, coverage of potential litigation costs, and the payment schedule should be obtained in writing. The PI should be certain that the payee of the study grant is noted in the document so the payments are not treated as personal income. Chapter 4 discusses some factors that deserve consideration before undertaking a contract with a sponsor.

CHAPTER 6

Staff Selection and Training

General Criteria for Selecting Staff • *Recruiting a Study Coordinator* • *Staff Training* • *Techniques for Facilitating Training and Employee Growth*

The PI of any project must have some assistance available for conducting drug research. Numerous regulatory and administrative tasks, as well as telephone contacts and completing CRFs, must be delegated to free the PI to concentrate on the medical aspects of the study. As was discussed in the previous chapter, each new protocol must be analyzed along the lines of budget planning to identify just what duties can be delegated. Table 7 contains a listing of common tasks that arise in protocols. A PI should attempt to determine exactly what skills are needed for a particular study and the percentage of staff time required to carry them out. Once the research-related tasks have been identified, the PI can decide whether they can be carried out by existing personnel or will require the recruitment of new employees. The PI must also decide whether he is prepared for extensive training of new personnel or wishes to hire highly skilled employees with some research experience. Inexperienced PIs are advised to employ those with specific drug-testing experience.

GENERAL CRITERIA FOR SELECTING STAFF

All staff must project an image of professionalism, friendliness, efficiency, and concern for individual clients. Research enterprises must convey these messages in every contact because, like other services, a single negative experience can undo 10 to 20 excellent ones.

Experience in the health fields by formal training or previous work experience is a very valuable asset in an employee. This experience provides an understanding of illness and health care systems that is not easily learned in a short period of time. The concept that the patient's

TABLE 7. Research Responsibilities That May Be Delegated to a
Trained Person

Communication functions
  Receiving and obtaining appropriate responses to telephone calls at all regular hours
  Screening potential applicants, recruiting while informing candidates about study
  Reminding enrollees of appointments, answering inquiries
  Making friendly calls to keep people in a study
  Setting up appointments
  Obtaining reports
  Screening reports for abnormalities
Administrative functions
  Assisting with preparation of the grant, budget, and IRB submission
  Preparing appropriate and timely reports for committees and sponsors
  Filling out CRF
  Keeping the research medical record
  Administering questionnaires
  Interviewing for side effects
Office technician functions
  Obtaining blood and urine samples and arranging delivery to the lab
  Conducting special tests (e.g., ECG, photography, audiometry)
  Leading patients from one laboratory to another
Professional functions
  Giving medication and injections
  Maintaining i.v. infusions
  Carrying out histories and physical examinations
  Controlling and dispensing medication
  Substitute physician for PI
  Specialist physician (e.g., ophthalmologist, dermatologist)

needs supersede the employee's "rights" is understood by nearly all health workers, but it is almost impossible to train new employees to accept such a premise readily. Health care is a confusing, often illogical, system that can be learned, but it is easier if the person has learned something about it before joining the PI's team. An employee's experience working with multiple doctors is also helpful in that he will have already familiarized himself with differences in style and manner among physicians. Such experience prevents the upsets that might otherwise come if the new employee were to encounter radically different personality types for the first time while on the PI's payroll.

EXAMPLE 1. Style

A study of ascites in hospitalized patients with cirrhosis provided randomization to continued (but failing) medical treatment and a LeVeen shunt, a surgical procedure. Although potential patients were abundant *(one each week), a nurse totally failed to recruit patients. Her replacement recruited approximately one patient a month, leading the 15 centers in the project. The two nurses were equally competent and professional. The successful one was confident, worked hard to find all possible patients when they arrived in the hospital, and served as a highly effective interface with them. She successfully eliminated the many hassles of a VA hospital by facilitating medicines, appointments, hospital admission when necessary, and waiting time. The unsuccessful one was timid, unsure of the study, and unsure of her role. Two different personalities produced very different outcomes.*

Research experience is very valuable and should be deliberately incorporated at some level in the organization. The authors have observed that fabrication of data tends to occur more often when no one on the team has had such a background. This background helps the entire staff keep its mind on the truth requirement of research, rather than on the recruitment-retention emphasis that is regularly reinforced.

References should always be carefully checked for interpersonal relationships, evidence of honesty and integrity, and high reliability. If a staff member is not available to a patient, or is casual about appointments, patients will be inclined to perform in a similar manner.

RECRUITING A STUDY COORDINATOR

Large studies utilize a full-time research assistant who functions in many different capacities depending upon the PI, the protocol, and the duties that can be appropriately delegated. Many protocols are successfully completed by the efforts of the PI and the study coordinator (SC),

TABLE 8. *Characteristics Desirable in a Study Coordinator*

College education, preferably in science or health care
Previous experience in some aspect of research
Previous experience in some aspect of health care, possibly in the PI's own hospital if recruitment is to be carried out there
Great human skills even under duress (e.g., no tendency toward temper outbursts)[a]
Willingness to work irregular hours
High reliability[a]
Middle-of-the-road dress and appearance
Background free of dishonesty[a]
Record of attainment in some field

[a]Essential.

who, combined, literally perform every function. Table 8 lists some characteristics to be considered in choosing an SC.

The adherence to protocols and the interaction with the many regulatory people and other professionals is better handled by a mature person more often found in a college graduate than in one without advanced education. Friendly, exuberant, youthful enthusiasm for life has almost invariably been a characteristic of the most highly successful study personnel. Independent of sex, age, and background, this is a valuable consideration. Successful service to clients involves high reliability in meeting personal commitments and the occasional necessity to meet someone at irregular hours to accommodate an unexpected crisis. Again, the authors have found that well-organized, committed persons can manage these things despite their own personal lives, young children, or moonlighting jobs.

EXAMPLE 2. Mister America

A highly successful study coordinator was an all-state athlete, loved people, and had a degree in business administration. His first job was recruiting people for a 1-year study of an agent to dissolve gallstones. His zest for life, enthusiasm for his work, use of a great deal of personal contact, and willingness to talk and meet with people and their families made him the nation's leader in the recruitment and retention of people in this difficult study. His personal qualities and effective use of the many required facilities of the hospital led to this success.

STAFF TRAINING

Regardless of their background and previous experience, all staff members need formal orientation to the PI and his philosophy of research as well as to the specific protocol. Although existing qualified staff can conduct portions of this orientation, it must meet the standards of the PI. The PI should schedule this orientation on the first day or two of employment. Table 9 indicates important areas that must be covered.

ORIENTATION OF THE STUDY COORDINATOR AND OTHER ADMINISTRATIVE STAFF. The research orientation, which requires two or three hours, sets the high standards to which the PI aspires and allows no misunderstanding of the overriding importance of truth, honesty, and full disclosure. A detailed presentation of the IRB process, the informed consent process, and the rights of subjects can be amplified

TABLE 9. *Orientation of Employees to the Research and the Protocol*

Research orientation
  Process of IRB and informed consent
  Rights of subjects
  Confidentiality
  Team honesty
  Defining delegated responsibility
  Use and abuse of PI's authority
Protocol orientation
  Review and understanding of plan of study
  Division of labor
  Adverse event management
  Relationship with the sponsor
  CRF and research record-keeping procedures

with examples from the PI's experience and discussed. The issue of confidentiality as it relates to the subject and sponsors' trade secrets must be discussed. The need for truth in the research process to supersede recruitment pressures should also be discussed with examples pertinent to the present protocol. Making some reference to the inevitable omissions, inconsistencies, and unkept appointments that are common to the research setting and suggestions for keeping them to a minimum assists in building a good relation between the SC and PI. All employees should be aware that their work will be subjected to continuing quality assurance.

Each PI and SC combination functions differently with regard to the responsibilities of each and the SC's use of the PI's authority. This should be defined and limited and an SOP (standard operating procedure) written that defines the delegation of authority and responsibility. This SOP may change from time to time to account for additional training, increasing confidence in the staff, or changes in methods of conducting the research.

Protocol orientation is carried out by the PI and the study team separately from the sponsor's training visit(s). Its purpose is to allow the new employee to obtain an understanding of the team's recruitment methods and study procedures unique to the site. A clear discussion should be undertaken of the division of labor, exactly who will be responsible for each of the many duties, and the limits of that delegated authority applicable to the particular protocol under discussion.

Each employee with protocol responsibilities must learn them. This is most commonly accomplished in a preceptor relationship with someone who fully understands the duties of the position. For this reason it is often advisable to have a mechanism in place to cross-train employees so they are familiar with a number of positions on the team. The preceptor might be the PI or an existing staff member who has carried out this function previously. Sometimes the CRA of the sponsor can identify a local group conducting the identical protocol who can provide this preceptorship. The employee should witness the specific duties that he will perform, subsequently perform part and later all of them under direct guidance, and finally perform the duties independent of the preceptor. His work then should be reviewed for completeness, with an opportunity to amplify or address problems. Each employee's responsibilities may be expanded one by one as the specific duties are learned and executed successfully while maintaining the standards of the research team. Specific training issues relevant to staff members of professionals with more limited roles are discussed below.

The sponsor's role in orienting the research team is to provide training for staff members involved in patient care, diary review, pill counts, and CRFs. The sponsor's orientation ordinarily will focus on the company's policies on safety monitoring and reporting as well as CRF completion. The sponsor's CRA may also provide suggestions on recruiting and data management that have proven successful at other sites. This training is of great benefit as a supplement to the PI's more comprehensive orientation.

EXAMPLE 3. A Great Study Coordinator

An outstanding study coordinator graduated from high school, took up serious drinking, and eventually recovered through medically related programs. He became an alcoholism counselor in a unit that performed research studies, participating in recruitment in some of these. After five years of this work, he applied for an SC position. His understanding of research was gained through five years in apprenticeship, but hard work was required to learn some of the special skills of drug administration, venesection, and processing of specimens. The characteristics that made him a superb SC were sincerity in every transaction, complete commitment to the subjects in his studies, total belief in the research and its integrity, and love of helping people. He used the authority of his PI to great advantage for his clients.

TRAINING OF THE SECRETARY-RECEPTIONIST. This person is invariably already present in the organization but if he is hired as a new employee, interpersonal skills, knowledge of the medical process, research experience, and a genuine desire to help people are characteristics that should be sought. Since this person is the first contact with a patient or possible client, it is very important that he be oriented to the PI's standards. This is best done by role playing both in person and over the phone.

Common problems that must be attended to in this orientation include how to satisfy a talkative, curious person while other calls are waiting (call back at an appointed time, or have another knowledgeable person call back); how to indicate he does not know the answer to a particular question or cannot give medical advice; how to calm an angry person; what sort of personal data about a caller is useful in making the enrollment decision; how to determine that the doctor is urgently needed by a caller, and how to determine that he is not; and, finally, how to improve recruitment from the initial contact.

This person must understand that he is the initial contact and that judgments about the entire program will be made on that first impression. Presenting a professional image should be a job requirement, and the employee should know at the outset whether his salary and evaluations will be affected by his performance in that area.

A separate function, usually assigned to the receptionist, is the expeditious arranging of visits, starting with the very first. Again, role playing in the orientation is helpful. The new employee should have an opportunity to practice making friendly contact at the first visit, indicating, for example: "I'm Gloria, and I will usually be answering the phone and will be talking with you about appointments, etc. I want you to know that I am here to help, so call me if things come up, if you need help in changing appointments, or if you need the doctor. Here is a card with my number and here is Dr. Iber's answering service, which can reach him or whatever doctor is covering for him at night." In this orientation, it must be emphasized through discussion and example that the patient's time is important and must not be abused.

ORIENTATION OF TECHNICIANS. The most important point to communicate in the orientation of technical personnel is that the patients are doing the research team a favor by being in the study and that promptness and consideration on the part of all personnel are urgent to the entire operation. A PI should be alert for signs of resentment that the research duties involve extra work and should address any such behavior promptly.

ORIENTATION OF PROFESSIONALS. Full-time nurses, physician assistants, dieticians, psychologists, and physicians are sometimes recruited to join a study team, but part-time or fee-for-special-service arrangements are much more common. Often the choices of available persons are limited, but when choices are available previous research experience and willingness to give service, even out of routine hours, are important considerations. As with all staff, they must project a friendly, professional manner and enjoy people.

The orientation and training are often more difficult in the latter two groups because of two problems. First, the PI may presume that professionals already know many of the things about which orientation is, in fact, needed and, second, the professional receiving the orientation may resist any perceived attempts to limit his freedom of action. Many professionals accustomed to the independence of private practice may not be aware that research requires much more detailed documentation than they may employ with their practice records. Some may not be willing to offer the additional flexibility in scheduling needed to accommodate strict visit windows of protocols. A PI who is selecting and orienting professionals to join the study team should make some assessment of their familiarity with research regulation and willingness to conform to it. A true "free spirit" who resists or ignores all regulatory requirements will only cause great aggravation for the PI and other team members.

As with the other team members, the PI must take the time to outline his expectations and those of the sponsor. It is useful to review the protocol, how it is set up, how it is to be performed, and the individual tasks expected of each person. Since doctors and nurses sometimes are reluctant to participate in detailed orientations involving all employees, it may be necessary to meet with them separately and review the objectives of the study as they pertain to their tasks. A simulated case or situation remains one of the best teaching tools followed by observations of actual performance.

Professionals are usually hired for a very specific action, such as an ophthalmological examination, diet interview or instruction, conducting physical examinations, or dosing a group of subjects. They need be oriented only to that which they do and be given copies of the protocol should they wish to learn more or answer basic inquiries from subjects. Because of their limited involvement, however, they should be encouraged to refer all questions they do not understand to the study physicians or the full-time staff. It is essential that they receive some orientation as to what their records and reports should contain. Physicians seeing patients for study purposes who do not expect to see the patients privately may not see the need to retain copies of their evaluations in their own records. The authors have employed endoscopists who did not retain copies of their endoscopy reports as an audit trail. Since such a practice is not acceptable from a regulatory point of view, it is worthwhile to clarify the documentation requirements at the outset.

TECHNIQUES FOR FACILITATING TRAINING AND
EMPLOYEE GROWTH

Group discussions of the progress of the study are valuable for improving both quality and morale. Most of the full-time team should assemble for such meetings, which should be leisurely. Lunch purchased from study funds is a good investment, allowing the employees to discuss how the study is progressing and to identify necessary improvements. At this time meritorious accomplishments by individuals can freely be cited, but individual derelictions should not be revealed, since these are better discussed in private. A one-page summary of the most positive suggestions should be prepared to set the stage for the next discussion.

Employees can be asked to develop SOPs for areas in which variability or deficiencies are noted. Should a large number of people participate in blood drawing, for example, and potassium levels are found to be quite variable, an SOP for drawing and separation of erythrocytes may be in order. Such an assignment offers an opportunity for the employees to vent their frustrations and suggest improvements that will be satisfactory to all.

Review of inspections by CRAs, quality assurance, and the FDA is highly valuable. Again, the staff should be highly praised for the good outcomes, and any problems should be tackled collectively so that solutions can be identified.

Citations of superior ideas or effective performance with a small award or letter to the team improves morale. The following are a few examples: By making home visits, Cyndy retained a subject inclined to drop out in the last 2 weeks of a 52-week study. Duane computerized all of the follow-up appointments so each staff person can receive a printed weekly schedule. Phyllis contacted 36 former arthritis patients by phone and has interested 10 of them in the study.

Not singling out employees publicly when an error has been made, and using individual names when praise or noteworthy accomplishments occur are recommended. Offering encouragement to do better, recognizing accomplishment, and understanding shortfalls all encourage employees to make their subsequent performance surpass previous efforts. Where feasible, cross-training employees in several areas of the research operation will allow them to learn the impact of their performance on that of their co-workers.

Research is of necessity a team effort. The morale and competence of each and every person involved with the study will greatly influence the subjects' perceptions of the research experience. It is the PI's role to provide his staff and associates with the necessary orientation and, where appropriate, guidance to fulfill their responsibilities effectively. The personal satisfaction they will enjoy for carrying out those functions well will have a positive impact on both the study as a whole and the research care of the subjects.

FURTHER READING

American Hospital Association, *The Management of Hospital Employee Productivity: An Introductory Handbook*, American Hospital Association, Chicago, 1973.

Journal of Health Administration and Education (quarterly journal published on this topic).

Quatrano, L.A., and Clary, L.S., *Utility of Student Selection Criteria for Predicting Academic Outcome in the Health Administration Field: Literature Review and Recommendation*, Association of University Programs in Health Administration, Washington, D.C., 1976.

CHAPTER 7

Other Preparatory Activities

National Regulatory Requirements • State, Local, and Institutional Regulatory Requirements • Fiscal Issues • Malpractice Insurance Coverage • Special Problems If Patients Are Housed

In complying with the many regulatory activities associated with clinical research, the investigative team will be involved primarily with the sponsor and the IRB. The sponsor ordinarily coordinates all communication with the FDA, such as the filing of the IND itself, submission of the investigator's credentials to the IND, and reporting of adverse experiences while the study is under way. There may be other local regulatory committees or agencies, however, with whom the investigator may need to deal directly for some studies. Authorizations may be required from some of these committees or agencies before the IRB will approve a study. Since many of these have similar or less stringent requirements than those of federal agencies, the investigator frequently can oblige all of their requirements with a limited amount of paper work.

Since the requirements of these committees or agencies can vary markedly from locale to locale, this chapter will provide a brief overview of the issues involved with each. The PI should always contact the responsible local personnel to learn the requirements unique to his institution or community.

All research submissions will require a protocol that provides a detailed description of the inclusion and exclusion criteria for subjects. The aim of the research must be formulated and some consideration rendered on how many subjects will be included. If analyses are to be undertaken in a serial fashion to determine when sufficient numbers of subjects have been obtained, this should be so stated. An outline of the standard elements of a research protocol is included in Chapter 8. Chapter 22 outlines the contents of the standard *curriculum vitae* format in which all investigators will be required to list their credentials. Investigators should be prepared to receive many requests for additional details or clarification. Although it is understandable that a PI may become frustrated with these requests, it is important to realize that many committees have a multidisciplinary membership, with professional training and interests quite different from that of the PI. Information that a PI may not have considered it necessary to include in a submission may not be readily obvious or available to professionals outside of the PI's particular specialty.

NATIONAL REGULATORY REQUIREMENTS

An IND is required to conduct research on a new entity, a new combination of commercially available drugs, treatment of a disease for which the drug is not currently approved, or a new release form of an available drug. The sponsor generally files the IND for a new drug. An investigator also may be the holder of an IND. An investigator may choose to file an IND himself for products of limited commercial value, such as orphan drugs for which the manufacturer is unwilling to serve as the sponsor. Any licensed physician may file an IND. The Form FDA-1571, which is the IND exemption form, may be obtained from the Public Health Service, Forms and Publications Distribution Center, 12100 Parklawn Drive, Rockville, Maryland 20857.

Investigators conducting research on controlled substances must have the appropriate DEA licensure that covers research activities.

STATE, LOCAL, AND INSTITUTIONAL REGULATORY REQUIREMENTS

Some states have state bureaus of food and drugs that require notification that research on investigational products is taking place. The IRB can usually provide information on their requirements, as some documentation of IRB approval is often required.

Research on specialized products may require the approval of various institutional committees in addition to the IRB. Investigation utilizing ionizing radiation or radioisotopes in other than routine uses must be conducted under a special license. Special committee review is not ordinarily required if the protocol involves the use of diagnostic quantities of radiation, since the risks and benefits of these procedures are ordinarily taken into account by the IRB. However, any unapproved uses of these procedures will likely require radioisotope or nuclear medicine committee review. Universities, most hospitals, and some individuals may have licenses for human use. A collaborator who has a full license may be recruited to assist with the study if necessary to satisfy committee requirements. Generally, an investigator should receive prior special instruction in the use of radioisotopes and their safe dosing and disposition. These applications are complex, requiring many calculations as to the dose being delivered to each organ in the body. It is usually cost-effective to obtain consultation in the preparation of materials for committee review.

The approval of the hospital's biomedical engineering office may be required to undertake research on new devices or equipment. These committees or offices generally have flexible submission requirements and can accept for review the same package of materials prepared for the IRB.

The majority of sponsors and the FDA recommend that the pharmacy department supervise the dispensing and storage of investigational products where feasible. Many institutions have this policy as well. Investigators should contact the research pharmacist before initiating the study to devise procedures that will meet the team's needs and allow patients easy access to the medications. There is often a charge for these services, which must be included in the study budget.

Many institutions and sponsors restrict the selection of local laboratories. Sponsors require that the laboratories selected for the study have College of American Pathologists (CAP) or state certifications. A PI must ascertain whether the results of urinalyses or other tests normally performed in his own office will be acceptable as study data.

Some institutions may have procedures in place to prohibit initiation of studies unless approvals have been obtained from the appropriate administrative departments and hospital chiefs. Such procedures are established to assure that the study funds are being disbursed through the hospital's grants management section and that the chiefs of the services whose patients will be involved have been notified of the study.

Investigators not on the staff of an institution who wish to conduct research involving its patients are usually required to obtain authorization from the responsible chief of service before the institution's IRB will review the protocol.

FISCAL ISSUES

Financial pressures are increasing on all types of health care organizations. Many administrative units look upon drug study sponsors as endless sources of revenue. Charges for fund management (overhead) may be modest (0 to 8%) or massive (up to 40%). Some units add facility costs (rent) and benefits for all program personnel as extra charges and may deduct unemployment charges and income tax from the subjects. These policies should be learned before the final budget is prepared, since they can alter the income for a project by as much as one-third.

MALPRACTICE INSURANCE COVERAGE

Malpractice policies do not often describe coverage for research activities in sufficient detail. Coverage policies for the screening process, the care of study patients after they have completed therapy, or care of patients who do not qualify are often vague. It is worthwhile to address this in writing with the private or institutional carrier at the outset. Providing a copy of the sponsor's indemnification policy is usually helpful.

Under state law, normal subjects participating in research may be considered temporary employees. Such a designation requires that appropriate taxes and unemployment insurance fees be paid for each subject. However, it does permit any injury claims to be processed as workmen's compensation cases.

SPECIAL PROBLEMS IF PATIENTS ARE HOUSED

Local ordinances governing sleeping density, fire safety, and food provision and storage may be a concern if subjects are being housed overnight. Hotels and hospitals should have passed the necessary inspections already. Setting up a study in a gymnasium or some other facility not intended for overnight use may run afoul of local regulations and should be investigated with local inspectors.

Clearly, this list of regulatory undertakings can appear overwhelming to an investigator anxious to get his new project under way. However, for the majority of investigations, the IRB approval will be the only documentation required. Many of the local requirements will be handled as a matter of course while preparing the budget or deciding where study supplies should be stored. Many other institutional committees can be satisfied by providing IRB submission documents. If properly prepared, these will be sufficiently detailed to accommodate any number of requests. Finally, many investigators will likely begin new projects with the best of intentions, only to receive notification that they have failed to comply with some regulatory or institutional requirements of which they were unaware. When such notifications are issued, it is best to make an effort to comply as expeditiously as possible, using, whenever appropriate, written documents already on hand describing the study.

The Institutional Review Mechanism

This section describes the process of institutional review, an essential regulatory requirement that must be completed before initiating a clinical trial. Suggestions for facilitating the review process are included.

CHAPTER 8

The Institutional Review Board Process

An institutional review board (IRB) is a multidisciplinary research review committee whose primary purpose is to protect the rights and welfare of research subjects. These review committees must have at least five members of varying backgrounds who can provide the breadth of scientific expertise and sense of community values required to evaluate protocols in many subspecialties of medicine and social science. Their membership ordinarily includes physicians and administrators from the board's parent institution, social science and nursing representatives, and unaffiliated community representatives from the clergy, academia, and local patient population. Although the majority of IRBs are affiliated with hospitals or academic institutions, a small number of pharmaceutical firms and contract agencies have chosen to establish independent IRBs to conduct reviews of protocols for practitioners unaffiliated with research institutions. Since IRB approval of a protocol and consent form must be secured before any research involving human subjects may be undertaken at any health care facility, these committees significantly affect the speed with which new research ventures may be initiated. The purpose of this chapter is to provide the overview of the IRB process needed for an investigator to achieve prompt IRB approvals and to comply with all applicable federal regulations.

Investigators conducting clinical trials have scientific and professional goals that can easily conflict with their immediate patient care responsibilities. The IRB review mechanism was established to provide a forum for health care professionals and interested community members to assist investigators in assessing the potential benefits and risks of a given project. The potential risks to the subjects are often substantial and the benefits uncertain. An independent assessment of the relative value of each risk is of great importance to both individual subjects and society at large. The IRB review provides assurance that new avenues of scientific inquiry are pursued responsibly.

In reviewing new protocols, IRB members consider whether appropriate preliminary research has been conducted to validate the objective of the present study. They also assess whether the study has been designed to fulfill its objective with the least possible risk to subjects. The IRB also brings to this review a perspective on local standards of care as well as compensation for research participation. The board evaluates the risks and benefits associated with the study to reach a conclusion regarding its appropriateness. The IRB's deliberations culminate in a discussion of the informed consent process in which the committee considers the setting, timing, and documents that can best be utilized to secure meaningful informed consent.

IRBs conduct this highly responsible work amid conflicting pressures from investigators desiring prompt approvals and regulatory agencies favoring greater supervision of study procedures and the informed consent process. The scope of responsibility assigned to the IRB varies with the institution and the views of the committee members themselves. It may be limited to review of the initial application and subsequent annual updates or involve extensive safety audits of patients' records and actual participation in the consent process. Whatever its mandate, it is highly likely that the IRB conducts these functions with extremely limited staff support. With this in mind, the investigator who prepares a careful and timely submission will find that his application will proceed through the IRB process much more smoothly and that the experience will prove a rewarding one.

JURISDICTION

Institutional policy determines the circumstances under which an IRB must review a protocol involving its facility, records, or personnel. Although the federal regulations require that an investigator obtain approval from only one IRB meeting the agency's criteria, the investigator must, nevertheless, comply with the requirements of all the IRBs having jurisdiction over the project. Each committee's bylaws will specify the conditions under which it chooses to review protocols somehow connected with its facility, namely, when (1) the research will involve patients under the care of the institution, (2) the research will be conducted by professional or support personnel acting in their official capacity within the institution, (3) the institution's name will be used in any reports or publications of the research, (4) the research will involve the records of the facility, and (5) the research will be conducted at the facility.

Copies of the IRB's bylaws or comparable policy statements are made available routinely to investigators. Some IRBs will also provide these copies to the sponsor upon request. Investigators unaffiliated with an institution who wish to conduct research involving its subjects are usually required to secure authorization from the appropriate chief of service before the IRB will review the project.

Overlapping jurisdictions can cause considerable delays in securing all required approvals of protocols involving more than one local facility. Multiple reviews place the investigator in the awkward position of having to reconcile possible opposing views of different committees. Although committees do have the latitude to enter into arrangements with other IRBs to accept one committee's review of a project, they will likely only consider such an arrangement if they are very familiar with both the investigator and the cooperating IRBs. Nevertheless, any investigator facing this prospect should contact the IRB chairperson he knows best to discuss the possibility of securing cooperative approval of the protocol. Broaching this subject with sufficient notice and a genuine willingness to conduct the IRB process efficiently and meaningfully will often motivate that chairperson to intervene on the investigator's behalf with the other committees. Such cooperative arrangements can usually decrease by up to two months the time required for the IRB process.

IRB MEMBERSHIP

Under current federal regulation, IRBs must contain at least five members with diverse backgrounds that reflect the cultural makeup of the community and represent the disciplines in which research is most commonly conducted within the institution. These members must display a knowledge of local standards of professional practice, prevalent community attitudes, and local laws and regulations to engender respect for the board's recommendations and decisions. Both sexes and more than one profession must be represented in the membership. An IRB must also include at least one member whose primary expertise is in a nonscientific area as well as one member who is unaffiliated with the institution and is not in the immediate family of any employee of the institution. IRBs that routinely review research conducted on a vulnerable category of subjects, such as the economically disadvantaged, should include in their membership representation of this category of subjects. In practice, most IRBs contain more than the required number of members to provide the necessary diverse representation and even include a number of persons who have never been involved in medical research and strongly oppose any nonessential manipulation. Committees also recruit consultants to issue opinions on any proposals that the membership does not have the competence to evaluate independently. The consultants' recommendations are then taken into account by the committee in voting on the proposal.

In signing the FDA 1572/3 form, the FDA secures the investigator's commitment to assure that the IRB that has reviewed the research proposal is in compliance with the FDA regulations governing the composition and functioning of IRBs. If the PI is not comfortable that the committee reviewing his work meets FDA composition requirements, he may review the membership and procedures of the IRB to note any deficiencies that could discredit the review. In such rare cases, alternative review arrangements or consultation with the committee chairman may be in order. In circumstances where the committee's procedures and membership composition are not provided to the investigator, some sponsors and physicians request a written statement from the IRB that the committee is operating in compliance with FDA regulations. Studies reviewed by an inappropriately constituted IRB can be disqualified from inclusion in a regulatory submission.

THE REVIEW PROCESS

Protocols that involve minimal risk to subjects, such as studies collecting small samples of blood from healthy subjects, or involving noninvasive measurements, may be reviewed by an expedited procedure. The nature of this expedited review mechanism will vary with the IRB, although most committees delegate the responsibility for these reviews to a few reviewers or to the chairman. The list of research activities that may be reviewed under an expedited procedure was first published by the FDA on January 19, 1981, and is available from pharmaceutical sponsors or the IRB. Protocols involving the administration of any medication to subjects do not fall in this category.

Projects requiring consideration by the full committee will be reviewed at regularly scheduled meetings, which usually are held at least monthly. Typical committees require that the materials for review be received for distribution at least seven to ten days prior to the session. Nearly all committees assign as primary reviewers of a project a few members who are charged with carefully reviewing the application and any relevant scientific references to highlight key issues for committee discussion. These reviewers are authorized to contact the investigator to discuss any questions regarding the study background and procedures. If a study is somewhat unusual and can best be presented by the responsible investigator, he may be requested to attend the meeting to brief the committee on the project. This presentation does not obviate the need for the investigator to record in the submission all details of the research and its rationale. It does, however, provide an opportunity for the PI to demonstrate an awareness of the ethical and safety concerns of particular importance. Sponsors are asked to attend IRB meetings for informational purposes only in extremely rare circumstances, since most IRBs feel very strongly that it is the investigator's responsibility to be sufficiently familiar with a study to present its rationale to both peers and lay personnel. Committees prefer to communicate with the sponsor only through the investigator and his staff.

Once the committee has deliberated on a particular protocol, it may choose to approve it without modification, conditionally approve it pending minor modification to the protocol and/or consent form (most common), defer the project pending further information, or reject it entirely. Investigators should be provided with documentation of the committee's decision and the conditions of approval, if any. The investigator must then notify the committee in writing of his intention to comply with these recommendations and secure written confirmation from the board that the project has been approved. Unless the committee's written procedures specifically indicate that a protocol can proceed after the investigator has indicated in writing his intention to comply with the approval conditions, a letter from the committee confirming the approval should be expected. Any modifications to the protocol that the board has recommended should also be communicated to the sponsor. The protocol that the sponsor files with the FDA must be the same as that approved by the IRB. Federal regulation prohibits the institution from overturning the committee's disapproval decisions. However, the institution's administration does have the right to disallow the initiation of protocols approved by the committee if the institution does not wish to support those research activities. Committees will, of course, reconsider protocols that have been revised to comply with the ethical or legal considerations raised in the review process. The circumstances under which protocols are likely to be disapproved are discussed later in this chapter.

TABLE 10. Components of the IRB Application

   I.   Purpose of study
  II.   Relevant background to support hypothesis and choice of study design
 III.   Type and number of prospective subjects and controls
  IV.   Locations of study and sources of subjects, including plans for payment of
        case identification
   V.   Duration of study and each subject's participation
  VI.   Names of medical personnel to be involved in study and, where pertinent for
        a highly technical portion, background (e.g., anesthesiologist)
 VII.   Procedures for obtaining subjects' consent and names of personnel to be
        involved in this process
VIII.   Description of study plan and methods
        A. Inclusion/exclusion criteria
        B. Study procedures
        C. Drug administration
        D. Data analysis
  IX.   Potential risks and benefits of the study for subjects and control group
   X.   Special precautions to be undertaken to minimize risks to subjects
  XI.   Provisions to maintain the confidentiality of research subjects
 XII.   Sample informed consent form, including compensation policy
XIII.   Supporting technical materials such as articles from professional journals and
        investigational drug brochures
 XIV.   Funding source

COMPONENTS OF THE APPLICATION

Table 10 contains an outline of the items included in typical committee applications. Some variations may be encountered. However, an investigator planning to initiate a new research project should be prepared to supply information on any of these areas. An investigator who approaches a committee with an incomplete research proposal is likely to be turned down or delayed because of missing information. The required elements of an informed consent document are included in the form of a checklist in Table 11.

THE COMMITTEE DECISION-MAKING PROCESS

The cornerstone of the IRB process is the risk–benefit assessment in which the committee defines and weighs the potential risks and benefits of the project to the individual subjects, scientific knowledge,

TABLE 11. Components of the Informed Consent Form[a]

Background
  *A statement that the study involves research
  *An explanation of the objectives of the research
  The reasons the subject has been asked to participate (e.g., he is a patient with hypertension)
  *An estimate of the duration of the subject's involvement
  The approximate number of subjects involved in the study (both at an individual site and in the study as a whole)
Procedures
  *A description of the research procedures
  *Identification of any procedures that are experimental in nature
  Any important disqualifying factors that the subject should report in the initial interview
  Any anticipated circumstances under which the study could be terminated without the subject's consent
Description of potential risks of study
  *A description of the potential risks of any procedures
  *A description of the potential toxicity associated with the study and control drugs
  A statement that the study may involve risks to the subject or to the subject's unborn child that are at present unknown
  Any additional costs the subject may incur in participating
  The consequences of the subject's decision to discontinue participation and any termination procedures that may be required to assure safe exit from the study
  A statement that any significant new information developed during the course of the study, which may affect the subject's desire to continue, will be communicated to him
Description of potential benefits of study
  *The potential benefits to the individual subject
  *Any anticipated advances in medical knowledge
  *Any anticipated benefits to the general public health
  *Honoraria to be paid to the individual subject, including the conditions under which these will be provided
Alternatives to participation
  *A description of any alternatives to participation that the subject may wish to consider for treatment of his condition
Confidentiality of records
  *Whether confidentiality will be maintained in all scientific reports or publications
  *Whether the sponsor will have access to the subject's record, including his name and other identifying information
  *A statement that the FDA may review the subject's records (the FDA has this authority under current regulation and requires that subjects be apprised of the possibility of inspection)
  Whether the IRB will have access to the subject's record
  The measures to be undertaken to preserve confidentiality (e.g., codifying research records and eliminating identifiers)
Compensation policy
  *The details of any medical treatment and/or compensation that will be provided if injury should occur

(continued)

TABLE 11 (Continued)

*The name of the research team member who can be contacted for further
information
Contact information
  *Name of individual to contact in the event of a research-related injury
  *Name of individual to contact with questions about the research and the subject's
  rights
  Information on whom to contact in the event of a medical emergency, including an
  evening telephone number, if needed
Conditions of participation
  *A statement that participation is voluntary
  *A statement that refusal to participate will not result in any loss of benefits or
  services to which the subject is otherwise entitled
  *A statement that the subject may withdraw at any time without penalty
Signature section
  *Space for the subject's signature and date
  Space for a legally authorized representative to indicate his relationship to the
  subject
  Space for the signature and date of the team member obtaining consent
  Space for the signature of a witness
  Space for the pediatric subject to sign if required
General format
  The title of the study listed at the top of each page
  The pages numbered "Page __ of __" for clarity
  Space for the subject to initial each page if required

---

^aThis checklist contains all elements of an informed consent form currently required by regulation (21
CFR Part 50) with annotation by the authors. These elements constitute the minimum content of any
consent document being utilized for clinical research. The "Additional Elements of Informed Consent," which the regulations stipulate should be included in some circumstances (determined by the
investigator and IRB), have been included along with suggestions for format or content enhance-
ments that have been utilized with success by the authors in the past. The eight standard elements of
an informed consent form have been broken down into separate items where appropriate and have
been identified with an asterisk for easy reference. The items designated with an asterisk must be
included in all informed consent forms subject to FDA review. The remaining items need be included only as deemed appropriate by the investigator or his IRB.

and the general public. IRBs enjoy a broad mandate to include a variety
of factors in making this decision. Some considerations are as follows:

1. The selection of subjects represents that of the disease under
   study.
2. The inclusion/exclusion criteria set appropriate safety limits
   for participation.
3. The measure proposed to assess the research hypothesis is
   valid and safe.
4. The numbers of patients and the estimated sensitivity of the
   measure can test the hypothesis.

5. The procedures employed in the protocol reflect the standard of care in the community.
6. Confidentiality of research subjects is suitable for the sensitivity of the data being collected.
7. The safety measurements are appropriate for the risk to which subjects will be exposed.
8. The remuneration offered to subjects is not so great as to cause a person to place himself at risk for the coercive payments and reflects the policy of the institution.
9. The procedures for informed consent allow for a meaningful exchange between the subjects and research team and usually include a written consent document.
10. The research team is qualified to undertake the study.
11. The study is in compliance with all applicable laws.

These deliberations result in approval, disapproval, or a statement of the conditions under which the committee will allow the project to proceed.

IRBs may decline to approve a protocol in its original form for any number of reasons. Committees may disapprove protocols that are not scientifically valid because of sample size, methods, or subjects. Scientific concerns of the study may be addressed either by altering its design or requesting that the board solicit comments on the design from consultants in the field. IRBs may also disapprove protocols that involve risky, uncomfortable procedures that would not otherwise be appropriate for the patients' care or do not include sufficient provisions to monitor subjects' safety. For example, one study proposed by one of the authors was approved by the committee on the condition that the study be conducted in a hospital setting with a physician skilled in resuscitation present for the entire period. Should an investigator find it infeasible to institute the modifications required, he has no alternative but to withdraw the protocol from consideration. Alternatively, if the investigator does not consider these recommendations medically or scientifically valid, he should contact the committee chairman to discuss whether the opinions of independent specialists in the field could be solicited to comment on the committee's views.

IRBs continue to have strong views on whether subjects should receive remuneration for their involvement in a study. While it has become widely accepted to offer subjects some compensation for travel expenses incurred at each visit ($5–$15), payment of bonuses to subjects who successfully complete a study remains a much more controversial practice. It is not common to reimburse subjects for time lost from work due to study visits unless the subjects are normal, healthy volunteers who are in effect functioning as short-term employees of the research facility. The policies acceptable to individual IRBs can best be learned from discussions with the chairperson and the IRB staff. Some IRBs strongly object to providing patients with any remuneration beyond the potential medical benefits they may expect to derive from the study. Although the final decision rests with the IRB, a proper defense can be mounted for bonus payments that will balance somewhat the inconvenience of a demanding study. While patients should not be offered inappropriate inducements to participation, neither should worthwhile research be rendered invalid because subjects are not adequately motivated to comply with the treatment program.

Other less common reasons for rejecting a research proposal include a lack of confidence in the investigator's ability to conduct the study safely and effectively or the personal biases of the reviewers. These objections are best resolved by discussing with the chairman possible strategies for addressing the board's objections. For example, new investigators may satisfy the committee's concerns by recruiting an established coinvestigator to join the study. Most committees are anxious to cooperate with investigators to develop a method of executing the protocol that meets both scientific and ethical concerns. Engaging in these informal discussions with the committee chairman and members allows less experienced investigators to take advantage of their considerable expertise in reviewing protocols in a variety of disciplines.

STRATEGIES FOR SUBMISSIONS INVOLVING SPECIAL POPULATIONS

Research involving children, prisoners, the poor confined to shelters, and the mentally impaired is evaluated with particular attention to the unique vulnerabilities of these groups. Research involving these groups can seldom be defended unless two conditions exist: (1) The disease under study occurs disproportionately in the target population, and (2) the research cannot be conducted without recruiting from this group. If these criteria have been met, the investigator should present a persuasive risk–benefit assessment that will acquaint the committee with the justification for conducting the study in this population and the steps being taken to preserve the autonomy of this disadvantaged group. The authors have undertaken research in adult depressed, schizophrenics, and memory-impaired patients as well as research in alcoholics who were acutely psychotic with delirium tremens. In each of these complex cases, the committee was presented with a particularly extensive information package that included consultants' reports supporting the value of the research. The committee was also offered a presentation on the specific procedures that would be instituted to safeguard the rights of the research subjects. In one proposal, a videotape of the research team conducting the informed consent process with a schizophrenic patient was included in the submission. The consultant for the committee was satisfied that the proposed procedure constituted meaningful and appropriate informed consent. In many of these studies, the committee granted permission for the team to enroll the first five or ten patients in the study and report these findings to the committee for a decision as to whether the project should be allowed to continue. At the conclusion of each project, the committee was provided with extensive follow-up data that demonstrated the advantages of the research to the patients. These reports were employed by the committee in evaluating future similar protocols. Any protocol involving subjects considered economically or socially disadvantaged or mentally impaired should include specific safeguards to preserve their autonomy.

In studies involving these special populations, the method by which informed consent will be solicited is of particular importance. In pediatric research, for example, the IRB will determine whether any members of the study population are old enough to provide their assent to participate in the study. (This assent does not supersede the legal requirement that the patient's parent or other legally authorized representative, defined by state law, grant consent for participation on the child's behalf.) The investigator can greatly aid the process of determining whether some provisions should be made to seek the children's agreement to participate by offering his own opinion on the matter in the application itself. The intent of the regulations is to offer children an opportunity to participate in the consent process as soon as they have reached an age at which they could reasonably be expected to comprehend the events taking place. The assent requirement ideally should not be waived unless the study is complex and offers the prospect of direct health benefits that are not available outside of the research setting. Similar considerations apply when developing consent procedures for prisoners and the legally incompetent.

FACILITATING THE REVIEW PROCESS

The complete and orderly review of a protocol and an opportunity to modify the informed consent document are prerogatives that the IRB takes very seriously. Committees expect to receive the required documentation well ahead of the meeting. This review period assures that the members have an opportunity to discuss the studies informally with the investigator or conduct whatever personal research may be required to determine the merits of the project. Occasionally an outside consultant is utilized, and sufficient time must be allotted for him to render an opinion. It is unlikely that committees will ever respond favorably to requests for a specially convened meeting or exceptions to the standard review mechanism for reasons other than patient safety or a patient's urgent need for an investigative drug. Most have been pressured into arranging such reviews at some time in the past, only to discover that the project in question was, in fact, not ready for immediate initiation. Expressed desire to circumvent the routine review mechanism will be perceived as an effort to deprive the committee of the opportunity for a thorough review and is not likely to be received favorably.

In contrast, the investigator who is motivated and submits materials for review on schedule and in the desired format is likely to encounter few delays in securing approval. Committee chairmen and their support personnel are anxious to provide orientation and will often provide sample applications for perusal. Particular attention should be paid to the application format, the style and standard wording of the informed consent document, and the types of supporting materials required. The investigator and his staff have the clear responsibility for seeing that these materials are provided in a neatly typed format, with the requisite number of copies and support documents.

Most application forms do not include specific sections in which the investigator can comment on the ethical issues relevant to the study. However, the investigator should prepare his application to address major ethical issues and gain the board's confidence that he has carefully considered the ethical implications of his work. For example, an investigator proposing a study of a new ulcer medication that requires weekly endoscopies, when other similar protocols require them only every two weeks, should be prepared to discuss why the more frequent testing is appropriate. While the committee may not concur with the investigator's rationale for the design, it will, at least, be reassured that the patients' welfare was considered in developing it. Committees will often reward such conscientiousness by contacting the investigator during the meeting to resolve any objections expeditiously.

Methods for securing the subjects' informed consent deserve similar review. Although committees are coming to expect that prior written informed consent be solicited from subjects where feasible, regardless of the degree of risk associated with the study, such a policy may not be uniformly applicable to all proposals. For example, severely injured patients who must be approached for consent immediately upon admission to the emergency room may not be able to give valid informed consent in a time of such considerable stress. In such cases, it is worthwhile to explore with the IRB whether arrangements could be made for a family member to consent to the study on the patient's behalf, with provisions for the patient to grant consent himself as soon as he is considered well enough to do so. In considering these alternatives, it is worthwhile to keep in mind that the purpose of the consent process is to allow the subject sufficient opportunity to make a voluntary decision to participate after having weighed the potential risks, benefits, and inconveniences involved. Subjects should be given the opportunity to make this important decision in an environment that is free of duress, coercion, or any personal factors that might limit their ability to make an independent choice. Methods to secure informed consent that are compatible with the written regulations but not their intent fail to serve the desired purpose of preserving subjects' autonomy.

If a protocol is being conducted in multiple centers, many funding sources require that the identical protocol and informed consent be employed at all sites. Notifying the committee of this restriction in the transmittal documents will allow the board to assure that any revisions it requires in the consent form are suggested only when necessary to assure accuracy.

Committees will often agree to review draft protocols that include the maximum number of procedures that subjects may be asked to undergo. If the methods of evaluation, types of subjects, maximum dose of medication, and invasive procedures have been established, such a draft can be acted on by the committee. If the final protocol then involves fewer samples or a lower dose of medication, these changes can ordinarily be approved by the chairperson as an amendment *unless they substantially alter the design or risk–benefit assessment.*

Industry or academic pressures to initiate new protocols rapidly may cause investigators to misuse the committee's time and limited resources in reviewing projects of little interest or merit. Some investigators develop long-term relationships with certain pharmaceutical sponsors and, hence, find it difficult to refuse any protocol presented by their representative. Thus, they submit an application to the committee that has been less than thoroughly prepared in the hope that the project will be rejected. If the PI fails to express his objections to the sponsor directly, the committee is placed in the awkward position of seeming to support different research standards from those of the physicians who would actually be conducting the project. Such a burden not only wastes the committee's time but also gives the pharmaceutical sponsor an unrealistic representation of the standards held by actual investigators in the field.

Carelessly prepared protocols and consent documents also subject the IRB to the inconvenience of serving as the proofreader or investigator of last resort. Expecting the IRB to point out typographical errors or ethical concerns that should have been apparent to the investigator upon careful review prolongs the approval process and shifts costs and responsibility to the IRB inappropriately. The investigator who insists that his associates prepare submissions carefully will encounter fewer delays in securing committee approval.

CONTINUING REVIEW

Review of ongoing studies is required at intervals of no less than one year. The frequency with which the IRB wishes to receive updates on the investigation is specified in the initial approval consistent with the perceived degree of risk to subjects. Ordinarily this process consists of a review of the investigator's report of the number of subjects enrolled in the study, a summary of any adverse experiences (including

---

Title of Protocol: Use of Drug X in Treatment of Alcohol Withdrawal

Committee Number: 85-412

Committee Approval Date: October 15, 1985

Total Number of Patients Studied: 44 (The first patient was enrolled on November 1, 1985.)

Adverse Effects: Three patients had a single seizure; all patients recovered.

Change in Protocol: No patient may remain in Alcoholism Unit more than 7 days so protocol has been modified to cease giving experimental medicine on the 7th day rather than when patients are discharged from the hospital. Thus, when patients are transferred within the hospital and a new team of physicians takes care of them, they are no longer on this study protocol and may be given any medications that the physicians feel appropriate. This modification was approved by the committee on December 15, 1985.

Results: An abstract submitted to the American Psychiatric Society Meeting on the first 20 patients is attached. Subsequent analyses have not been carried out because the studies are still in progress.

Continuation: The protocol is to be continued until 100 patients have been recruited.

FIGURE 7. Sample annual report.

TABLE 12. Reports to Be Sent by Investigator
to Institutional Review Board

Required
  Annual report
  Final report
  Reports of substantial adverse events
  New information from sponsor affecting safety
  Requests for protocol modifications
Suggested and optional
  All FDA 1639 reports of adverse experiences
  Abstracts of data
  Published reports of data
  Interim reports prepared for sponsor

their outcome), and the investigator's impressions of the study as of the renewal date (see Figure 7). Some committees conduct a review of a selected number of subjects' records either during or at the conclusion of the approval period to confirm the accuracy of the investigator's report.

Since it is desirable for the committee to learn of any new findings affecting the study as soon as they are discovered, sending interim reports to the board when information is accumulated is an excellent practice. (Table 12 contains a list of reports of interest to an IRB.) Many of these can be adapted for IRB submission from data provided to or by the sponsor. For example, reports describing individual or summary adverse experience data can easily be modified for forwarding to the committee chairman. Interim updates to the investigational drug brochure should be forwarded to the board with all changes from the previous version highlighted. In the ongoing investigation of a drug, new findings often emerge from long-term laboratory or animal studies simultaneously being conducted by the sponsor. If new reports of carcinogenicity or teratogenicity in rodents, for example, are issued by the sponsor, these data may well influence the subjects' decision to participate and the IRB's decision to continue the project. The committee should be notified of these findings promptly with a proposal of the desired method for communicating them to subjects.

Often data are summarized for other administrative purposes, such as preparing a report for a grant, or preparing an abstract for a meeting. Sending the IRB this information as an interim report is an excellent practice. Similarly, sending the IRB a copy of reports of adverse reactions completed for the sponsor is strongly recommended. This communication assures the IRB that the investigator is making every effort to keep the members informed.

REPORTING OF SIGNIFICANT ADVERSE EVENTS AND EMERGENCY USES OF INVESTIGATIONAL DRUGS

Life-threatening adverse experiences, including those causing syncope, cardiopulmonary arrest, arrhythmia, marrow depression, substantive liver or kidney function changes, overdose, congenital anomaly, cancer, psychosis, or death (due to *any* cause) should be reported immediately to the IRB chairperson and the sponsor by telephone, with written follow-up within five working days. Other serious adverse experiences that are permanently disabling, require hospitalization, or require prescription drug therapy also should be reported promptly to the sponsor and the IRB. Minor adverse experiences are best reported in the periodic summaries sent to the committee.

In rare medical emergencies in which the physician concludes that an investigational therapy is the only possible treatment available for an illness or disease, he may administer the investigational product to the individual patient and notify the IRB within five working days of his action. Where possible, it is preferable to contact the IRB chairman by telephone to discuss the case in question and secure verbal permission to proceed with the intervention. This provision is applicable to investigational treatments for rare diseases for which no protocol is currently active at the institution. It also applies to the administration of medication to a patient who does not meet the inclusion/exclusion criteria of the protocol that is currently ongoing.

MODIFICATIONS

Any proposed changes to the protocol must receive the approval or acknowledgment of the committee before being implemented. If permitted by the board, modifications that are clearly administrative in nature and involve no additional risk or inconvenience to subjects may be implemented without specific approval as long as the committee is notified of the changes. For example, a modification involving additional analyses on samples of blood already being obtained in the protocol ordinarily requires only notification to the committee rather than actual approval. Similarly, modifications that decrease the risks to subjects may be implemented prior to review by the board provided the committee is notified of this action within ten working days. Such occurrences are rare but may be justified in projects involving considerable risks to subjects. The majority of modifications to a protocol will require some committee action. Proposed changes to a protocol most often are reviewed by the expedited procedure described above and reported to the committee members at the subsequent meeting. Any modification proposals submitted to the committee must include an assessment of how the change will affect research subjects and a revised consent form, if applicable.

Medical treatment of an intercurrent illness or of symptomatic complaints does not constitute a modification and may be conducted without committee approval by a qualified physician consistent with good medical practice. (The consultant should be sufficiently familiar with the protocol to avoid using agents that might interact with the study medication.) Appropriate testing of individual subjects to diagnose abnormalities revealed either during screening or during the study does not require committee approval.

FINAL REPORTS

A final report must be submitted to the IRB within three months of the study's conclusion. This report should be prepared in the committee's desired format, which will ordinarily include a summary of enrollment activity, the outcome of any adverse experiences, and the investigator's conclusions about the research. Figure 8 contains a sample format which includes the information required by many IRBs. It is valuable to list the subjects who fail to complete the study and the reasons for their discontinuation. Summaries of all substantive adverse experiences and their outcomes are also of great value to the committee in determining the appropriateness of future similar studies.

IRB ACCESS TO SUBJECTS' RECORDS

As the primary advocates of human subjects' participation, IRBs should have access to any documentation needed to review the details of the subjects' involvement in the study. Board members may make it a practice to review the records of a percentage of the subjects screened for or participating in a study. They may also choose to interview a percentage of the subjects to verify that the informed consent process has been conducted appropriately. IRB members are fairly sensitive to the need to preserve confidentiality of the identity of research subjects. Should they request lists of the names and hospital numbers of an investigator's study participants, they will routinely make arrangements to seal or destroy these lists after use so they are not readily accessible in the IRB files.

Title: Drug Y for Chronic Musculoskeletal Pain

Committee Number: C41-35

Committee Approval Date: December 10, 1983

Date First Patient Enrolled: 1-19-84

Date Last Patient Completed Study: 12-31-86

Total Number of Patients Enrolled: 185

    Ages 18–40   83
         41–60   72
         over 60   30

Results: The clinical abstract that was included in report to the committee on 11-5-85 revealed significantly better relief of pain with Drug Y vs. placebo in bursitis patients and patients with hip replacements. The drug was not found to be significantly better than placebo in treating athletic injuries.

Dropouts and Reactions:
Enrolled: 185 subjects
Completed: 154 subjects (no adverse effects noted)
                 2 subjects who developed skin rashes.
Discontinued: 21 subjects did not return for interview and examination.
                 4 subjects discontinued medicine for upset stomach.
                 4 subjects had intercurrent illness and were advised to discontinue the medication before the month completed. No side effects were noted.

#13 A 26-year-old man with an ankle sprain from basketball developed stomach intolerance with vomiting during 2nd week. Stopped medication after call to study center, improved by 2nd day, restarted medication and after 4 days symptoms recurred. Believed to be a definite reaction. (The code was broken when the study was completed; the patient had received Drug Y.)

#19 A 55-year-old woman 2 months after hip replacement. Almost daily calls about study to center. Third day complained of stomach upset, stopped medicine, went back on codeine from regular doctor. Still had stomach upset on calls 7 and 21 days after cessation of medicine. Believed to be possibly related to drug. (Code indicated placebo.)

#104 70-year-old woman with hip replacement 1 year previously. Nausea and vomiting during 3rd week, stopped medicine and promptly got better. Did not return to drug. Possibly related to drug. (Code indicated placebo.)

#177 35-year-old man with traumatic arthritis in shoulder from auto accident. From 2nd week until the end of the study said stomach did not feel right but took drug anyhow. Two weeks after the study ended, felt better. Probably relate i to drug. (Code indicated Drug Y.)

#37 31-year-old, bursitis known psoriasis. Psoriatic lesions became worse during study, but completed the study with no specific therapy. Unrelated to the drug.

#106 42-year-old man bilateral hip replacements for aseptic necrosis, last one 11 months ago. Developed mild maculopapular rash at waistband and in

FIGURE 8. Sample final report.

groin. Distribution suggested contact, drug continued, rash continued throughout study. Phone call 60 days later indicated rash gone, probably due to changed laundry detergent. Nonrelated to drug.

#14 62, 100, 135 developed, respectively, otitis media requiring antibiotics, uterine hemorrhage requiring surgery, a left cerebral vascular accident requiring hospitalization, and severe urinary tract infection requiring antibiotics. None were thought related.

FIGURE 8. (Continued)

The expertise of an institutional review board arises out of many years of evaluating protocols in a variety of disciplines. IRBs take their responsibility to the research subjects, investigators, and institution quite seriously and can offer unique insight into local regulations and practices applicable to clinical trials. Since pressures for prompt approvals and limited administrative support pose significant barriers to this important interaction, the investigator who has the good sense to use the committee's time efficiently is much more likely to find that the board shares with him new perspectives that can enhance the quality of his research efforts.

FURTHER READING

Code of Federal Regulations, Title 21, Parts 50 and 54.

Engelhardt, H.T., Jr., Free and informed consent, in: The Foundations of Bioethics, Oxford University Press, London/New York, 1986, pp. 250–335.

FDA Information Sheets on the IRB process. Available from the Office of Health Affairs (HFY-1), Food and Drug Administration, Room 14-95, 5600 Fishers Lane, Rockville, MD 20857.

Levine, R.J., Ethics and Regulation of Clinical Research (2nd ed.), Urban and Schwarzenberg, Baltimore, 1986.

Levine, R.J., and Holder, A.R., Legal and ethical problems in clinical research, in: The Clinical Research Process in the Pharmaceutical Industry (G.M. Matoren, ed.), Marcel Dekker, Inc., New York, 1984, pp. 67–89.

Mahoney, D.M., Protection of Human Research Subjects: A Practical Guide to Laws and Regulations, Plenum Press, New York, 1984.

Meisel, A., and Roth, L., "What we do and do not know about informed consent": An overview of the empirical studies, J. Am. Med. Assoc. 246:2473–2477, 1981.

President's Commission for the Study of Ethical Problems in Medicine and Biomedical and Behavioral Research, Making Health Care Decisions: The Ethical and Legal Implications of Informed Consent in the Patient–Practitioner Relationship (Vol. 3 and Appendices), U.S. Government Printing Office, Washington, D.C., 1982.

Sheldon, M., Truth telling in medicine, J. Am. Med. Assoc. 247:651–654, 1982.

Thomson, J.J., The right to privacy, Philos Public Affairs 4:295–314, 1975.

A three-part videotape series on "Protecting Human Subjects" can be obtained from the Office for Protection from Research Risks, NIH, Building 31, Room 4B09, 9000 Rockville Pike, Bethesda, MD 20892. The tapes trace the development of regulations governing clinical research and show the IRB process for a particular protocol.

The Recruitment Process

Recruitment distinguishes successful from unsuccessful investigators in clinical trials. Subjects' motivations for participating in research protocols are explored and methods for distinguishing the research interaction as a positive health care experience are presented.

CHAPTER 9

Recruitment

Reasons Patients Enter New Drug or Device Investigations • The Clear Advantages of Entering Research Protocols • Planning Recruitment Strategies: Setting Goals and Developing Alternatives • Steps in Recruitment • Obtaining Subject (or Referral Source) Interest • Screening • Enrollment • Compliance and Retention • Completion, Debriefing, and Separation • Techniques That Enhance Recruitment and Retention of Patients • Special Considerations with Elderly Patients

The recruitment of adequate numbers of qualified patients most distinguishes the highly successful from the unsuccessful principal investigator (PI). All PIs undertaking drug or device investigation have made some sort of preliminary study to estimate the numbers of available patients with the desired condition, but the new PI often falls short on recruitment because eligible patients do not enroll in the expected numbers, physician colleagues are not cooperating to the expected degree, patients once enrolled drop out in inordinately high numbers, or other unanticipated problems arise. This chapter presents many ways to enhance recruitment and to encourage subjects and colleagues to take part in a particular study. The enrollment chapter reviews carefully how to select prospective research subjects for participation in a particular protocol.

Research may or may not involve direct treatment benefits to the subject. Studies in which patients may be offered treatment of their disease may involve a new agent for a condition for which a superb treatment is already available (e.g., penicillin for pneumonia). The new agent may be a replacement for an existing therapy with many side effects (e.g., methotrexate for psoriasis) or may be the only hope for patients for whom all existing treatments have failed. Recruitment for this type of research, particularly if the new therapy has a lot to offer the patient, is relatively easier than recruitment for research in which the only benefits will accrue to society.

Research in which the subject will receive little direct benefit always involves some risk to health and poses some inconvenience. The magnitude of each of these must determine the recruitment strategy and the manner in which the study is presented to subjects. A fully informed subject learning of the risk and the inconvenience would probably never participate in such a study unless the finite advantages to him were clearly delineated.

REASONS PATIENTS ENTER NEW DRUG OR DEVICE INVESTIGATIONS

All patients who enter a research trial must anticipate a clear benefit to themselves or they will not enter and continue. It also has been the authors' observation that patients with a reasonable health outcome and an excellent relationship with their physician do not undertake research unless advised by that physician to do so. The following are several reasons that patients choose to undertake research:

1. Patients may be dissatisfied with the *status quo* of their medical care, be it current relationships with health providers, current therapy, or current results. Thus, they seek alternatives and will respond eagerly to responsibly presented ones.

2. Patients who have experienced therapeutic failure with existing treatment will often consider investigative alternatives.

EXAMPLE 1. A Painful Lesson

Our group defaulted on a protocol testing a marketed hemorrhoidal preparation in acute hemorrhoidal pain. We were simply unable to recruit adequate numbers within the budget that we had available. Radio announcements and notices in employment locker rooms targeting bus and truck drivers failed to gain the numbers that were required. We learned that the protocol was subsequently placed in an obstetrics clinic and the protocol involving 100 subjects was completed in 4 months. The obstetrics patients were enthusiastic about the protocol because they had obtained little relief from OTC preparations and were willing to consider the alternative posed by the study.

3. Patients who fear the loss of a satisfactory relationship with the physician-investigator in whom they have confidence and trust are usually willing to participate in research. This phenomenon explains the recruitment successes of physicians recruiting from their own practices. The better the relationship, the more assured recruitment will be.

4. Patients may deny or avoid treating current health problems out of fear of the diagnostic process, the cost, the possibility that no organic illness will be found, or, worse, the possibility that the symptoms suggest cancer. A screening evaluation for a study represents an opportunity for the patient to have his affliction evaluated without having to face many of these difficulties.

5. Patients, particularly those who are poor or who have had unsatisfactory interactions with health providers in the past, are often intimidated by the medical system and the arrogance of health personnel. Reversing the patient's position from a supplicant seeking aid to a highly desirable participant with something to contribute often leads an otherwise apprehensive patient to come for screening.

6. The modest (or occasionally substantial) payment for the study is particularly meaningful to some subjects and serves to motivate them. Surprisingly, this factor is not limited to those in need but may appeal to a "thrifty person" who feels good about getting paid for something he was going to do for nothing anyway.

7. Loneliness, a feeling of powerlessness, or lack of excitement often leads people to participate in study after study. Every study team can cite a few persons who regularly seek the extra attention and prestige that go with being a study subject. To a small degree, this is a motivation found in all study participants.

EXAMPLE 2. Dependency

An unemployed man, seemingly insecure about nearly all aspects of daily life, was noticed to appear in three separate studies for evaluation of new agents for duodenal ulcer. Inquiry throughout the large city indicated that he had been in at least seven trials in a three-year period, remaining eligible because his ulcer did not heal. Following the interview, it was clear that being in drug trials gave him a sense of worth that he did not achieve in any other situations in his current life. The need for bolstering of self-esteem that led this man to seek so many ulcer trials might have superseded his desire for a cure. Although it was never established that he had neglected to take his medication, this person's dependency on the doctors and the trial staffs proved a problem and made him a very poor subject for future studies.

8. An adventuresome, risk-taking spirit believing firmly in American technology and being convinced that the new is so much better than the tried and true often solicits research participation. Although this attitude is diminishing in the United States, it is still encountered and makes the informed consent process difficult. This subject tends to appear in many studies.

EXAMPLE 3. Loyal Entrepreneur

A successful business manager noted for his entrepreneurial approach to new ventures learned of a new antismoking drug through his business research. He went to extraordinary means to enroll in a study to test this drug and arranged to continue the agent long after the study was ended. In the end, the drug was found to have no merit.

THE CLEAR ADVANTAGES OF ENTERING RESEARCH PROTOCOLS

Each potential applicant must be presented with an advantage for his participating. Research offering a potentially better treatment for disease, particularly when a well-characterized outcome can be expected, has clear health advantages. Many current effective treatments of chronic disease such as cancer, arthritis, hypertension, and angina have side effects that lead those with disease to have an interest in alternative treatments, even unproven ones. Table 13 lists other advantages of participating in a clinical trial.

The very nature of protocols, which require standardized and frequent observations to follow outcome, provides the patient with a better assessment of therapeutic result, more safety checks, more attention from the physician and staff, and more access to the medical system. The screening process provides an excellent overall health assessment, and this information, as well as any other testing done, is available to the physicians caring for the patient. The physicians undertaking the research, the consultants, and the laboratories are usually among the best in the community and provide state-of-the-art diagnosis and ad-

TABLE 13. Advantages to the Subject in Research Participation

---

Possible therapeutic advantage
Better outcome of disease
Closer monitoring than in routine practice
More objective outcome assessment
Getting attention for other ailments
Better physical and laboratory health check
Superior physicians, labs, and testing
More contact with the providers
Access to contacts for future health information
Remuneration
The opportunity to make new friends
Contributions to society

---

vice. As a part of the process of encouraging continuation in the study, the attitudes of health providers shift from acting as though they are doing the patient a favor to seeking to please the patient who is doing them a favor. This shift is reflected in waiting time, friendliness, and overall efficiency in using the patient's time. There is often some monetary reward and there is some understanding on the part of the participants of their contribution to society through the value of the research to future patients.

PLANNING RECRUITMENT STRATEGIES: SETTING GOALS AND DEVELOPING ALTERNATIVES

The protocol must be reviewed carefully to determine exactly what types of patients are needed for the investigation. Age, sex, stage of the disease, and restrictions on the use of other medicines during the study period must be clearly defined. A knowledgeable physician working with the disease under study must advise on the availability in the community of patients who meet these criteria. The exclusions of the protocol must then be reviewed carefully and the bother factor assessed. By the latter is meant the degree of interruption to regular life that the protocol entails—specifically, the number of trips required for testing, evaluation, repeat X rays and laboratory tests. On the basis of all of these considerations, an estimate must be made of the numbers of eligible patients available and the fraction of that population that must be enrolled to complete the contract successfully. Usually actual statistics of an HMO or a large specialty practice, hospital outpatient records, or drug sales information can be gathered to provide credibility to the estimate.

From these data a plan is developed that identifies the location of eligible patients. Exactly how these patients will be reached and what will encourage them to enter the study must be considered. The steps in recruiting a study population outlined below should be developed for the particular study being considered. This plan should be quite specific and should be ready to implement as soon as the contract has been awarded. As a part of this plan, criteria for failure of the initial recruiting strategy should be outlined (e.g., a minimum of three persons per month must be enrolled). If the recruitment goals fail to be achieved in two successive months, an alternative plan must be implemented. Since many initial recruiting strategies have some weaknesses, it is advisable to develop the alternative strategy at the outset.

Alternative planning must be implemented quickly when the initial plan is found to have failed. Usually the pool of eligible patients must be enlarged (e.g., new centers or hospitals must be added) or the strategy to reach patients must be modified. The investigator who has already thought about an alternative plan and budgeted for it as a contingency will be pleased at the favorable reception this sort of planning receives from the sponsor.

EXAMPLE 4. Recruiting by Radio

Recruitment of patients with radiolucent gallstones for a one-year trial of dissolution agents was undertaken by writing every 60 days to each of the physicians in the city of Baltimore. Education exhibits, lectures to doctors, and personal appeals to a few close associates who identified possible patients in their practices brought little success. A direct appeal to the patients by radio announcements of the study, using the public service provision to have these carried at no cost to us, resulted in an immense response from the patients. Although only about 5% of the patients who responded were eligible and about half of these enrolled, the recruitment with this alternative plan was highly successful, whereas the initial plan had failed.

STEPS IN RECRUITMENT

Table 14 indicates specific steps of the recruitment process that need to be addressed. Although these are presented as individual steps, they may all be occurring simultaneously or several may be accomplished in a single transaction. As much detail as possible on the inclusion/exclusion criteria is needed to identify the best possible sources of subjects. Thus, recruitment of patients with biopsy-proven cirrhosis with unresponsive ascites largely must be limited to hospitals and specialists' practices, whereas patients with early liver test abnormalities could be recruited from any number of sources. A protocol that excludes all women who are physiologically capable of having a child, for example, is poorly targeted if recruitment includes a women's college. On the other hand, birth control testing may prove highly successful in such a location. Common sources for patient recruitment are presented below.

1. Patients currently in the PI's practice are readily identifiable and are one of the easiest groups to recruit.

2. Patients currently under the care of a colleague with whom the PI has a good working relationship may be willing to participate if encouraged by their physician to do so. This is a particularly important source of patients in studies where the patients must be hospitalized. Usually patients under the care of another physician with whom a

TABLE 14. Steps in Recruitment

Identifying appropriate subjects for targeting
Obtaining subjects' or referral source interest
Screening
Enrollment
Compliance and retention
Debriefing

---

special relationship has been established before the study are not likely to participate without their physician's approval. This is more fully discussed in the chapter on physician relationships.

3. Screening areas such as emergency areas or walk-in clinics in hospitals, community health facilities, and health maintenance organizations (HMOs) can identify suitable patients. These facilities are often overworked, understaffed, and quite limited in the work-ups that they can make available, due to reimbursement policy. Often in return for working up referrals, they will provide possible patients. A busy staff person often provides the referral and usually is given some reward for this extra effort to continue the motivation. Thus, delivering some snacks to the staff or offering individual finders' fees of $5 to $20 is common practice.

4. Screening of hospital admitting or discharge diagnoses, laboratories for key tests, or radiology department reports (for ulcers) permits identification of target patients. No confidentiality issues will be raised if prospective patients' physicians are contacted. Most hospitals have research committees to provide policy and guidance on contacting patients with a given finding who are identified from hospital reports. Usually a low-pressure letter or phone call indicating that the individual has been identified as possibly suitable for a given study (e.g., a new drug to treat his condition) and that the patient can contact the PI or his staff at a certain telephone number if he wishes any further information is considered appropriate. Sometimes a flier with a postcard that the patient may return will produce even less pressure for the prospective subject.

EXAMPLE 5. Hepatitis B Research Program

A highly successful recruitment program for hepatitis B patients rejected by the Red Cross from giving blood worked in this way. The Red Cross, unwilling to reveal names to the research team, sent subjects a brief notice with a postcard. The notice said that the condition for which the

Red Cross blood donors' program had rejected them was under active investigation at the local university to determine the significance of the abnormality to the patients and their families. Patients were instructed to fill in their addresses and telephone numbers and to return the postcard if they wished more information on the program. More than 95% of the cards were returned, for the notice addressed exactly that which was of concern to them. An information sheet on hepatitis B was provided that discussed its importance to the patients and their families. The protocol was outlined, highlighting the advantage that all services were free of cost as long as hospitalization was not required. Some 70% of the eligible patients came in for further testing and about half of these were enrolled.

5. Direct contact with the target patients also can be effective. Notices placed in pharmacies, notices handed to certain types of patients by the pharmacist, and advertisements in church or neighborhood newspapers can be utilized. Mass media contacts and appeals are costly, but sometimes the advertisement qualifies as a public service announcement, which is nearly cost-free. All notices should be brief and should indicate that a new treatment is to be provided for the targeted condition (e.g., ulcer, skin rashes, gallstones). The sponsoring agency should be indicated (e.g., State University School of Medicine, Seymour General Hospital) and one or two advantages such as free evaluation by a gastroenterologist or the remuneration being offered should be presented. The ad or flier should clearly indicate and repeat at least twice how to reach the research team. It is also important that the treatment not be presented as safe and effective if it is still under investigation, since current regulation prohibits commercializing investigational products in any way.

EXAMPLE 6. Reaching the Subject

A protocol required acute injuries of muscles or ligaments to be evaluated and treatment to be started within 12 hours before any other medications were employed. Initial efforts through doctors' offices and emergency rooms failed. It also was not possible to enroll occupational clinics in this study, for they did not want their employees to miss additional work. Successful recruitment was obtained by putting one-page fliers up on playgrounds where young men of the desired ages (over 18 years) were working out. The response from this facility enabled the study to be filled in about two months.

6. Increasingly, hospital departments. clinics, and outpatient sections are willing to take on protocols collectively to make additional money. In this circumstance, the protocol is accepted by the depart-

ment (or the division) and all possible patients, no matter who sees or reviews them, are compared for eligibility with a wide variety of professionals becoming recruiters. These units are usually able to recruit more rapidly because the collective commitment to the protocol leads to its more rapid completion. Increasingly, university departments are undertaking this form of collaboration to attain good recruitment results and additional income.

EXAMPLE 7. Togetherness

New antibiotic research in specific bacterial infections was largely an individual investigator's responsibility until a few years ago. In the older system, when suitable patients were identified, the PI talked with the patient's physician to request permission to speak with his patients about the study, even if he was an associate in the same division of infectious disease. The PI usually obtained only a small fraction of the eligibles because so much time was lost in the communication process that the patient became ineligible. The division then took on responsibility for all antibiotic protocols. Now all eligible patients are approached as soon as their eligibility is established. All infectious disease consultants now share in selection of protocols and recommend them to all of the private physicians. This change has increased recruitment almost tenfold and has improved the recruitment and conduct of new antibiotic studies.

In a general way, the PI, losing as little time as possible, must reach the appropriate population that both qualifies and is motivated to participate (Table 13). It is of value to reach patients before a close patient–physician relationship is established. Direct advertisement through notices or through the media reaches the patient who is dissatisfied or who has failed to make a contact about his symptoms. A highly effective program provided in newspapers, radio, and, occasionally, television includes a list of common ulcer symptoms, followed by the statement: "If you have these, get evaluated free and get paid for receiving treatment." Responses to such advertisements can be impressive.

OBTAINING SUBJECT (OR REFERRAL SOURCE) INTEREST

Once the target group has been identified, a reasonable assessment of which factors will most influence the group must be made. These should be heavily featured in the recruitment notification whether verbally or in writing. Thus, a new agent much in the newspapers could be stressed (e.g., "The new antibiotic noted in the *Wall Street Journal*,

June 8, 1987 is the one we are using"). If the study features extra amounts of tests (which some possibly consider burdensome), such as unnecessary endoscopies for healing of ulcer or gastritis, one could present this in recruitment as follows: "Ulcers will be carefully observed by repeated endoscopy to assure that healing has occurred." If the payment is interesting, it might be stated, "Subjects who complete six or more months on this new agent will be paid $500."

EXAMPLE 8. Timely Recruitment

A protocol requiring acute infectious diarrhea within 24 hours of onset proved most troublesome to fill except during the summer. Patient-finding fees to local practitioners, HMO referrals, and emergency room referrals were ineffective because these patients did not go to these facilities in any numbers. The most successful approach was to engage the pharmacists in eight local pharmacies to hand out a flier to anyone who bought over-the-counter antidiarrheal preparations. This was highly successful when the prevalence of diarrhea was high.

When the PI is completely convinced about the value of undertaking a study, then the patients and associates who have contact with this PI will be inclined to share his views. As part of the process of recruitment planning, the PI should perform an analysis in which the PI and recruitment staff specify those features of the protocol and study that have clear advantages to the patient and those features that are of concern. The many details of more careful observation present such a striking advantage for many patients that often they will see the benefits of undertaking the study. The team should analyze carefully those parts of the protocol that are of concern and, with the sponsor, devise ways of altering the techniques of testing or safety monitoring to satisfy the team's objections in order to generate enthusiasm for the protocol.

EXAMPLE 9. Better Endoscopy Procedure

Ulcer protocols required endoscopy initially and at frequent subsequent visits, and this produced a problem because it required several hours to recover from the diazepam used for the procedure. However, shifting to a pediatric endoscope (9 mm versus 12 or 13 mm) and using meperidine analgesia with Narcan reversal to nearly eliminate recovery time led to a much wider acceptance and almost totally eliminated dropouts.

Displaying enthusiasm for the study is particularly important in inpatient studies, where the team may need to rely on a number of personnel to refer subjects. Ideally, the PI should issue initial announcements about the study, publicizing it at grand rounds or in other available forums and contacting colleagues to inform them that the study is getting under way. The team should have already decided upon a clear mechanism for receiving referrals so this can be presented to interested colleagues at the outset. Once the PI has secured the support of the referral sources, it is best to establish the study coordinator, resident, or fellow as the primary contact through which all referral information will pass. This individual will likely have more time than the PI to establish a relationship with employees or physicians in other areas of the hospital who might be motivated to refer subjects. His continuing presence in those offices or facilities can then serve as an effective reminder of the study. The study contact should be provided with a beeper or answering service to assure his easy accessibility to referral sources. He should also have access to all current study information and any interim updates that may be provided by the sponsor. Presenting new information or informing referral sources of how far the study has progressed can often be effective in rejuvenating interest in a study. Scheduling occasional snack sessions with particularly cooperative clinics is also an inexpensive and effective way of showing appreciation. Responses to any referral calls or requests for information should be predictable and prompt so the physician or employee making the call will not find it burdensome. Coverage by another research team member should always be arranged if the primary study contact will be unavailable. The PI should also be certain to reinforce the credibility of the contact person as the study's advocate, making sure that his subordinate has immediate access to him for any questions or problems a colleague or patient may raise.

In any communication with subjects or referral physicians, the first sentence must succeed in gaining and maintaining interest, or the interested party may be lost. Therefore, presentations must be structured carefully. If a patient (or a physician) allows a recruiter to continue beyond the opening remark, there is an excellent chance of successful recruitment. Physicians who refer patients, even ineligible ones, should be complimented and thanked profusely for their assistance. Physicians who refer a large number of patients or display interest in the study should receive an occasional thank-you call from the PI.

SCREENING

The nature of the performance of screening can do a great deal to assure that the patient joins the study. Identification of patients is commonly done by someone other than the study staff; screening always involves the study staff directly and may be the patient's first introduction to exactly what the study team is like. The very first impressions of the staff and the PI set the tone as to whether the patient can entrust his health problem to them. A patient should emerge from a screening session feeling very positive vibrations that are the result of the friendly, concerned, efficient, and professional atmosphere to which he was exposed.

There are always entry requirements that must be met, including verification of disease state (e.g., positive laboratory test, examination, or special procedure) and verification of certain exclusions. In addition, baseline observations such as normal biochemistry, audiometry, and examinations of the eyes are usually required.

It is important to identify those criteria that most often are the basis of screening disqualification (such as age under 60, ability to get to a laboratory weekly between 8:00 and 9:00 a.m., interdiction of other medicines during the study) and review these over the phone so that persons who cannot meet these basic restrictions are screened out before their first visit. Those who are scheduled to visit the office then are limited to a group more likely to remain eligible. All patients appreciate being spared unnecessary visits. Two types of attitudes are in order in the screening contacts: (1) an eager desire to have this person in the study because he is so pleasant, cooperative, and fun to work with and (2) a hope that he meets the full eligibility requirements. If the disease criteria are met, the team must explain that, before starting, some safety checks are necessary. If the need is expressed in this way, people will accept a little more delay and bother because they know the screening process is being conducted for their benefit. The team should go to extraordinary ends to minimize the time and bother of the delay between establishing disease state eligibility and completion of the many safety and baseline checks.

Frequent sources of delays are the return of necessary laboratory tests (sometimes performed in a single lab for the entire country) or obtaining a consultant's confirmation of normal eyes and ears, or the magnitude of an abnormality. By working with consultants and labs, it is usually possible to identify those who can see the patient the same day that other screening is done. Most patients who submit to screening are highly inclined to undertake the study. Efficiency in screening is an excellent method to assure enrollment and retention. If a standard laboratory required for testing cannot offer timely service, parallel duplicate tests may be obtained and enrollment may be completed on the basis of local results. Discrepancies between local and national laboratory results must be discussed with the sponsor.

The professional tone and friendliness set by the PI and his staff during the screening period largely assures enrollment. Extra effort and dollars invested in setting this initial tone make many other parts of the study easier.

ENROLLMENT

During recruitment and screening, the PI and his staff have the opportunity to instruct the patient on the nature of the study and what is required. The patient needs only the formal informed consent process (see Chapter 10) and an opportunity to have his questions answered. It is, indeed, infrequent that patients completing screening fail to be enrolled if the pitfalls have already been identified and discussed.

COMPLIANCE AND RETENTION

In the screening process, the PI and his staff have devoted some time to studying the protocol and requirements regarding patient compliance with medication, the many return trips, and the many activities that the patient must voluntarily perform. With such preparation, few subjects should find it necessary to withdraw because they were unaware of the commitment involved.

Careful planning allows the PI and his staff to increase compliance quite markedly by education of the participant and frequent reminders in the form of letters, phone calls, or devices, with specific motivation through extra attention and specific payments. Certain things, like keeping of diaries, bringing back empty bottles, keeping appointments, and reporting symptoms, are recurrent problems in all study clinics and almost can be eliminated by skillfully prepared education, awards, or phone calls that both show concern and serve as reminders. In complex studies, it is often worthwhile to offer patients a small ($3) bonus for every pill bottle they bring in on a visit. Developing checklist forms or a diary facilitates better compliance than providing the patient with no written instructions. Costly appointments with consultants are often better kept with a reminder call. Sometimes reimbursing patients for cab fare for an important visit even if a cab is not used is often all that is needed to guarantee attendance.

The generalization that is useful here is that the PI and his staff should know the patients well enough to understand what motivates them and pleases them and strive to meet those needs.

COMPLETION, DEBRIEFING, AND SEPARATION

Well-run clinics obtain 15 to 30% of their subjects from previous clients and from word of mouth. It is of great value to the study and to future studies done by the same team if every patient becomes an advocate of the team's studies and is willing to participate in further studies and to assist in recruiting his friends. To this end, the same respect for the patient's time in screening should be achieved in termination. The patient should be offered the option of having the useful lab tests sent to one or more physicians of his choice. Payment, if due, should be as prompt as possible and should always include a little extra, if only a warm thank-you note. A phone call to be certain the transition back to the patient's previous physician was trouble-free is valuable.

TECHNIQUES THAT ENHANCE RECRUITMENT AND RETENTION OF PATIENTS

Many techniques can be employed to encourage patients to join and remain in worthwhile studies. Several successful methods are listed as follows:

1. The PI must ensure that all staff and contacts, including receptionists, laboratory technicians, physicians, and telephone personnel, provide friendly, informed contacts that reflect the importance and uniqueness of the patient. Such professionalism is the underlying ingredient of all successful recruitment. Everyone having contact with the patient must have noticeable enthusiasm for the project. In the office, a single person can place the project in jeopardy if he conveys the attitude that the PI is abusing his employees by adding these research calls to a work load that is already excessive. All staff people need special training and monitoring in communicating with patients.

2. Thorough, competent professionalism must be presented. People with an illness like to feel they are placing their body's care in the hands of a staff competent to care for them. Thus, the screening contact, as the first that the research team may have, is important in projecting a proper image.

3. The research chart should clearly reflect those unique things that the patient expects in return for research participation. These may be a thorough review of his arthritis conditions for the benefit of his regular doctor or better control of his diabetes. The PI should assure that this contractual relationship is fulfilled so that the patient is not disappointed.

4. A few patients can easily be identified who have been through

the current research study or who have been involved in other research studies with the team. Staff members may inquire as to whether they would be willing to talk to potential patients about the fine treatment that they have received. Often potential subjects are reassured by someone who has worked with the same group.

5. A PI need not be modest about the unique advantages of the research (Table 13). In almost all situations, the study population does better than patients who are not under protocol study largely because they get more attention and close monitoring of the major abnormality. Confidence in the team must be transferred to the patient, and it starts with the team's being confident in itself.

6. The PI can be used effectively in aspects of recruitment. Most people want better medical care and believe that the doctor has something to do with that. Further, if the patient spends some time with the doctor, the former is given a feeling of importance. However, it is important not to mislead the patient on how often he will see the doctor if everything is going well.

7. The team should demonstrate to each patient his uniqueness to the study. Specific items of concern to the patient (e.g., new grandchild, new job, or wife's illness) or items of pride (e.g., gardening or cooking) should be noted in the study chart so the patient can be asked about them on the next visit or telephoned about them. Displaying this interest will assure far greater compliance. In long studies, a birthday card should always be sent and some little remembrance provided if the occasion coincides with a visit to the clinic.

8. If any staff person detects anxiety about an unrelated health area ("I have this rash"), the symptoms should be evaluated promptly by the PI whenever possible to offer reassurance and instill confidence in the study. This permits the physician to identify possible reactions.

9. A patient's caution in making an enrollment decision may indicate that the patient is not yet certain of the motivation of the PI and the study staff and, therefore, does not want to enter. This can be overcome by discussion, showing the thoroughness of the protocol procedures, and perhaps arranging a meeting with an alumnus of the program. Caution reflecting indecisiveness or possible depression needs to be recognized because such subjects are poor choices. They have a high incidence of side effects and drop out more frequently.

10. Providing a description of what will be done for the patient in screening even if he chooses not to enter the study is an important recruitment device. This reassures the patients that the tests that are ordered as part of screening are their property and can be used to their benefit. Getting difficult and sometimes costly health care for someone who cannot cope with a new problem (e.g., a prompt referral to a

university or Veterans Administration clinic for removal of a basal cell carcinoma of the skin) goes a long way toward establishing trust with that subject if he is still eligible. It also may reassure several other reluctant ones who will hear about the services provided for the skin cancer.

In many recruitment systems, a number of employees have some responsibility for providing study-related information to subjects. The PI should be certain that all who answer the phone are fully knowledgeable about the study. If there is need for a prolonged discussion and the receptionist cannot spare the time, an exact time at which the staff member can call back should be arranged and adhered to. Answering devices usually are not successful screening aids. Renting a paging beeper to simplify contact is often a good investment.

SPECIAL CONSIDERATIONS WITH ELDERLY PATIENTS

Many of the recruiting concepts already discussed are applicable to the elderly population. However, certain differences can be identified that must be recognized and planned for to assure the investigator's recruiting success with this population. These major differences have been summarized in Table 15. One difference that needs special emphasis is the typical interposition of third parties into the decision-making process between the investigator and the patient. These third parties generally claim an advocacy role for any variety of reasons, some formally by legal guardianship or power of attorney, some by virtue of a long-established relationship (e.g., a family physician, lawyer, or family member), and some by virtue of the fact that the elderly person is receiving support or services from an organization or agency. The presence of these advocates must be acknowledged and dealt with regardless of the patient's ability to make decisions for himself.

In general, a successful elderly recruitment strategy incorporates the following guidelines:

1. The team must systematically identify organizations or activities known to reach or care for large numbers of elderly patients (see Table 16). An effort can be made to collaborate with these programs, not only to reach the elderly patients but also to allow the research activity to gain credibility.

2. Each organization should be approached at the executive level. Medical directors or executive directors of agencies interested in maintaining a high community profile will often be anxious to cooperate with the local medical community. These organizations should be

TABLE 15. *Considerations in Recruiting Elderly Patients as Compared with Younger Adults*

The elderly are perceived as more vulnerable; hence, there is more concern about their participation and more of an emotional reaction to the prospect of conducting research in this population.

The elderly often have many advocates—physician, family members, and multiple senior organizations and agencies—who feel they have a role in participating in the elder's decision to participate in a clinical trial. The involvement of these advocates must be anticipated and efforts must be made to offer them an accurate assessment of the project's benefits so they may encourage participation in a worthwhile project.

The elderly are far more likely to have developed a long-term relationship with a physician to whom they look for assistance in making the decision to participate. Many are quite dependent and will not proceed without permission from their physician.

Many elderly are socially isolated and, hence, are more difficult to reach. They also are less likely to have an informal support system that facilitates participation in any activity, much less a clinical trial.

The elderly are likely to have different motivations for participating. The social nature of research is likely to be more important.

The inconvenience of participating is a great deterrent to elderly patients. Special efforts must be made to minimize unnecessary visits or requirements.

---

sought out and sold on the benefits of supporting a research activity as well as the benefits that may accrue to the patients from participating in the research. Patient advocates may be persuaded to become advocates of the research as well. If involvement on the first project proves a mutually positive experience, additional studies usually can be placed at the facility following simple notification. Securing permission to initiate the first study is the most difficult task and, hence, the project

TABLE 16. *Organizations or Facilities That May Be Contacted for Assistance in Recruiting Elderly Patients[a]*

Nursing homes
Adult day care centers
Communal dining locations
Meals on Wheels
Churches with active senior groups
Senior centers
Geriatric evaluation units
Pharmacy outreach programs
Blood pressure screening programs
Various patient support groups (e.g., Alzheimer's disease, Parkinson's disease, stroke rehabilitation)
Foster grandparent programs

---

[a]These same organizations can also hinder recruitment if their involvement is not anticipated and properly managed.

must be selected carefully. The authors have found that organizations were most receptive to Phase IV trials when approached for the first time.

3. Once permission to undertake the study has been obtained, the PI should not seek the organization's approval to enroll individual patients in the study. Most often the organization does not have a formal role in the consent process. Seeking its permission wastes time and undermines the essential role of the legal guardian or the patient himself. Additionally, in this era of readily perceived costs of financial and malpractice liability, administrators can say no too easily. These persons should not be accorded a decision-making role. Instead, they should be asked to permit the use of the facility or their patient rosters for research purposes. Reimbursement for the direct costs of the research activity such as clerical time and effort, supplies, and rental fees should be discussed. Assurance that the research staff and activity being conducted within the facility are covered by the researcher's IRB approval and malpractice policy often can allay any liability concerns.

4. The family should not be neglected or ignored, even with patients who are fully active and competent. The family very often is called upon to help bear the hassles of the protocol such as transportation and medication compliance. While the family may not have control over the patient's decision, it can functionally veto the decision by refusing to cooperate at critical moments.

5. The team should make an effort to do whatever is feasible to minimize the inconvenience of participating. When conducting a blood pressure protocol in the elderly, the authors transported the staff to a local senior center to perform the procedures required for each visit. This arrangement obviated the need to arrange additional transportation since transportation already was being provided by other service agencies. This approach required planning and discussion with the senior center staff, as well as detailed scheduling, but yielded much higher enrollment and compliance rates.

Successful drug and device research is like most other service industries. The client's needs and wants must be identified and the team must endeavor to fulfill these in the best possible manner. When the whole staff resolves to make each clinical transaction pleasant for the subject, the success of the venture is assured.

FURTHER READING

Bok, S., The ethics of giving placebos, *Sci. Am.* **231**:17–23, 1974.
Brody, H., *Placebos and the Philosophy of Medicine*, University of Chicago Press, Chicago, 1980.

Graber, G.C., Beasley, A.D., and Eaddy, J.A., *Ethical Analysis of Clinical Medicine: A Guide to Self-Evaluation*, Urban and Schwarzenberg, Baltimore, 1985.

Jonsen, A.R., and Perkins, H.S., Conflicting duties to patients: The case of a sexually active hepatitis B carrier, *Ann. Intern. Med.* **94:**523–530, 1981.

Leslie, A., Ethics and practice of placebo therapy. *Am. J. Med.* **16:**854–862, 1954.

Manoff, R.K., *Social Marketing: New Imperative for Public Health*, Praeger Publishers, New York, 1985.

National Center for Health Statistics, *Health, United States*, Public Health Service, U.S. Government Printing Office (PHS 86-1232), Washington, D.C., 1985.

Siegler, M., Searching for moral certainty in medicine: A proposal for a new model of the doctor–patient encounter, *Bull. N.Y. Acad. Med.* **57:**56–60, 1981.

Critical Decision Points
in a Clinical Trial

The intellectual, professional, and moral dilemmas that arise in the key areas of protocol execution are presented. Since the quality of the research and the satisfaction of the investigator, his staff, and the patients are closely related to successful completion of these functions, methods for conducting the study efficiently are described.

CHAPTER 10

Informed Consent: Decision amid Uncertainty

Types of Patients • Formal Consent Procedures and Documentation • Role of the Investigator • New Information • Peer Participation in the Informed Consent Process • Evidence of an Adequate Informed Consent Process

The line between what is known and what is not known about a drug and study is blurred and hence is a difficult one to draw. Informed consent is the process by which the patient and research staff come to a common understanding about what the uncertainties might be. The informed consent process is not a formality or an empty gesture designed to satisfy risk and liability management. It is an interaction—a dialogue intended not only to satisfy the medicolegal requirement but also to use the uncertainty of the research process as a basis for developing mutual trust and an alliance with the patient. This working together in dealing with the uncertainty of the research is the first step in bringing the patient into the research team (i.e., having the patient give his consent to participate).

The informed consent process is an ongoing one and occurs during each and every interaction between the staff and the patient. The patient gives his consent to participate in the research process on the basis of the broad impressions and specific information received from the research staff in an informal manner. The consent signifies that the subject has assimilated the information and is willing to be studied. It begins with the first recruiting contact and ends when the patient completes the study. At any point in the research process, the patient may withdraw his consent and terminate his participation in the protocol. The informed consent process can best be carried out in a context of easy communication between the patient and the research staff. If the relationship is poor or tenuous, the informed consent process may be hindered. A trusting relationship must be present for an effective in-

TABLE 17. *Relationship Barriers to Effective Informed Consent*

Socioeconomic differences
Foreign language barriers
Cultural stereotypes
Presumptions of knowledge of the other party's motivations (e.g., assuming money as
  the incentive)
Communication style differences (many subjects are nonverbal and express themselves
  through their bodies rather than words)

---

formed consent process to occur. Language difficulties, socioeconomic
or cultural barriers, or assumed motivations are common obstacles to
proper informed consent (see Table 17). Many subjects lack the ability
to express themselves and, hence, depend on nonverbal expression for
better understanding.

EXAMPLE 1. *Aspects of Informed Consent*

*A chronic dosing study on diazepam offered subjects $1200 for 24 days
of confinement, drug ingestion, and blood testing. A new subject answering an advertisement learned about the $1200, 24 days' confinement,
and ingesting of diazepam in a phone interview and presented himself
for a screening physical exam. He met many of the staff and favorably
judged their concern about his welfare from the screening interaction. He
asked to see the facility where he would remain for 24 days. During that
visit he saw a study in progress, watched a meal, noted the rooms and the
recreational facilities available. He was not selected for the study because of his uncertainty about the long confinement but almost immediately undertook a shorter study. Each such interaction is a part of informed consent.*

An informed consent process that is tailored and individualized to
meet the patient's needs during the research recruiting and screening
process is likely to be more effective both in informing the subject and
in gaining cooperation. Thus, each staff member must view his role as
significant in the informed consent process. Should it appear that a
patient does not understand even the simplest concepts or potential
inconveniences, the staff must try to clarify them with the patient. This
approach usually prevents the possibility of a patient's feeling "ripped
off," victimized, or blind-sided by hassles or side effects at a later time.
For example, the telephone recruiter needs to make it clear to a particular patient that he will have a two-hour drive each and every time he

comes for a visit should he become eligible. While emphasizing the hassles of each visit, the recruiter may also point out the clinic's liberal, flexible scheduling policy and payment for expenses. The recruiter should also express the clinic's appreciation of the interest the patient has displayed and how much the clinic wants him to participate in the protocol. Also, while emphasizing the real risks of the study, the investigator may tell the subject about the precautions taken to minimize the risks or to detect their occurrence as soon as possible by frequent visits and lab tests. The issue of balancing a realistic presentation of risks and hassles of participation with the positive aspects needs to be emphasized because an incorrect perception in either direction is not in the interests of the investigator or the subject. Too much emphasis on risks may cause patients to underestimate the magnitude of the study's benefits and, hence, may lead to poor enrollment. Too much emphasis on the benefits of the study may produce dissatisfied patients and high dropout rates.

EXAMPLE 2. Missing Items in Informed Consent

An informed consent form cannot cover all things that individuals hold highly important. In the live-in facility that the authors use, two pay phones are available for 20 to 40 persons. One subject left a study because he could not use the phone for his one-hour nightly call to a friend. Another subject left a study because the shower time was too brief (10 minutes). Both were irritated that the item that upset them most was not presented in the informed consent.

The authors have found that stool and urine collections, number of venipunctures, limitation of activity or food intake, prolonged waiting time, and amenities promised but unavailable are more important than almost anything else. No informed consent process can be totally satisfactory in addressing at the outset all the concerns of particular importance to individual subjects. However, an effort should be made to discuss aspects of the study likely to be of concern to a broad spectrum of subjects.

A good staff and subject relationship is a necessary but insufficient condition for establishing an effective informed consent process. Staff orientation that addresses the types of information each staff member is qualified to convey and the limitations of his role, including his inability to answer certain questions, makes the staff member an effective agent in the process. Staff and investigators who admit the limitation of their personal knowledge and acknowledge the limits of the state-of-the-art data greatly help the patient deal realistically with the inherent uncertainties in the research and serve to further a trusting, frank relationship with him. For example, each person procuring a screening blood specimen should be able to convey to each patient the risk of phlebotomies and even the effects of the medication on the blood draw (e.g., slow clotting). However, questions about generalized bleeding problems would probably be best addressed by a more medically knowledgeable staff person. The well-trained, well-oriented phlebotomist knows when and to whom to refer this type of question. Utilizing these simple approaches will greatly reassure the patient and provide a progressively sophisticated information base about the risks and benefits of research participation.

The well-trained staff is also alert to gauge and judge the patient's receptiveness and capacity for new information. For example, an experienced telephone recruiter who notices that the patient required having the directions to the clinic repeated four times will make a note on the screening sheet of this fact and may even suggest that the patient's hearing be formally assessed. Knowing this fact at the outset will help the research staff address the issue and make a special effort to ensure that the patient hears the information being presented. In this way, the informed consent is individualized without being patronizing or demeaning to the patient.

The staff also has available different materials using different media to aid in the transfer of the information. Written materials, pictures, and videotapes all can be used effectively depending upon the patient's receptiveness. The information base that patients use to give their consent will vary from patient to patient. Some require a lot of information; some require very little.

TYPES OF PATIENTS

Experienced investigators and staff encounter different types of patients. Each type requires a slightly different approach (Table 18).

EARLY DECIDERS. Patients who make "snap" judgments or early deciders will give consent for almost anything on the basis of very little factual information. Several reasons account for this. First, the patient may have decided that he can "trust" the investigator and can depend on him and, thus, personally needs to go no further in gathering information to make the decision to participate. Second, the patient may have no idea of what information he is lacking. Hence, he does not know how to ask for it or how to use it in his decision making. Third, the patient is so motivated to participate (e.g., for financial or personal

TABLE 18. Types of Patients

Patients who make "snap" judgments—early deciders
  Childlike trust of the investigator
  Inadequate knowledge/experience
  Monomotivated
Legalistic nit-picker
  Medically sophisticated participant
Detail person, compulsive information-gatherer
"I'll need to ask my wife, girlfriend, mother, next-door neighbor before I can decide"
  type
Patients with handicaps or special needs

---

reasons) that knowing the facts only confuses him and slows the process down. While not using the full range of information available to make the decision, these early deciders, nonetheless, have made their decision to participate. The staff has the task of ensuring that the patients at least know about the potential pitfalls of participation. These patients are such willing participants that the staff must be careful to take the time necessary to question them to ascertain how much information they have retained.

Overly dependent subjects should not be left in this vulnerable state because they may come to feel like helpless victims of the investigator rather than participants. An experienced staff can draw these subjects into the consent process with offers of reassurance that it is all right for prospective subjects to ask many questions. The staff should also take the initiative to communicate the fallibility and uncertainty of the research process. For example, the following statements have proven useful in establishing meaningful communication: "There is no guarantee that these small risks of death will not happen. I wish I could guarantee it," or "I wish that I could give you a medication that was sure to be free of side effects, but I can't. In fact, that is one of the reasons we are doing this study—to help us find out whether the drug helps people more often than it harms them." These interactions help the patient and the investigator to form an adult participatory alliance.

The subject who has very little lay medical knowledge or experience in any health care setting needs to have much factual information presented in ways that do not make him defensive about his lack of knowledge. If he becomes defensive, he is even less likely to ask for and may even resist learning new information since it would only confirm his lack of knowledge. Patients can be offered tactful support with reassuring statements such as the following: "I know you probably have some questions but, before you ask them, let me answer some of the usual questions asked by nearly everybody that considers this study" or "Most people wonder about just how bad the side effects will be." Sometimes another subject is able to communicate with an insecure subject better than the staff can.

The monomotivated subject sees only one side of the risk/benefit equation and needs to have the risks personalized and crystallized for his comprehension. Using the second person when talking about risks and the third person when talking about benefits helps personalize the risks. For example, potential risks can be described as follows: "You will experience nausea and vomiting after administration of the drug." In discussing potential benefits, however, the PI may explain: "Patients receiving active medication may benefit from faster healing of their ulcer disease." Translating the probabilities of risk into meaningful numbers can be done by use of a comparison to the million-dollar Lotto games. "You are less likely to get a fatal blood reaction than to win the lucky Lotto game, and you know you always hear about someone's winning a million dollars. To win, you have to be very lucky, and to get the blood reaction, you have to be very unlucky, but it can happen."

LEGALISTIC NIT-PICKER. This type of patient will ask questions that will make the staff defensive even though the patient may be asking more out of his own need for protection and a feeling of trust than out of hostility toward the staff. This patient asks questions or makes statements like the following:

1. How can you assure that my records will be confidential? Will I be a case written up in the literature?
2. How can you tell which side effects are drug-related and, hence, paid for by the sponsor?
3. Is it okay for my lawyer to read this informed consent?
4. You know, these consent documents never hold up in court, and if I am injured I don't know what I'll do.

Such questions or statements need to be listened to and handled objectively. Patients who make these comments should not be rejected on this basis alone. The statements are merely requests for something more—information, certainty, trust, reassurance. Responses should indicate that it is commonplace for patients to ask these questions, that it is all right to worry about these concerns, that it is all right for the patient's lawyer to look at the consent form, that not everything is known about the drug (that is why it is being studied), and that not all questions can be answered with certainty. Complete reassurances about any risks should not be given unless the investigator is absolutely certain that they will not occur. Mistrusting patients are not likely to respond to any reassurances offered and will gain respect and trust only if the investigator is blunt, open, and honest about what is or is not known and what contingency plans are available if the subject is injured. Only rarely will the patient make further inquiries if he has been handled in this forthright manner. Those patients who have reservations to the point of having their lawyer review the informed consent usually will not participate and usually never even consider participation in the first place.

EXAMPLE 3. Fears

The statement "sudden death is possible" appears in a number of informed consents. Slightly less than 50% of the time that this statement is used, a subject will ask for further explanation of just what the likelihood is that this will occur. An excellent open dialogue usually follows, with our PI or another study physician stating calmly that: (1) it is possible; (2) it is rare; (3) our resuscitative training and equipment are present to make death even more unlikely. We do not remember anyone's leaving after such a discussion.

On the other hand, studies with radioactivity (Cr-51 red cells or C-14 metabolic tracers) have had dropouts after a good open dialogue on the risks.

THE MEDICALLY SOPHISTICATED PATIENT. These patients generally are a delight to work with but at times can cause defensiveness in staff members, who may feel ill-prepared to answer the insightful and difficult questions that are asked. These patients are best handled by employees who know the limits of their knowledge and are not afraid to expose their ignorance. Investigators caring for these patients will often be confronted by their own ignorance as well as that of the state-of-the-art knowledge. An open exchange on the uncertainties present will help make these patients feel comfortable placing their care in the hands of the investigator. Well-informed patients can become very valuable persons in the research process, offering insight into subtle side effects and helping other patients get through the study. They must be recognized early so that they are not permitted to inadvertently slip into a subversive, competitive role with the investigator, or a glib "know-it-all" role that threatens staff members and other patients.

EXAMPLE 4. Tit for Tat

A highly intelligent pharmacy manager regularly undertakes studies out of a feeling of loyalty to the industry from which he makes his livelihood.

For each study agent, he reads widely, often educates the research staff, and also intimidates them by displaying his knowledge, asking questions to which he already has the answers, or correcting their replies to other subjects' questions. This energy has been converted to a useful function by appointing him to the IRB as the subjects' representative. In return, he has been able to improve written informed consent documents and has privately helped many subjects understand the research process.

COMPULSIVE INFORMATION-GATHERERS. These patients have endless questions about the study. They delay their decision to participate by asking for more and more progressively less relevant information. These patients fail to see the forest while looking at the branches of the tree! This kind of patient can be handled by allowing him a reasonable time to reflect on each question and then establishing a time limit for his decision. Reorienting the patient to the substantive issues, providing feedback, summarizing the salient features of the study, and outlining the specific areas of uncertainty will help keep the patient focused on the decision at hand.

THE INDECISIVE PATIENT. The indecisive patient views himself as incapable of making the enrollment decision. Unlike the early decider who wants the investigator to decide for him, an indecisive patient wants his significant other or committee of others to decide for him. While most patients check with their spouses regarding participation to be assured that there is no serious discordance, this type of patient does not want to face the consequences of deciding for himself. The staff must avoid being involved, reinforce the position that the patient himself must decide, and point out that while input from his family and friends is important, they are *not* the ones participating in the study!

PATIENTS WITH HANDICAPS OR OTHER SPECIAL NEEDS. Illiterate, deaf, vision-impaired, and memory-impaired subjects, or subjects who comprehend English poorly pose problems that are not barriers to communication if an understanding staff person will work with them to help overcome the handicap. A staff member may read the informed consent document to a subject to be sure that it is understood and then verify comprehension by asking the patient questions on key points. A translation of the document into the patient's native language can be supplied if available. Procuring a translation and having an employee who can communicate with non-English-speaking subjects are advisable if the team will be seeing a large population of subjects of a particular nationality. A written document always should be provided to the subject so he can have a family member or friend read it to him subsequently if he wishes. The possibility of having a family member available for the interviews can also be discussed. Subjects with handicaps or comprehension problems should be identified during the initial screening and a note made in the chart to the effect that the problem was observed. Special efforts made to assure comprehension should be noted in the chart as well. In deciding whether to include subjects requiring highly individualized attention, the team should be certain to identify the type of assistance that will be required for the patient to understand the study and participate. The team should enter such subjects only if it has the time and energy that will be required to assure the patients' safe participation.

The staff has the responsibility of ensuring that a reasonable amount of information is presented, received, and retained by the patient. The required minimum information is formalized in the informed consent document, which has been reviewed and approved by the IRB. (The elements of informed consent are outlined in the chapter on the IRB process.) The signing of this document should not be viewed as the informed consent process but as a formal, ritualized, legalistic event that standardizes and validates the entire preceding informed consent process in the public's eyes. A signed document does not automatically mean that informed consent has been given. However, each participant in a study must nevertheless have a signed informed consent document in his record.

Many studies are single- or double-blind placebo-controlled. Patients will often ask during the consent process about the justification for placebo, particularly in studies involving a diseased population. The experienced investigator is prepared for this question and has prepared his staff for it as well. The staff and patient must convey that the use of placebo is not a deception against the patient but is a feature of the study that involves an agreement by the patient (and the research team if double-blinded) to remain ignorant for the purpose of gaining more objective and certain knowledge of the agent under study. The patient must be informed that placebo will be used sometime during the study. Because some patients may withhold symptoms for fear of being on placebo and risking being told "it is all in your mind," the staff should let it be known that many patients have all kinds of symptoms while on placebo and that the investigator is just as interested in those patients on placebo as those on active medication. If the study is double-blinded, the staff may explain that the investigator will be placed in the same position as the subject of reporting many possible drug-related events that occur in patients on placebo.

FORMAL CONSENT PROCEDURES AND DOCUMENTATION

Having stated that the signing of the informed consent document is a ritualized process, the authors do not wish to convey the impression that the ritual is a trivial matter. The ritual of signing the informed consent document helps to convey to the patient the significance of his decision to participate. The ritual also indicates to the patient that he is no longer considered a private patient but a research patient accepting the shared risk and liability of participation. The ritual must also involve the principal investigator in ceremonial as well as substantive ways. The PI should meet with the patient at least at some point after the patient has consented to participate and before he has completed a substantive portion of the study.

Physicians referring patients to the study should have available a description of the study (most likely the informed consent form) and current information about side effects or other safety issues. While these physicians can easily introduce the study to subjects, they should not be expected or asked to conduct the informed consent process. Securing informed consent is a study-specific activity that is the responsibility of the investigator and his staff.

Each staff member has a role in the informed consent process. The recruitment team informs the patient in a preliminary way about the study, the disease, the study location, and other elements, emphasizing that certain types of questions will be answered later by someone else informally or formally. Generally, this preliminary information is provided in layman's terms. The specific dates of screening or participation, location of the study, and remuneration are usually provided in a flier or written material as well.

The staff conducting the screening informs the patient further as he goes on in the process. The risks and benefits of the treatment are discussed. The hassles and risks of common procedures (e.g., EKG, endoscopy, and stress tests) are explained to the patient, using standard materials that can be obtained from various professional societies as a public service. The procedures that are performed should be documented in chart notes confirming that the patient was informed.

If the patient is interested and preliminarily eligible, the informed consent document can be presented to the patient for review. Generally, this is done in a private, quiet setting after the patient has had some positive contact with the staff and after the staff has ascertained his ability to comprehend the written document. Adequate time must be permitted for the patient to think about the decision. Premature presentation may have consequences that are counterproductive to the recruitment effort. It may preempt an open exchange of information, may suggest a mechanical and legalistic emphasis to the process, or may unnecessarily alienate the patient who has special needs, such as the subject who cannot read English well or needs reading glasses. Thus, premature delivery of the written document may scare the patient away. The staff must be sure to allow the patient sufficient time and privacy to decide with the facts in hand. The patient must be informed that he is permitted and encouraged to review and discuss the consent document with his family or with his personal doctor. The consent document may be taken home with the patient to allow him further time for reflection.

While the most up-to-date IRB-approved informed consent document must be used for signing by the patient, other materials can and should be used for educational purposes. The liberal use of progressively sophisticated materials and media that are presented at different points in the recruitment process is a sign of a well-prepared, well-oriented research staff. For example, a videotape of an endoscopy being performed may aid some subjects in understanding the inconvenience involved. This may be made available at a late stage of the recruitment process for those who desire it. Informing the IRB that these educational materials will be used may resolve some of the concerns the IRB may have about the phrasing of the informed consent document. Once the patient has read the informed consent form, the staff should present an opportunity for questions and answers. The staff, in turn, must ask some questions to determine the patient's degree of comprehension, while the patient should ask questions to clarify or elaborate on issues raised in the consent document. This question/ answer period is essential to the process. If both the staff and the patient are satisfied, the document can be signed and witnessed, if required. The meeting with the investigator may occur before or after the patient signs.

ROLE OF THE INVESTIGATOR

The investigator has the responsibility of setting the tone of the informed consent process. If the investigator sees the informed consent as "red tape" and an imposition of a legal constraint on him, the staff and patients will surely react to these feelings. These feelings are a threat to the relationship with the patient. The reverse is true as well. The investigator who sees the informed consent as a process and a means by which he and the patient form an alliance in the face of uncertainty is more likely to convey the essence of the informed consent process to the staff. The experienced investigator knows that informed consent is a means of dealing with the study's complex risk profile, which falls somewhere between the extremes of helpless chance and omniscient certainty. The investigator must choose the point on this spectrum that accurately reflects the amount of uncertainty inherent in a given protocol and give voice to it. For example, in Phase IV protocols, the investigators know a great deal about the drug and should be able to convey this to the patients. By conscientiously putting the risks of the study into perspective, the investigator can help the staff and the patients deal with the sense of fear and helplessness they may feel after learning how little is known about the risks of a Phase I study. It is equally important to give them assurance that they are not presented with an overly tidy disclosure that "covers all of the bases," which will lead them to conclude that there are no risks.

The experienced investigator sets up the consent process, participates in the process in a well-defined, yet limited, manner, and is accessible to the staff and patients for selected issues. The investigator must assure that the staff is properly oriented and prepared and that the preliminary information given to the patient is accurate. The research staff that prepares these materials usually cannot go wrong if the informed consent document is used as the basis. The investigator should train the staff to know and understand the elements of valid consent, to know what constitutes adequate information, to be able to convey it in simple terms, to be able to distinguish between persuasion and coercion, and to assess whether a patient is competent or not. The investigator can evaluate the quality of the consent process with periodic low-profile spot checks, witnessing the staff talking with actual patients, and discreetly questioning the patient about the consent process and content. Letting the staff know that an occasional "ringer" will be sent through the process may also be useful whether or not the investigator actually ever does use such a person!

The investigator also must act as the conduit of information about the study medication received from the sponsor. The investigator's brochure is usually the manner in which this type of information is transmitted by the sponsor. Contacting the sponsor's medical monitor for information needed to answer an individual patient's question also is very reassuring, for it conveys to the patient that the sponsor is involved and cares about his concerns.

An investigator's involved staff will anticipate the types of questions patients may ask as the study progresses. A method must be established to disseminate information received from the sponsor to all team members and, where appropriate, to research subjects. This is particularly true in long-term studies or multicenter studies as more experience with the agent is gathered.

NEW INFORMATION

Often new information occurs during the study and may be of such significance that an addition to the informed consent is necessary. Generally, the sponsor will provide this information on the basis of nationwide or worldwide performance and toxicity experience. The sponsor will also indicate whether the information requires IRB review. The PI must consider the sponsor's recommendation in the light of his own experience and his IRB's policies and should send the safety updates to the IRB for its records whether or not a formal review is requested. The PI must also decide the nature and degree of the increased risk and how best to tell the subjects. Patients currently enrolled in a study when the new information becomes available must be informed. Depending upon the IRB and/or sponsor's recommendations regarding the urgency, most often the information is such that the patient can be informed of the new development at the time of the next scheduled visit. If that visit is delayed, a special visit must be scheduled by the staff. At this visit, the patient is given the opportunity to give informed consent again. Generally, the staff's calm and reassuring demeanor and approach in handling the new information will allow the patient to consider the new findings without becoming alarmed. Though few patients choose to stop participation in the study following a report of new information, they nevertheless should have the opportunity to do so.

PEER PARTICIPATION IN THE INFORMED CONSENT PROCESS

Certain patients and situations require a little more effort and may require something not even the investigator can provide. Mistrustful or slow-to-trust patients are not likely to get ready reassurance from research personnel about whom they harbor some doubts. These patients, while interested in the research, feel more comfortable talking with an independent party about the research. This is readily and practically accomplished in a busy research setting by having the patient talk with eligible, current, or completing research participants. It is the authors' experience that peer participation is a valuable addition to the consent process and is much less cumbersome and more practical than a formal ombudsman role. For example, in the normal subject studies, the authors systematically attempt to mix groups of potential normal subjects to ensure that experienced subjects interact with the naive subjects. Peer participation probably occurs spontaneously in the waiting room as well. Concern about the spread of misinformation from peer to peer is appropriate, but if inaccuracies are observed, a review of the staff's informed consent process may be in order to ascertain whether the information was disseminated properly in the first place. Naturally, concern may arise that the naive subjects would be scared away by the factual lay descriptions of the reality of multiple phlebotomies or long-term studies. This is not much of a risk, however, since these subjects are not likely prospects for participation anyway.

EVIDENCE OF AN ADEQUATE INFORMED CONSENT PROCESS

The investigator can make some judgment about the adequacy of the informed consent process from what he overhears and from discussions with the patients. Another form of evidence is the "refusal rate," that is, the number of fully eligible patients who ultimately decide not to give consent. While the investigator may be genuinely disappointed that a patient has not entered, he may derive some satisfaction that in this patient's refusal there is evidence of a good informed consent process. The authors have experienced a predictable 3 to 5% refusal rate in standard normal subject bioavailability studies. Experienced investigators will usually share their assessments of refusal rates that can be expected with certain types of studies so that a new investigator can gauge how he is doing comparatively. Red flags that indicate difficulties with the consent process include a 100% acceptance rate, possibly indicating more coercion than persuasion; a high refusal rate, possibly indicating an unbalanced presentation of information; a high patient dropout rate, with patients stating that they were not told certain details or that they had not expected the study to be so difficult as it was, and similar problems. "Debriefing" the patient at completion of the study is a very opportune time to learn whether some of these problems are occurring. The authors use poststudy questionnaires that include questions about the consent process.

The informed consent process offers a worthwhile opportunity for the investigator and staff to establish a relationship of trust and mutual respect with the patient. While this process serves a necessary medicolegal function, its primary purpose is to provide the prospective subject with complete and realistic information about the risks, inconveniences, and benefits of participation. Since the subject and research team share in the uncertainty of the research process, this communication must occur in a setting that is conducive to free decision making. The quality of this decision making and the consent process itself are greatly influenced by the principal investigator, who sets the tone of the process and ensures that staff members are properly oriented before taking part in this important interaction. Of equal importance are the staff's professionalism and perceptiveness in identifying patients with special needs or barriers to effective communication and overcoming these to make the consent process a meaningful one. Once the systems for consent delivery have been developed and the staff trained, it becomes the PI's responsibility to monitor the process to make certain that his expectations are being met. Such conscientious efforts will result in meaningful interaction with the patients and thereby provide a positive introduction to the study experience for all involved.

FURTHER READING

Annas, G.J., Glantz, L.H., and Katz, P.F., *Informed Consent to Human Experimentation: The Subject's Dilemma*, Ballinger Publishing Co., Cambridge, 1977.

Barber, B., *Informed Consent in Medical Therapy and Research*, Rutgers University Press, New Brunswick, 1980.

Finkel, M.J., Role of the FDA in the clinical research process, in: *The Clinical Research Process in the Pharmaceutical Industry* (G.M. Matoren, ed.), Marcel Dekker, Inc., New York, 1984, pp. 450–464.

Levine, R.J., *Ethics and Regulation of Clinical Research* (2nd ed.), Urban & Schwarzenberg, Baltimore, 1986.

CHAPTER 11

Special Populations

Physical Problems Interfering with Communication or Participation •
Social, Cultural, or Economic Conditions • *Temporary Barriers to Full
Comprehension* • *Disease States Interfering with Comprehen-
sion* • *Special Status under the Law or in Current Ethical Thinking*

Certain patients cannot participate as readily in the informed consent
process because of a language or hearing defect or because their medical condition temporarily does not permit them to do so (e.g., unconscious patients). Other patients such as children, prisoners, or the mentally infirm may be less able to give their informed consent because
they are especially vulnerable to coercion or misinformation. This
chapter is concerned with some issues relevant to subjects who fall in
these categories and with possible solutions. Table 19 lists the types of
problems to be considered in the text that follows. The conditions
under which such subjects should be allowed to take part in a study are
clear-cut. They include the following: (1) The person must be able to
assimilate the study information and consent to participation. (2) The
person must be able to give consent legally. Various levels of interference with one or the other of these key conditions are presented in
Table 19.

Each year the American Federation for Clinical Research provides
a prize to investigators conducting research involving a difficult ethical
dilemma to which they considered possible solutions or which caused
them to forgo doing the study. This prize is called the Nellie Wester-
man Prize and the manuscripts are printed each year in Clinical
Research.[1]

PHYSICAL PROBLEMS INTERFERING WITH
COMMUNICATION OR PARTICIPATION

Blind patients present so many problems that it is probably best to
exclude them from participation. The reading difficulties, the difficul-

TABLE 19. *Problems Requiring Special Attention in the Consent Process and Enrollment Decision*

Physical problems interfering with communication or participation
  Hearing impairment
  Blindness
  Ambulatory handicaps
Social, cultural, or economic conditions
  Functional illiteracy
  Native language different from that of investigative staff, resulting in limited
    communication skills in English
  Homeless indigence
  Impecunious unemployment
  Employment in a testing company
Temporary barriers to full comprehension
  Use of alcohol or drugs
  Forgetfulness or confusion in elderly patients
Disease states interfering with comprehension
  Unconsciousness
  Severe illness requiring emergency treatment
  Diseases requiring medication that alters comprehension
  Diseases that themselves alter communicative abilities
  Mental illness in patients who are living free in community with or without
    medication
Patients accorded special status under the law or in current research thinking
  Minors below the age of consent
  Prisoners
  Wards of the court or patients of any age with a guardian
  Patients committed to mental institutions

ties with medication compliance, the completion of diaries, the logistics of visits and procedures, the difficulty of distinguishing drug-related eye events from other eye processes, and the difficulty to the patients of navigating in a new setting all make it unwise to include these individuals in the study. It is possible, however, to include such subjects in a few very limited circumstances when a very reliable, highly motivated support person is available to work with the patient in devising ways to make his participation safe (e.g., preparing taped instructions on proper medication compliance) while meeting the needs of the study. The inclusion of the blind patient is best limited to studies in which the demands of participation are minimal and sufficient data are available to confirm that eye toxicity is not a concern.

On the other hand, the problems of deaf patients generally are not so difficult to solve. Once the deaf patient is recognized, the staff usually can adjust its approach so that the patient can be reasonably informed and monitored throughout the study. Deaf patients often can be effectively paired with a partner to assure prompt communication in the event of an emergency. Assigning a partner will also facilitate the calling of the patients from one area to another while the study is being executed.

Other types of handicapped subjects, such as those with prosthetic limbs, should be considered individually to ensure that the staff is able to accommodate any special requirements for their safe participation.

SOCIAL, CULTURAL, OR ECONOMIC CONDITIONS

FUNCTIONAL ILLITERACY. The functionally illiterate patient should not be rejected from participation on that basis alone. However, special efforts must be made to identify these patients to ensure that they are fully informed. These patients often are not detected right away and can be well along in the recruitment process before their illiteracy is recognized. Many are literate enough to read simple fliers and instructions and to complete forms but cannot read the informed consent document with comprehension. These patients need to have the informed consent read to them completely. It then must be explained to them again individually, allowing ample time and opportunity for questions. Usually a witness must participate to ensure that the patient has been informed and to verify the "mark" or signature of the patient. Because most instructions on procedures and medication use are written, the staff must be committed to take the time and special effort with these patients as the study progresses. Assignment of a "buddy" or study partner is a method used by the authors to further guarantee that the patient gets the information necessary to make decisions. Many times this type of patient will come with a friend or partner already. Use of the illiterate or functionally illiterate should be limited to lower-risk studies.

NON-ENGLISH-SPEAKING PATIENTS. A subject unable to communicate in the language of the investigative staff presents serious problems of cooperation and safety. Although a translation of the informed consent document can be used on research of limited risk, there is no adequate way to ensure that the risks and benefits have been fully assimilated. The team may also have some difficulty in taking the history and securing accurate information on safety and compliance at on-study visits. When faced with such patients, the authors occasionally have found a bilingual friend who will assist the non-English-speaking subject. This is not generally recommended, however, since it is difficult to find a truly objective observer who will not interfere with the investigator–patient relationship. As with illiterate subjects, pictorial representations of the medication instructions and diary (e.g., putting a green circle on the calendar on the date that the subject is to start medication and a red one on the date that he is to stop) can be prepared to enhance their understanding.

HOMELESS INDIGENTS. These subjects are like prisoners in many ways in that they have very few options, have nothing to lose by participation, and, from their perspective, have very much to gain—food, shelter, and money. They also tend to have few advocates or anyone to look out for them. While their numbers are small for a variety of reasons, such as poor nutritional or health status, lack of a structured lifestyle conducive to keeping appointments, or lack of exposure to radio or newspaper advertisements, the few that do present themselves represent a challenge to the staff. The staff must be prepared to deal with these patients in the following ways:

1. The staff must personalize the risks for the subject in concrete and graphic terms.
2. The staff must have available many referrals to propose non-study options for the subject (e.g., lists of soup kitchens, overnight houses, and Traveler's Aid and Salvation Army locations). These options must be presented to the subject with enough clarity and detail that the potential subject sees them as options that offer him a real choice.
3. Staff members must be prepared to deal with their own feelings of helplessness and desire to allow the subject entry into the study, thereby creating subtle enrollment collusion.

The investigator must play an active role in helping the staff establish the best approach to deal with this group in relation to a specific study. Participation of these subjects is best limited to low-risk testing of generic formulations or marketed products where the likelihood of coercion is not so great.

IMPECUNIOUS UNEMPLOYED. Subjects from the ranks of the unemployed are frequent for they have the time, need the payments, and perceive they have little access to necessary medical care. However, alcoholics and street drug users are disproportionately represented in this group in addition to marginally motivated persons. The need for payment also may be so great that past disqualifying medical history information may be suppressed in order to gain acceptance into the study. Careful screening, including tests for drugs and alcohol, usually will allow one to select patients who will complete the study. There is always a question when dealing with willing but needy enrollees whether payment constitutes coercive motivation. This must be worked out by each investigative staff and its IRB. The authors have probably had more problems with subjects in this category than in any other.

EMPLOYEES IN A PHARMACEUTICAL COMPANY OR DRUG-TESTING FIRM. The scientist employees of a drug-testing firm are usually in a position to give valid informed consent. Other employees of pharmaceutical firms often are not able to do so and may be subjected to a great deal of coercion. The obvious pressures of a threatened loss of job or promotion advantage are of greatest concern in small companies where the influential decision-makers interact with all levels of staff. However, small departments within large organizations, particularly those involved in recruiting for the research, may feel some pressure to volunteer to participate. To ensure that such pressure does not compromise the validity of the consent process, it is best to exclude such individuals from participating or to restrict employees who are working on the particular research from volunteering for the study. Caution is in order, however, because the risk of abuse of the employee–supervisor relationship is very great when recruitment pressures are present.

TEMPORARY BARRIERS TO FULL COMPREHENSION

CURRENTLY MUDDLED BY ALCOHOL OR DRUG USE. This is a very important issue in that a research team will frequently encounter patients whose comprehension is affected by excessive use of drugs or alcohol or even abuse of physician-prescribed medications. The team may also be involved in research specifically studying these populations. At all times there are three issues involved. The overriding one is patient safety—namely, can the subject safely participate in the research? Sometimes experimental agents interact with alcohol or other sedative drugs to produce convulsions or other alarming side effects. The second issue is whether a person who is slightly confused from drugs can assimilate the information and give informed consent. This requires an individual judgment depending upon the complexity of the information, the risk of the procedure, and the extent of the drug's effects. Thus, a person drinking heavily during the Kentucky Derby can readily express his preferences for cigarettes and shoes in a sidewalk survey in exchange for a payment of $5 but may not be able to drive an automobile. The final issue concerns the sort of research subject the person will be. Will the use of drugs or alcohol (admitted or unadmitted) interfere with the research, preventing accurate reporting of side effects, compliance with medication and appointments, and accurate history-taking?

When investigations involve inebriated or drugged patients who must provide informed consent, many special considerations apply, depending upon the nature of the procedures and study under consideration. Observational research, measurement of tremor, EEG recordings, and Holter monitoring of the heart have been done with the permission of the IRB. The consent of the subjects was sought a day or two later when they were able to give valid informed consent. These provisions were allowed because the procedures involved were of minimal risk and possible benefit to the subjects. Other studies have necessitated the selection of an advocate such as the hospital administrator or a family member to provide informed consent. Two acceptable therapies for withdrawal have been compared in a randomized trial in an alcoholism unit with the permission of the IRB without specific informed consent. The IRB approved this comparison because substantive cost and safety differences between the two therapies could be identified that were deemed worthy of study in a controlled setting. In most instances, the patience and persistence of the staff will enable the patient to understand that to which he is committing himself and, thus, give informed consent.

A variation on this problem occurs when a person is in a drug study and becomes disoriented as a part of a study as an idiosyncratic side effect and wishes to leave the study immediately. Such patients are usually kept in the study even against their will until the effects have worn off in order to allow them to leave the unit safely and drive or undertake other hazardous activities. When procedures, such as endoscopy, that employ a lot of sedation are required, it is usually wise to build into the informed consent the notion that the patient may not be able to drive for a number of hours.

ELDERLY. There is the perception that drugs, even drugs likely to be used in the elderly, are not studied adequately in the aged population and that, as a consequence, older patients may experience a spectrum of adverse reactions undetected in younger patients. This may be due to age-related differences in drug metabolism and response, insufficient information about these changes, or the fact that the elderly have more concomitant diseases and, hence, use more drugs. Factually, older persons have a higher incidence of adverse reactions. For these reasons, the informed consent process in the elderly is very critical. The risks of participation may be greater for the elderly population. These patients need to be informed of that uncertainty. The societal benefits, however, may be greater with the increased participation of the elderly in the study. The informed consent process must be very carefully balanced lest the elderly be "scared" away or not fully informed.

Additional consent problems are present when the patient displays evidence of memory impairment and errors in judgment. Even in situations where the patient is legally competent, the family should be brought into the process to assist in the evaluation of the patient's ability to give consent and to participate in the consent process itself. There should also be family consensus that participation is advisable. Many family members are opposed to their loved one's participation until they are made part of the process and learn firsthand what the study is about.

Special care must be used to ensure that the aged patient has the privacy and time to make his own decision. It is the authors' experience that these patients can be very slow in making up their minds, and the staff must be advised not to pressure them to make a decision inadvertently. It is important to note, however, that the vast majority of elderly patients can assimilate information and give informed consent. Presenting written and verbal material to the patient and another member of the household and allowing the person to think about it for a day or two are methods that assist in the process. If a person is truly indecisive after this procedure has been used, the patient should not be allowed to take part in the investigation.

DISEASE STATES INTERFERING WITH COMPREHENSION

UNCONSCIOUS OR SEVERELY ILL PATIENTS. Unconscious, trauma, and severely burned patients should not be utilized in research without direct benefit to them except to the degree that the observations can be made incidental to their appropriate treatment. IRBs are most helpful in these decisions. Consent in research that uniquely requires this sort of patient can be handled by an advocate. In rare instances, the IRB may grant permission for a study to be undertaken without the subjects' prior informed consent if arrangements are made to secure consent as soon as the subjects are able to grant it. Sometimes the investigator may be able to limit the area of the research and, thus, gain permission to conduct the study. For example, one study compared bumetanide with furosemide in severe pulmonary edema in patients who could not grant informed consent because of cerebral anoxia at the time the condition was recognized. Responsibly showing comparability of the agents (at different doses) and a clear theoretical safety advantage in favor of bumetanide led a local IRB to accept a randomized study without informed consent. Failure necessitating withdrawal was clearly specified for each agent as a part of the approval process.

DISEASE REQUIRING MEDICATION THAT ALTERS COMPREHENSION. Subjects in this category require careful individual consideration. Issues such as what they can reasonably comprehend and the nature of the protocol merit consideration. Minor observational studies pose no problem, but major interventions are of much greater consequence if a patient cannot fully understand what will be involved in the study. Most doctors participating in evaluating acute abdomens or gastrointestinal bleeding patients encounter patients in practice who are making decisions about whether or not to have surgery at a time when they may not be prepared to consider the factors involved. When considerations other than the patient's own health benefit are involved, special precautions must be taken to ensure that the ingredients of a meaningful consent process are present. Arrangements can be made to have an advocate or family member available to give consent if the IRB will allow it. If patients must be interviewed at routine visits while they are under the influence of medication affecting their comprehension, the study procedures should take this fact into account. The interview process can usually be scheduled before new medication is administered, or, if necessary, subjects can be contacted at home later in the day to verify information provided at the office.

MENTAL ILLNESS. Chronic mental illness such as schizophrenia or depression is episodic and often recurs. With intermittent use of medications, however, patients so afflicted are quite well adjusted in the community and in their work. Surprisingly large numbers exist and many volunteer for studies. Every gradation of mental illness, from seemingly normal to psychotic, may be encountered. Some patients require medication daily to get through the day, while others have not been on medication in years. It becomes a sensitive judgment to determine which of these persons may be safely and appropriately used for a study and which may not. In a general way, patients requiring major behavior modifying agents for depression or schizophrenia should be considered mentally ill and should not be allowed to participate in long-term research protocols that are not specifically studying their condition or a related condition distinctly requiring those patients. On the other hand, they may be suitable choices for very limited studies of the relief of headaches, hemorrhoidal pain, or musculoskeletal aches. The problem diminishes as the interval for which they remain in remission increases. Patients with these conditions who are not on medication are legally competent and are suitable for many types of research. However, the informed consent process must be planned and administered carefully. There is extensive prejudice, even in the medical community, that subjects labeled with these diagnoses are not mentally whole. These prejudices may cause outside observers to question whether the consent process can be completely voluntary. The authors suggest that a member of the IRB be consulted who is conversant with the committee's views on research involving these subjects and can offer advice on how best to conduct the consent process.

Patients with these conditions who are considered legally competent can be suitable for many types of research. However, the informed consent process must be carefully and patiently administered. Even when an advocate or guardian is involved, the recruiter bears responsibility of being certain that the individual himself is willing to participate.

SPECIAL STATUS UNDER THE LAW OR IN CURRENT ETHICAL THINKING

Children, prisoners, pregnant women, patients institutionalized as mentally infirm, and nursing home residents are in varying degrees at risk for abuse of the consent process. Thus, there are major uncertainties about the ethical propriety and legal acceptability of conducting research on these groups. The ethical issues relevant to the participation of populations especially vulnerable to coercion or manipulation are quite complex. Although some of the groups listed above have been singled out by the various regulatory and funding agencies as deserving of special protection, it is clear that many of the other groups described in the earlier section may require similar protection at certain points in the research process. This section of the chapter will provide an overview of the issues of concern to regulatory agencies and IRBs charged with protecting the rights of these groups.

It must be emphasized that the conditions under which special populations should be allowed to participate in research have been explored at length by the ethical community and continue to be hotly debated. A detailed review of the literature is clearly a necessity for the investigator who expects to conduct extensive research involving these groups. The reader who has an interest in exploring these issues in greater depth is referred to Levine's excellent work, *Ethics and Regulation of Clinical Research*. That book contains a detailed discussion of the writings of the National Commission for the Protection of Human Subjects and includes a number of important references in the field.

CHILDREN. The DHHS has published final regulations governing the participation of children in clinical research (45 CFR Part 46). They were issued in March of 1983 and became effective in June of that same year. The FDA has issued proposed regulations governing research on this group, and its final regulations are expected to be similar to those of the DHHS.[2] In its recommendations suggesting conditions under which children should be allowed to participate in clinical investigations, the National Commission cited a number of factors that should be considered.[3] First, appropriate animal studies and studies in adults (if the condition exists in that population) or older children are in order. This recommendation is based on the premise that the least vulnerable population should be studied first before involving a younger group. Additionally, protecting the privacy of the subjects is an important concern. The regulations explicitly reflect the commission's recommendation that the assent of the children be sought for the research if they have reached the state of psychological maturity at which they can understand the choices presented. It also was recommended that the IRB assure that, when necessary, appropriate provisions be made to have an independent auditor monitor the consent process or to involve a parent or guardian in the research. Although the actual DHHS regulations do not specifically cover many of these issues, the commission's recommendations have greatly influenced current regulatory and ethical thinking and deserve exploration.

Since 1962, the FDA has required manufacturers to include in their labeling of nearly all new drugs a statement that the product is not recommended for use in young children and infants because little research has been conducted in these groups. Levine and Holder have pointed out that the cumbersome requirements governing investigation in children and pregnant women cause new medications to be administered to these patients in an unstructured practice setting rather than the more carefully controlled and monitored conditions offered by the Phase II and III clinical trial.[4] As a result, adverse reactions are detected much later than would be the case if the drugs had been studied in controlled trials. This conclusion might also be extended to the elderly.

THE FETUS OR THE PREGNANT WOMAN. DHHS has issued final regulations governing research on fetuses, pregnant women, and human *in vitro* fertilization (45 CFR 46.2). Since this is a rather complex and highly specialized area, the reader is referred to Lebacqz (1977) for a discussion of the ethical issues involved. In general, research involving pregnant women or fetuses may not be initiated unless appropriate animal studies and studies on nonpregnant individuals have been conducted. This requirement may be waived if the study involves minimal risk to the fetus and is being performed to meet the health needs of the fetus. Provisions must also be made to ensure that the investigators involved will play no role in the decision to terminate the pregnancy or to determine the viability of the fetus.

PATIENTS INSTITUTIONALIZED AS MENTALLY INFIRM. The DHHS published proposed regulations in 1978 governing the participation of patients institutionalized as mentally infirm. These were not favorably received by the research ethics community and are not expected to be revised or finalized in the near future. The National Commission did address the ethical issues relevant to this group and likened them to those applicable to the pediatric population. The commission has argued that investigators wishing to include this group in their study population must offer adequate justification for their involvement. There has long been concern in the research community that institutionalized subjects may be recruited disproportionately for studies because they are a convenient, readily identifiable population.[5] Particularly when a patient may not be capable of consenting to participation himself, special precautions ensuring that his right to free choice is protected are felt to be in order.

Research involving more than minimal risk is the area of greatest controversy. Studies involving more than minimal risk are generally thought to be acceptable if they offer the subjects the potential for direct benefits, provided that the consent guidelines discussed below are followed. When research involves more than a minor increment above minimal risk and does not offer the subjects direct benefits, the National Commission has advocated that the research proposal be submitted to a National Ethics Advisory Board following the IRB's review.[6] This national committee would be expected to determine whether the research will contribute to the understanding of a problem affecting the health and welfare of the vulnerable population. In such cases, the board would solicit public comment before making a final decision to approve the project.

The consent of institutionalized subjects who are considered legally competent should be obtained before they are enrolled in a study. If the subject is not legally competent, the consent of his legally authorized representative should be sought as well as the assent of the subject himself. This practice may require modification if an incompetent patient refuses to assent to participation in a study that offers him unique benefits not available outside of the research setting. In this latter case, the subject's welfare clearly is the overriding consideration.

PRISONERS. The DHHS has issued final regulations on research involving prisoners (45 CFR 46.3). Research on this group may be conducted if it involves minimal risk and concerns the effects of incarceration or other aspects of criminal behavior. The regulations also permit research to be conducted on prisoners if the research involves a condition which particularly affects prisoners as a class or if the research can reasonably be expected to improve the subjects' health and welfare.

In these latter instances, however, the secretary of the DHHS must be willing to authorize the research following IRB approval, a discussion of the study's merit with experts in the field, and publication of a notice in the *Federal Register* of his intent to approve the project. As with other DHHS regulations, these requirements apply only to research being funded by agencies within the DHHS. However, the FDA has issued these identical regulations for prisoners as well (21 CFR Part 50).

IRBs reviewing research involving prisoners must include a prisoner in their membership and maintain a majority of members who are unaffiliated with the prison. The IRB has the role of ensuring that the prisoners are not offered inappropriate inducements to participate, such as significant improvements in living, working, or eating conditions or promises that involvement in the study will have any influence on their parole. The prisoners also should not be subjected to risks that are greater than those that would be imposed on a nonprisoner population for the same study. Further, the IRB must ensure that the procedures for selecting subjects are equitable and free from the influence of prison authorities or other inmates. Specifically, DHHS requires subjects to be selected randomly from a pool of eligible candidates in most cases. Finally, the IRB must ensure that the information presented to the subjects is understandable and that appropriate provisions are made for any follow-up examinations or care that may be required.

Most investigators are not likely to conduct research involving prison populations, particularly since sponsors may have specific policies prohibiting their involvement in studies. Nevertheless, the special provisions that the DHHS has instituted to preserve the prisoners' autonomy may be of interest to investigators attempting to develop meaningful consent procedures for other vulnerable groups.

The research community has long been sensitive to the need to offer special protection to subjects whose ability to give free and informed consent may be compromised. Although a few specific groups have been singled out as deserving of special regulatory protection, it is clear that many patients face temporary barriers to comprehension that make them unable to participate fully in the investigator–subject relationship. As valuable as any regulatory protection might be, it is the investigator, with his personal knowledge of the patient and his individual circumstances, who can best guarantee that the subject's autonomy and right of free choice are respected in the research interaction. The team that addresses these vulnerabilities during the consent process and on-study interactions will make the study experience a much more satisfying one for both the subject and team members.

REFERENCES

1. Leikin, S.L., An ethical issue in biomedical research: The involvement of minors in informed consent and third party consent, *Clin. Res.* **31**:34–40, 1983.
2. Levine, R.J., *Ethics and Regulation of Clinical Research* (2nd ed.), Urban & Schwarzenberg, Baltimore, 1986, p. 242.
3. Levine, R.J., *Ethics and Regulation of Clinical Research* (2nd ed.), Urban & Schwarzenberg, Baltimore, 1986, pp. 242–256.
4. Levine, R.J., and Holder, A.R., Legal and ethical problems in clinical research, in: *The Clinical Research Process in the Pharmaceutical Industry* (G.M. Matoren, ed.), Marcel Dekker, Inc., New York, 1984.
5. Levine, R.J., *Ethics and Regulation of Clinical Research* (2nd ed.), Urban & Schwarzenberg, Baltimore, 1986, p. 260.
6. Levine, R.J., *Ethics and Regulation of Clinical Research* (2nd ed.), Urban & Schwarzenberg, Baltimore, 1986, p. 269.

FURTHER READING

Lebacqz, K., Reflections on the report and recommendations of the National Commission: Reflections on the fetus, *Villanova Law Rev.* **22**:357–366, 1977.

CHAPTER 12

The Enrollment/Continuation Decision

Significance of the Decision • Information Required for the Decision • Who Makes the Enrollment Decision? • Review of the Enrollment Information • Intentional Violations of the Inclusion/Exclusion Criteria • Enrollment Errors • Judging the Quality of an Enrollment Process • The Continuation Decision • Special Problem Areas

SIGNIFICANCE OF THE DECISION

This is the critical decision in the research process for both the patient and the investigator. It marks the transition for the patient from private or usual medical care to research care. The investigator is committing the patient to a course of action and therapy in the study by prescribing the study medication. Much of the "pressure" in the conduct of a study also centers around this decision. Rapid recruitment of an adequate number of patients who qualify is the name of the research game—good investigators recruit *enough good* patients for the study.

The enrollment decision should be made with several important concerns in mind: (1) a genuine concern for the safety of the potential subject, (2) an educated guess about the influence each individual patient will have on the validity of the study, and (3) an economic review, weighing speed of recruitment, evaluation of possible side effects, and likelihood of completing the study. Similar concerns apply at each on-study visit to evaluate the appropriateness of continuing an individual subject in the study.

INFORMATION REQUIRED FOR THE DECISION

The information used to make the enrollment decision should consist of routine, protocol-specific, and patient-specific components.

ROUTINE INFORMATION. General medical data such as demographic information and a basic history and physical exam should be collected and recorded routinely for general safety and liability reasons with a high degree of accuracy and certainty. The collection of this information may be delegated to motivated, trained, and supervised staff members. A medical history, including job history, hospitalizations, prescriptions and over-the-counter drug use, treatments, side effects, and habits, allows major judgments to be made regarding patient compliance, likelihood of experiencing side effects, and likelihood of completing the study. The review of habits should include alcohol use, smoking, and illicit drug use. This history forms the basis for progressing to the next steps in the preenrollment screening process.

PROTOCOL-SPECIFIC INFORMATION. Medical data specific to the study, such as a detailed stomach medication history or a gynecologic history, need to be collected with a great deal of care, specificity, and skill. A fair degree of sophistication in taking this history will ensure that important eligibility data are not overlooked. For a simple example: The patient being considered for an acute duodenal ulcer healing study reports taking Alka-Seltzer regularly. The experienced interviewer knows that Alka-Seltzer has a variety of preparations, some of which contain aspirin and some of which do not. Since the protocol prohibits recent aspirin use, the interviewer must try to get more specific information from the patient. Suggesting that he bring in the empty package of what he has used or having him review pictures in the product identification section of the PDR is useful in resolving, with a high degree of certainty, eligibility questions such as this. The well-prepared staff anticipates this type of difficulty and has these aids available at the onset of the screening process and has informed the patient in advance of the need to bring *all* medication into the screening interview. Improving the specificity of the information obtained from the patient *the first time* dramatically reduces the inconsistencies that sometimes appear when a patient's history is taken by a number of persons.

PATIENT-SPECIFIC INFORMATION. This is probably the most difficult of all preliminary data to obtain quickly and reliably, is usually not collected and recorded in a standard manner, and yet is valuable in making the enrollment decision. This type of information can be used to make predictions about a number of important issues.

First, though a patient may be medically eligible for the protocol, the PI must nevertheless assess his likelihood of entering the study. The authors have had the infrequent experience of having patients who are quite anxious to have the screening history, physical, laboratory, and procedures done and not so anxious to actually enter the study once found to be eligible. This phenomenon can be attributed less to the salutary effects of a valid informed consent process and more to the fact that the patient wanted the screening without ever intending to enter the study. With experience, such patients can be recognized during the early interviews.

Second, if entered into the protocol, will the patient comply with the rigors of the protocol and medication regimens? Since compliance is such a critical issue in judging the efficacy and safety of the agent, any clues that the staff can gather about the patient are important and should be passed on to the investigator.

Finally, if the patient is entered into the protocol, what kind of reporter will he be of any hassles, discomforts, and side effects? Since patients enter into clinical research for different reasons, their reliability and motivation to report subjective difficulties vary considerably. The rare patient who is anxious and somatizes everything may not be an appropriate subject. Neither is the normal subject who is so "macho" or nonverbal that he would never say a word about even the most severe pain or discomfort. Picking the "right" subject with the "right" symptom threshold is highly subjective and depends upon the availability of potential subjects, the investigator's prior experience with the particular subject, and the type of protocol being considered. For example, for comparative bioavailability testing of well-known products, one would prefer a subject with a very high symptom-reporting threshold for his study. For a Phase III or IV comparison of a new beta blocker in hypertensive subjects, one would prefer a verbal subject who can and will report minor symptoms to identify a possible advantage of the new agent. Realistically, an investigator is not often presented with this luxury of choice of subjects and must settle for a subject who approximates the ideal. Consciously thinking about and documenting the rationale for these choices helps the investigator do the screening better and prepare himself to comment upon any variations in population characteristics or side effect reporting among investigators. The authors have frequently been asked to suggest a reason that rates of side effect reporting were found to differ between investigators.

EXAMPLE 1. Variation

Two groups unrelated to each other undertook the identical protocol evaluating a topical salicylate versus oral aspirin. The efficacy of the two agents was approximately comparable in athletic injuries and acute bursitis but not in arthritis. However, the incidence of gastrointestinal side

TABLE 20. *Questions That May Be Asked to Elicit Patient-Specific Enrollment Information*

How is it that you are considering being in the research protocol?
How did you hear about this protocol?
What was it about what you read or heard that prompted you to come in today?
How does your family feel about your coming here today?
How does your doctor feel about your coming here today?
How do you plan to fit this protocol into your busy schedule?
How does your boss react when you miss work or are late for work due to illness?
How will you get to our facility from home/work and back?
Who, if anyone, usually goes to the doctor's office with you?
What aids do you use at home to help you remember to take your current medication?
    How does your family help you do this?
How do you feel about the prospect of being paid for your participation in the
    research?
How much/how soon had you hoped you would be paid for your participation?

effects was 24% at one investigative site and 4% at the other. At the site with the higher figure, it was significantly higher with aspirin than with placebo. In preparing these data for publication, it was soon apparent that the site with the higher yield of side efects was recruited almost entirely from the personal practice of the PI. He saw the patients frequently and met with them during the study. The lower incidence occurred in a group of persons recruited from playgrounds with athletic injuries, who were younger and were reviewed much less thoroughly. The marked difference in the subjects influenced the results as to side effects.

Conducting this selection process consciously also allows the investigator to compensate for enrollment trade-offs in the form of closer behavior observation in the care of the nonverbal subject or more structured symptom reviews with the anxious somatizing subject. Patient-specific information of this type is best elicited by the use of open-ended questions asked by a variety of staff members in low-key, nonthreatening ways.

Preliminary information also needs to be corroborated by observation, again made by the greeting staff. Table 20 lists some of the questions that may be asked to elicit this information. Some of these questions may be asked as part of the receptionist's attempt to put the patient at ease. Others are best asked after a positive interaction with the patient is well under way with the research nurse or coordinator or after the patient is considered eligible for entry into the study. Table 21 lists some behavioral observations that may be clues to research behavior.

TABLE 21. *Observations That May Yield Patient-Specific Enrollment Information*

Arrival observations (usually made by the receptionist)
    What form of transportation did the patient use—private car, taxi, bus, etc.?
    Did the patient complain of parking—access, costs?
    With whom did the patient arrive—family, spouse, friend?
    Was the patient prompt and on time? If late, what was the explanation offered?
Waiting room observations
    What did the patient do while waiting—read the patient educational materials,
       fidget nervously, talk with staff or other patients, chain-smoke, etc.?
    How did the patient interact with accompanying persons while waiting?
    Did the patient seem to get more comfortable with the passage of time or number of
       visits?

WHO MAKES THE ENROLLMENT DECISION?

The enrollment decision is made by the investigator and should be considered the same as the act of prescribing and dispensing a medication. The enrollment decision requires thoughtful review of the available information, including staff input on the patient's personality and reliability. The review of the patient's data and the decision to include him should be documented thoroughly. The enrollment decision cannot be delegated to another individual other than a coprincipal investigator except under very limited circumstances. In studies with clear objective inclusion/exclusion criteria and a population that is not severely ill, the PI may establish eligibility ranges for laboratory and diagnostic tests and permit a clinically trained staff member (e.g., a nurse) to enroll subjects whose data fall in those ranges. Such a mechanism is acceptable only if these criteria are written and a system is in place for the PI to perform a timely review of the staff member's decisions. An investigator also must anticipate the times when he will be unavailable on either a scheduled or an emergency basis. During these times, it is preferable not to enroll new subjects in the study unless the PI has a collaborating investigator quite familiar with the study who can function on his behalf. Coverage arrangements nevertheless must be made for those subjects already in the study. If a physician not involved with the study must be asked to cover for the PI, he should have a background and skills similar to those of the PI and should be oriented to the study. The IRB and the sponsor should be notified of the fact that the person is in charge for a specific period of time. Other regulatory issues must be addressed as well if the coverage is scheduled for more than a few days (e.g., 1572/73 forms must be amended and forwarded to clients).

REVIEW OF THE ENROLLMENT INFORMATION

PURPOSE OF THE REVIEW. Prior to making the enrollment decision, the investigator must review and spot-check the information after the staff has preliminarily sorted through the candidates. The investigator may choose to verify personally with the patient and/or staff only the most salient features of the history or occasionally even the more mundane bits of information. This review and spot-checking serves three important purposes. First, it is a quality check in very specific terms on the preenrollment screening process and on the adequacy of its documentation up to that point. The check provides staff with immediate feedback from the investigator and gives the investigator the chance to orient and focus the staff on the priorities of the protocol. This staff–investigator interaction regarding a specific patient is an invaluable and necessary process if the staff is to assimilate the investigator's values and standards. Second, it identifies any omissions or inconsistencies in the information base that must be resolved prior to enrollment. Third, it ensures the genuineness of the enrollment decision and firmly and clearly identifies the investigator as the responsible person for the decision *and* for the preenrollment process.

FACILITATING THE REVIEW. The staff must be sensitive to the work style of the investigator and prepare information for review in a manner that makes the best use of the investigator's time. The authors have found that review of the information may be best accomplished in a two-step process. Physical exams, laboratory information, chest films, and similar items are reviewed as they arrive or in a batch by the PI or his designate to ensure the timeliness and completeness of the lab results and to screen them for normalcy. The few abnormal ones are shown promptly to the PI, who makes a disposition. Once reviewed, the information is then placed in the patient's record. If the patient remains eligible at this point, the entire chart is then presented to the investigator for a final review of all the gathered information prior to the enrollment decision. The systematic review of components of the patient's chart enables the staff to feel comfortable with the automatic progression and entry procedures set up by the PI and staff. Staff concerns about patient compliance, symptom reporting, or completing the study can be voiced at the final review. The staff can further facilitate review by a liberal use of tabs and "flags" that guide the investigator to the areas of concern.

INCONSISTENCIES AND OMISSIONS IN THE INFORMATION BASE. During the course of the review of the enrollment information base, the investigator may discover omissions or inconsistencies in the data base. Since the investigator generally has limited time available, it is often helpful to have the patient's record prereviewed by a knowledgeable staff person to highlight the omissions and inconsistencies. This will greatly facilitate the physician's review and will help the staff anticipate what may be required next. This prereview, if entirely normal and without questions, concerns, or comments, may be used by the staff to advance the patient in the process *without* specific review by the PI. A patient must not progress, however, if the omissions and inconsistencies have not been clarified. These often require the review and judgment of the investigator.

Inconsistencies are a fact of life when patients are involved and when more than one person is gathering the data. They arise from the multiple but necessary sources of information needed for the decision, overinterpretations of available facts (e.g., patient's history of "tube surgery" is interpreted as tubal ligation by the staff), a lack of clarity in documentation, a lack of specific detail, or a lack of attention to the timing of a historical detail. The inconsistencies also stem from the patient himself, whose recollection of events may be poor.

The majority of inconsistencies are trivial but become particularly glaring when they appear in relation to criteria that affect the patient's eligibility for the protocol. The issues most often troublesome are dates of onset and duration of prior medical conditions, prior medication use, prior therapy of alcohol and drug abuse, prior medical conditions such as asthma or chest pain, and contraceptive use.

The investigator has the final responsibility to resolve any inconsistencies in the enrollment information base prior to making the enrollment decision and to document as part of the enrollment decision how they were resolved. The investigator must attempt to establish the most reasonable workable interpretation of the best available facts and make any necessary judgments about the accuracy or reliability of the patient's reports. Inconsistencies can be resolved by talking with the staff or the patient as necessary. Sometimes an eligibility question is of such importance that the patient's entry must be delayed until the old records have been reviewed. A well-trained staff will routinely request these records at the first visit.

Omissions in the enrollment information base are also a fact of life. Some, such as height or weight omissions, are a result of sporadic breakdown in the data-collection process. Others, such as lab results, are systematic and are related to the timing of the investigator's review in relation to the staff's receipt of the information, to the demands of patient convenience and compliance, or to the demands of the protocol "windows." Omissions due to sporadic breakdowns in the data-collection process are infrequent in a well-run facility and when they do occur can be traced to a particularly hectic screening session or some

other isolated reasons. Frequent omissions of this type suggest a need
to evaluate the staffing pattern or screening sequence in order to reduce
the frequency of this problem. Omissions of this type can be resolved
by obtaining the sponsor's conditional approval for the patient to enter
the study contingent upon the procurement of the missing information
by the time of actual enrollment into the study. The staff should be
alerted to this circumstance and should notify the investigator of the
availability of the information for his review prior to dispensing or
dosing of any medication. All of this should be documented in the
patient's chart and countersigned by the investigator at the earliest
convenient time.

Omissions resulting from systematic problems are the bane of an
investigator staff's existence and represent a major challenge to their
creativeness, persistence, and ingenuity. Prompt identification and resolution of systematic deficiencies will allow the team to keep the patient happy, the protocol inviolate, and the PI placated.

Since the enrollment decision is based upon the specific eligibility
criteria established with patient safety or scientific considerations in
mind, information required to determine the patient's eligibility must
be available for review *prior to dosing* the patient. The review and
analysis of a large number of abnormal safety or diagnostic tests to
establish whether the patient meets the protocol requirements and general health requirements for safe entry are functions for which the
physician is uniquely qualified. While a PI may choose to establish
written procedures so the staff may enroll subjects with entirely normal
or routine results following a preliminary medical exam, the physician
must recognize his responsibility for the action delegated to the staff
and for reviewing their actions as promptly as possible. The significance of this review and entry decision must be emphasized in the
recruiting process. There should be very few exceptions to the requirement that test results be available prior to dosing. Those that are
granted are generally known and approved in advance by the client and
the IRB and are allowed because it is common practice to begin therapy
presumptively while awaiting test results. Examples include biopsy
results, culture and sensitivity results, and special laboratory test results. If those exceptions are part of the protocol, there are usually
explicit instructions on how to deal with the results once they are
known.

EXAMPLE 2. Sloppiness

*A college student who had successfully completed several bio-
availability studies applied for still another. His baseline chemistry re-*

sults did not return in hard copy, but one of the recruiting staff telephoned the lab and reported that the test results were normal. On the strength of this telephone report, the patient was entered as a normal subject. When hard copy appeared, he had early hepatitis with elevated AST and ALT, as well as positive test for hepatitis B at the time of dosing. This single erroneous report exposed a number of patients and staff to hepatitis B, placed the subject at risk, and resulted in the testing of a drug in an unqualified subject. The breaches of responsible behavior are self-evident in this example.

With the realities of heavy or conflicting schedules, it is recognized that the investigator may not always be available to physically review all of the documents generated during the screening process at the time that the patient is in the facility waiting to be dosed. A telephone review of the final test results required for dosing or the use of delivery services to allow review of the patient's record can certainly be employed to minimize inconvenience to both the PI and the patient. With proper orientation of staff and a good system for alerting the PI by phone of lab results or any other final test results needed for dosing, inconveniences can be minimized without loss of quality or safety. Additionally, written guidelines may be established for review of laboratory data and delegation of responsibility for reviewing and highlighting abnormalities of particular concern so these can be prioritized for the PI's attention. Any enrollment decisions made by telephone should be documented as such and countersigned by the investigator upon his return to the facility.

Another way of coping with omitted data is to establish a "conditional approval" mechanism. A conditional approval by the investigator indicates that his review of the available information declares the patient eligible for enrollment, contingent upon the receipt, review, and normalcy of the omitted bit of information. If this is agreed upon at the outset, the research nurse needs only to document the conditional approval and the receipt, review, and normalcy of the information, and proceed to dispense or administer the medication. The investigator may then countersign the nurse's note and indicate total approval at the earliest convenience.

It is not acceptable to send a patient home with medication and instructions not to begin the medication regimen until the PI or his staff has received outstanding test results. Patients rarely comply with such an instruction, and the risk of subjecting a patient to investigational drug therapy is not justified. If the patient can conveniently pick up his study medication once the report has been received, an honorarium provided to defray parking or travel expenses should greatly minimize

any potential inconvenience. If necessary, express mail to his home can
be used for delivery.

INTENTIONAL VIOLATIONS OF INCLUSION/EXCLUSION CRITERIA

POSSIBLE ADVERSE CONSEQUENCES OF VARIANCES. The protocol is a
contract involving the investigator, the patient, the FDA, the client, and
the IRB. This document represents the investigator's commitment to a
particular methodology for selecting patients with a selected disease
and administering a specific therapy on an established monitoring
schedule to determine safety and efficacy of the treatment modality.
Any variances in adhering to the inclusion/exclusion criteria established may have several negative consequences.

1. Variances undermine the confidence and trust that the patient,
   the FDA, the sponsor, and the IRB have in the investigator's
   ability to conduct the protocol as written, agreed to, and approved. This loss of trust is often the most long-lasting and
   damaging consequence to the investigator and may exclude him
   from further participation in clinical trials. This loss of trust
   biases all subsequent interactions with the parties.
2. They can jeopardize the individual patient's safety.
3. If a patient's data are disqualified because of the protocol variance, there will have been no benefit to counterbalance the patient's risks in participating in the study; hence, the decision to
   enter the subject will not have been ethically justified.
4. A large percentage of entry violations could jeopardize the integrity of the entire study, since these could reduce the statistical power of the study to such a degree that the study objectives could not be rigorously met. If an entire study is jeopardized, the cumulative risks of all participating patients would
   not result in any benefit to the public at large and could not be
   ethically justified.

POSSIBLE JUSTIFICATIONS FOR INTENTIONAL PROTOCOL VARIANCES.
The realities and complexities of the clinical research process, the
uniqueness of the individual patient, and the limitations of even the
best-written and conceived protocol very occasionally create a need for
a protocol variance.

A variance may be appropriate if it is clearly minor and does not
alter subject safety (see Example 3, below). Knowing whether a vari-

ance is major or minor often is not easy. The harder it is to figure out, the more likely it is that the variance is major. The investigator may determine that the variance is minor on the basis of his assessment that there is only a small increment in the theoretical risk to the patient's safety. The investigator may base this on a very thorough and precise knowledge of the patient (e.g., patients who have been under his care for 10 years). In general, the less that is known about the patient, the less likely any variance can be considered minor. The theoretical risk to the patient's safety must also be considered in light of both the individual patient and the drug's toxicity profile. Unless the investigator has worked with the agent in depth and has performed some of the toxicity studies, the best way to assess safety risks is to contact the sponsor's medical monitor, who should have an intimate knowledge of the drug and the latest information regarding its experience in human subjects. In general, the less that is known about the agent, the less likely a variance will be judged minor. This means that during late Phase III or IV studies more variances may be acceptable to the medical monitor. Contact with the medical monitor before entry of the patient with a minor variance is very important for other reasons as well. Prior approval by the client will often determine whether the investigator receives payment for the patient should the patient not be considered evaluable for some reason at a later date. Prior discussion with the client facilitates the development of an approach that can be taken with the individual patient to reduce these added risks or monitoring of these risks. These precautions, set up and taken proactively, help maintain the trust and confidence the patient and staff have in the investigator's ability to safely and expertly conduct the research.

EXAMPLE 3. Minor Variance

A protocol required a normal chest film within the last three months. A 31-year-old subject had a film taken and confirmed as normal with a written report 106 days prior to planned dosing. Though eligible in every manner except this, he was not willing to have another chest film. The medical monitor agreed that this person could be enrolled.

A variance may be appropriate if it is minor and does not affect the statistical evaluability of the patient—that is, if the variance is thought to have a low theoretical risk to the protocol's integrity and does not violate its intent. This assessment cannot be made without a conversation with the sponsor's staff unless the investigator designed the protocol. The designers of the protocol should be fully aware of the strong and weak points of the protocol's design. They should be aware of what regulatory constraints may have been placed on the protocol. These are things that are not normally known and dealt with every day by the investigator; thus, the investigator must talk with a knowledgeable scientific representative of the sponsor. Sometimes the sponsor may be reluctant to share all of this background information through its monitoring staff, who may insist on rigid adherence to the "letter" of the protocol without an obvious rationale. This may be dealt with by talking with the senior staff or talking with other investigators who may share insight into the situation. The ultimate issue is evaluability of the patient's data. If the evaluability criteria are explicit, well known, not likely to change as a result of changes in state-of-the-art knowledge, and articulated up front, the determination of whether or not a variance is trivial is easy. When the criteria are not so well formed, the significance of a variance cannot be assessed and, hence, may be sufficient to result in disqualification of the patient's data. If there is a doubt, enrollment should not be permitted.

Enrolling a subject who has provided historical information suggesting an exclusion criterion of minor significance may be warranted to preserve the integrity of the preenrollment screening process. A process that proves too restrictive and predictable may encourage patients to withhold information (either inadvertently or intentionally) that could be thought to exclude them from participating. This circumvention removes the investigator's opportunity to consider the complexities of each potential subject's health status and individual risk–benefit assessment in deciding whether he or she can safely participate. A common example would be the recovered alcoholic with a proven history of sobriety and without clinically significant abnormalities in any diagnostic or laboratory tests. The investigator's intimate knowledge of the patient's psychological and medical history and the potential benefits of participation for this individual may warrant contacting the sponsor for special permission for the patient to be included in the study. This justification can never apply to the enrollment of any patient with a major protocol violation.

EXAMPLE 4. You Are Told What You Want to Hear

Most bioavailability protocols exclude all over-the-counter medications for the two weeks prior to dosing and all caffeine-containing foods and beverages for 48 hours before actual dosing. These exclusions are established to avoid drug interference and high levels of caffeine, even though 80% of Americans have measurable caffeine in their blood at any given time. Many subjects upon interview at the entry to the study 8 to 12 hours before dosing will admit to a violation—one acetaminophen, some chocolate, a cola beverage, or (even more taboo) a single portion of beer. If all

*such persons are excluded, the group is conditioned to suppress the
information. We have usually individualized this to allow credible con-
fessed intakes of caffeine and even one beer or acetaminophen tablets
more than several days prior to the time of dosing and have treated these
as minor but permissible variations. On infrequent occasions, we have
had completed patients with such recorded information disqualified and
not paid for by the sponsor.*

In some protocols, the financial costs to the investigator as well as
the risks undertaken by the patient in the preenrollment screening
process are substantial. The rejection of a patient at this point in the
process for a minor variance could result in an unnecessary waste of
limited research resources. The financial rationale is employed more
frequently when the study budget is "tight" at the onset of the protocol;
nonetheless, while it is a real consideration, finances should not interfere with the judgment of whether a variance is minor or major.

The justification that patient accrual is slow is rarely voiced explicitly, yet it is one of the more common reasons investigators commit
protocol violations. Poor enrollment performance must prompt a review of the individual investigator's recruiting techniques and patient
population by talking with the other investigators or with the sponsor.
If the proper patients are not to be found by that investigator, the investigator must withdraw from participation in the protocol rather than
enroll ineligible patients.

If enrollment is slow for all investigators, the sponsor may need to
review and redesign the whole protocol and solicit IRB and FDA approval for the "looser" eligibility criteria that would be applied to a
whole new population of potential subjects.

WHEN ARE VARIANCES ACCEPTABLE? Enrollment variances are acceptable when the justification of enrollment outweighs the potential
negative consequences of enrollment. This balance can be assured in
the following circumstances: (1) The decision to enter patient with
protocol variances is made thoughtfully and proactively. (2) The decision and rationale are fully documented at the time of enrollment. (3)
The decision has been approved by the sponsor and with the knowledge of the patient. (4) Special precautions that reduce the safety risk to
the patient are taken prior to and during the conduct of the study.

EXAMPLE 5. Minor Variation, Safety Monitoring

*A 23-year-old woman being considered for an acute duodenal ulcer pro-
tocol was found on screening endoscopy to have an appropriate ulcer in*

*size and location and was eligible according to all criteria with the ex-
ception of a hematocrit of 28. The stool occult blood tests proved negative, the smear was compatible with iron deficiency anemia, and the
patient had heavy menstrual bleeding by history. The medical monitor
permitted the patient to enter the study, provided the patient agreed to
have hematocrit and stool occult blood testing at each visit (even if not
required by the protocol) or more frequently, received special education
regarding signs and symptoms of gastrointestinal bleeding, and agreed to
have the heavy menstrual bleeding evaluated. The patient healed her
ulcer and corrected her hematocrit in the next eight weeks.*

ENROLLMENT ERRORS

OBVIOUS ENROLLMENT ERRORS. In the flurry of activity surrounding
the screening and enrollment process, errors will occur that will result
in the entry of a patient who fails to meet the entry criteria. Sporadic
errors must be expected in a process of such medical and administrative complexity. These errors may result from errors made by the
staff in data collection or interpretation or from information not revealed or accurately reported by a patient prior to entry. It is essential
that the staff be oriented to the need to note openly and take immediate
action when any such errors are discovered. Specifically, the details of
the violation should be gathered and the medical monitor contacted to
discuss whether the patient should be allowed to remain in the study.
The critical factors involve the patient's response to the study medication and whether inclusion of the patient's data can be justified by the
study design. If no such justification exists, the sponsor will request
that the patient be discontinued promptly and appropriate follow-up
care be arranged. In a study of a new agent for preventing ulcer recurrence, for example, a patient who was found after entry not to meet the
protocol criteria for history of ulcer disease would likely need to be
withdrawn once this information was learned since it could not be
adequately demonstrated that he or she had the condition being studied. While many new investigators and staff may harbor concern that
such errors will negatively affect their image with the sponsor, the
contrary is usually the case. The demonstrated openness in acknowledging the oversight lends credibility to the process by which the study
is being conducted and can be used positively to point out the integrity
of the operation. With the many recruitment pressures facing both investigators and the research staff, it is important to emphasize that such
errors must be reported promptly when observed. The clinical trials
process now includes a number of checks and balances, such as com-

pany monitors, quality assurance teams, IRB members, and FDA inspectors, all of whom have access to an investigator's research records and opportunities to contact research subjects in some circumstances. The likelihood that such errors would go undiscovered is slim. It would certainly be preferable for the sponsor to learn of the violation directly and in a timely manner.

EXAMPLE 6. *Careful Staff Work Renders Patient Ineligible*

A study on prevention of ulcer required that a verified ulcer be healed in the previous six months. Endoscopy or X ray could be used to establish the presence of the ulcer, but a repeat endoscopy by the study was used to establish that healing had occurred. A patient was entered into this study on the basis of a written X ray report and a compatible history. Subsequently, old X rays were obtained that indicated a diverticulum of the duodenum was present and was unchanged. In a report of a single barium meal, this had been erroneously reported as an ulcer, which seemed very unlikely. This thorough review made the patient ineligible for the study. The medical monitor concurred in the decision to remove the patient from the protocol. The monitor approved payment to the investigative team of all their costs for chemistries and endoscopies invested in the patient.

Enrollment errors arise most commonly in situations where the subject is not known to the investigator prior to his or her inclusion in the study, where the relationship with the patient is not yet completely open and trusting, where the time from screening to entry is brief, and where the patient may have a strong personal motivation to withhold information relevant to the conduct of the study, such as a history of drug or alcohol abuse. Information of this kind is developed by repeated observation and interaction with the subject and as a result of the development of greater trust between the investigator and/or staff and the patient.

EXAMPLE 7. *Screw-Up*

A study of a new agent required that female patients practice an acceptable method of contraception and have a pregnancy test at each evaluation visit. A patient enrolled in the study failed to have a pregnancy test on a second or third visit. When tested eight weeks later, she was found to be pregnant. The patient was promptly discontinued from study, but her unborn child may have been exposed to as much as three months of a new drug. She was followed by the study team through the pregnancy and gave birth to a normal child. Apparently this resulted in no harm but the potential was great. She had been on the experimental agent.

When an enrollment error is discovered, the PI should review the comparative risks and benefits to the patient and study population, as outlined earlier in the context of the enrollment decision. Since the patient is already on the study medication without apparent adverse effects or consequences, the question of whether the patient should be discontinued is somewhat difficult. The sponsor should be contacted and given the opportunity to participate in the decision. The outcome of the decision should be documented in the patient's record with a rationale for the decision and any measures that must be taken to guarantee the patient's safe withdrawal from, or continuation in, the study.

JUDGING THE QUALITY OF AN ENROLLMENT PROCESS

An investigator's recruitment and enrollment process must be conducted in a genuine manner that meets three important criteria: (1) evidence of progressive selectivity based on medically or scientifically valid reasons for exclusion at the various stages of the process; (2) absence of collusion with and/or coercion of the prospective participant; and (3) methods for evaluation and self-correction of the process.

SELECTIVITY. Progressive appropriate selectivity is required to assure the genuineness of the recruitment process. Both subjects and the research staff must see evidence of selectivity in enrollment for specific studies to credibly support the stated importance of the information being provided and collected. If these data are not used in the enrollment decision, the necessary feedback to the prospective subject and research staff fails to occur.

Inappropriate selectivity must also be guarded against for social as well as scientific reasons. Race or socioeconomic status is rarely a reason to exclude patients from participating in clinical research. The demographics of the study population of the investigator should reflect the general population cared for by the investigator or reflect the demographics of the community in which the investigator is actively recruiting.

To ensure progressive appropriate selectivity, a proactive step-by-step screening process should be outlined by the investigator and shared with the staff. The investigator should specify what he wants to screen out, how it is to be screened out and based on what information, and when in the process it should be screened out. For example, a Phase I study of a new agent excludes women of childbearing potential. The investigator may state to the person conducting the telescreening that all females should be excluded. Alternately the investigator may indicate that the telescreener may permit only women more than 50 years old to proceed in the screening process. The investigator may also tell the telescreener to permit only women who state they have had surgical sterility to proceed in the screening. Regardless of where the threshold is set, if it is set clearly, the adequacy of the telescreening process can then be judged because there are subsequent checks of the process as the screening continues and the information is corroborated. A telescreening person who permits the progression of too many obvious exclusions should be reoriented. Frequent team meetings early in the protocol enrollment process can allow these issues to be identified and addressed clearly and quickly.

COLLUSION. The issue of collusion is of critical importance to subject safety. A collusion between the subject and the recruiter/enrolling physician may form as a result of an implicit understanding and merger of mutual interests—"I need to be in a study" matched with "I need you to be in this study." This collusion begins by an action, demeanor, or words indicating to the subject those criteria that may affect eligibility and discouraging him from communicating potential variations to the screening staff or physician. Failure of the research or recruiting staff to respond to patients' clues that suggest the presence of certain disqualifying factors fosters an environment in which accurate medical information is not likely to be revealed. The potential for this collusion can be minimized by structuring the recruitment process to include multiple steps. For example, a telescreening function to eliminate candidates with obvious excluding criteria can be carried out quite well over the telephone by a capable secretary or receptionist. This role can also include documentation of any potentially significant information noted during the telephone conversation.

It is also essential to instill in each of the research team members a clear understanding of the purpose of the specific trial being conducted and clinical trials in general. With the constant recruiting and data-management pressures facing research staff, the recognition that the results of a clinical trial may be used by practitioners around the country as a basis for prescribing medication may be obscured. Staff members who recognize that their individual decisions contribute significantly to an enterprise with potentially broad medical implications may be less likely to respond to these minor pressures with techniques such as collusion. This orientation must be complemented, however, with an atmosphere that allows errors or collusive behavior to be noted and constructively confronted. The investigator's demeanor will largely determine the character of the enrollment process in this setting.

EXAMPLE 8. Foolish Enrollment

A chronic alcoholic man of 58 years has compensated cirrhosis, portal hypertension, and malnutrition when drinking. He willingly accepts the bother of protocol studies and usually prefers those that require him to be in the hospital. Recently, he completed a three-month binge and as he recovered learned of a five-year study of sclerotherapy for varices. He was quickly enrolled. The dependent nature of this subject does not make him representative of the preferred test population. Although his enrollment swells the numbers, it does not aid the evaluation.

COERCION. Coercion is often in the eye of the beholder. The fine line between reasonable inducement and coercion may not be clear at times. More often the patient's personal circumstances influence his decision more than the staff's presentation. For example, large study payments may represent such an inducement to an indigent patient that the patient minimizes or ignores the risk of the study. The staff needs to be sensitive to this issue and help the patient to assess the balance more appropriately and truly exercise his informed free choice. Evidence of the exercise of free choice can be found in the reasons for the patient refusal. Cumulative detailed data about the reasons for patient refusal to enter the study are often used to buttress arguments that there is no substantial or systematic coercion. Analysis of dropout rates and reasons can also be similarly used. Debriefing of the participant after the study also can be useful in determining if the research process has been coercive to him.

EVALUATION AND FEEDBACK. The recruitment/enrollment process must include an opportunity for evaluation and self-correction. A mechanism for providing feedback at specific checkpoints must exist in order to allow the recruiter to screen out and block the entry of similarly unreliable or noncompliant subjects in the future and to allow the investigator to reassess the appropriateness of the enrollment decision at a later time. In facilities that offer subjects an opportunity to participate in multiple studies or continue into long-term studies, some attention must be paid to purifying the pool of available potential subjects, since it is these selected repeat subjects who often show new patients the "ropes." Experienced subjects also can quickly learn the general enrollment criteria established for a particular protocol.

The feedback can be accomplished informally by sharing information among the research team. Notations in the participant's chart can be made to indicate whether the subject should be considered for additional studies. The authors used a system of notations on the subject's

TABLE 22. Categories of Reasons for Nonenrollment

Demographics
Medical—inclusion/exclusion criteria
Psychosocial—unreliable, potentially noncompliant, drug or alcohol user
Patient refusal—refused appointment, failed to keep appointment, rejected study after
  informed consent process.

---

problem list to transmit this information succinctly. The authors also used "incident reports" that became part of the participant's record. These incident reports could be completed by research coordinator or investigator and detail the circumstances and recommended actions.

In most instances, a selected case study method or error-analysis method of system evaluation is adequate and provides timely information for the whole team to use to adjust or correct the system. For facilities or investigators conducting numerous protocols, regular review of the quality of the enrollment process is needed. If problems are revealed, the PI should attempt to determine whether they are the result of the design of the system or random chance.

The data base necessary to assess a preenrollment screening process need not be large and must be organized by study and by patient. The basic information consists of the patient's identifying information, reason for nonenrollment (see Table 22 for a simple system), and optimally the step in the screening process at which the exclusion was made (e.g., telemarketing step or investigator's final review). This data base will more than meet the regulatory and clients' requirements and will provide the basis for evaluating the screening process. This can be accomplished by a manual two-card system. For every patient considered for screening for a study, the receptionist should complete the patient's identifying information on two index cards (one for the protocol file and one for the alphabetical patient file). Both can be attached to the patient's record and subsequently split when a final disposition is made. There should be only two possible outcomes—enrolled in a study or excluded (see Chapters 17 and 21 for a discussion of card systems and records for excluded patients).

Once the patient is enrolled in a study, certain information needs to be collected about that study population. High drop rates, failure to return after the initial visit or receipt of drug, and rates of a subject's failure to comply with the visit schedule are some data that raise "red flags" about the adequacy of subject selection and the enrollment process.

THE CONTINUATION DECISION

The continuation decision is similar to the enrollment decision, involving many of the same considerations that were involved in the enrollment decision. Specifically, in light of the patient's experience with the medication: Is the patient still likely to experience greater benefits than costs of participation? Does the patient wish to continue in the study? The investigator's response to these questions should be documented and should be the determining factor in whether or not the patient continues in the study.

The continuation decision should be made at any time there is new relevant information related to the patient's safety or adherence to the protocol. Each scheduled visit, review of lab/procedure results, patient contact, or lack of expected patient contact should promote a review of the patient's status in the study and a conscious decision to continue or discontinue the patient.

The continuation decision should be made on the basis of the following information: (1) compliance with medication, procedure, and visit schedule; (2) adverse events noted during therapy—interval history, physical exam, procedures, and lab results; (3) patient's wishes—the patient's continuing informed consent and agreement to participate; (4) wishes of the research staff—the staff's continuing willingness to deal with the patient and his idiosyncrasies.

The continuation decision must be coordinated with the dispensation of the medication. The dispensation of additional medication at the patient's current visit constitutes the research equivalent of a prescription and should be documented in the patient's file as such. Ordinarily the investigator's decision to continue a patient in a study occurs at two points in each routine visit, preliminarily following the clinical assessment made when the visit occurs, and subsequently when the results of the laboratory or other reference tests are returned and available for review. The results of all protocol-required tests must be evaluated with the view that changes in the patient's medication schedule may be required or special precautions or observations instituted if these results prove significantly abnormal. Documentation of these qualitative assessments demonstrates to sponsors and regulatory agencies the attention to patient safety and protocol compliance that guided clinical management decisions.

SPECIAL PROBLEM AREAS

DEFINITION OF THE CRITERION "WOMEN OF CHILDBEARING POTENTIAL." This enrollment criterion is included in many early phase studies until sponsors have satisfactorily compiled the results of their teratogenic studies and can provide data on the likely effects of the drug on a fetus. The guidelines the authors use are as follows:

1. The strict definition of "not of childbearing potential" refers to women who have been surgically sterilized, women who are postmenopausal, or women who are infertile.
2. Some studies allow the inclusion of women of childbearing potential who are using a clinically accepted method of contraception. Abstinence, foam, cervical caps, or coitus interruptus are not considered acceptable forms of contraception. The condom, diaphragm, oral contraceptive, intrauterine devices, and tubal ligation are acceptable methods of contraception.
3. Women with infertility are permitted to enter the study provided they are willing to use an effective form of contraception during the study, or have been evaluated by a fertility expert and have been found to be infertile, and have been so for greater than five years. (Documentation should be available.)
4. Women who are perimenopausal are eligible for participation if there is hormonal evidence of lack of ovarian function (e.g., elevated FSH/LH and low estriol levels). Postmenopausal women (e.g., no menses for greater than one year and symptoms of estrogen withdrawal) are permitted to enter the study if allowed by the protocol.
5. A pregnancy test should be performed prior to enrollment of any woman of childbearing potential. It should be repeated at each visit if there is uncertainty about the effectiveness of the contraceptive method. Pregnancy tests should be performed at the end of the patient's participation in the study.
6. Women of childbearing potential who have partners with a vasectomy are eligible for participation, provided an acceptable method of contraception listed above is used during the course of the study.

ALCOHOL/DRUG ABUSE. Nearly all protocols exclude patients with active alcohol or drug problems. Two years free of the habit by history is usually considered as inactive and such subjects are used unless specifically forbidden. Efforts to identify these individuals prior to entry are made during the routine interview and physical screening process and by direct questioning. When the potential participants are new and without a prior relationship with the investigator or staff, information of this nature may not come to light during the first visit. Hence, the enrollment decision is made with the best information available at the time.

Once the enrollment decision is made, the staff should still be alert to the continuing possibility of alcohol/substance abuse. If suspicions arise, the participant should be positively confronted and, at this point, he may feel comfortable enough to admit to the usage and amount. If denials occur and suspicions are high, the participant may be asked to submit to a urine screen. As further information is developed that confirms the suspicion that the participant has been denying the substance abuse, the investigator must decide whether further participation is safe. The sponsor should also be involved in this decision. This decision should be based on the potential for interaction with the study drug *and* based on the participant's potentially unreliable reporting of safety-related events. Consideration must also be given to the possible confounding effects of alcohol or other drugs of abuse on the interpretation of adverse events or laboratory abnormalities. Regardless of whether the alcoholic participant is dropped or continued in the study, the participant should be referred for ongoing treatment of the problem.

"RECYCLING OF PATIENTS." Many drug development and other studies deal with illnesses of a chronic nature such as hypertension, chronic peptic ulcer disease, or angina. The chronicity of these illnesses in patients means that upon completion of one study, many patients may be eligible for another similar study. Sometimes this is by design, such as an acute duodenal ulcer healing study followed by a chronic prevention of relapse study in the same patients. In such cases, it is openly recognized and approved by the client and the IRB that the patient will enter sequential studies. What are the other circumstances when patients may be entered sequentially into multiple studies? The investigator who considers the enrollment of patients like these must assure himself of the following:

1. The patient does, in fact, have the condition under study that is intended for the protocol. Patients with continuing unresponsive conditions despite conventional therapy may not have the correct diagnosis, may have a severe variant of the disease and should be excluded from the protocol on that basis for safety or statistical reasons, or may choose to go from study to study by not taking medication.
2. The patient receives poststudy follow-up care of the continuing medical condition. An investigator's intentional or neglectful maintenance of a pool of suboptimally managed patients for the purpose of retaining their eligibility for a future protocol cannot be condoned.
3. The interval (washout) between the administration of different

investigational materials is consistent with the client's expectations and current practice. The authors adopted a 30- to 45-day washout interval when none was specified by the protocol. The washout interval is necessary to avoid a delay phase effect on efficacy of sequential administration of medication, to be able to clearly define drug toxicity relationships, and to ensure that the long half-life metabolites of the first agent do not interfere with the metabolism of the second agent. The interval period would not be in order if the two studies utilize the same investigational agent and have been reviewed by the FDA with the knowledge that one study is a short-term study and the other is a follow-up study. Because of the research context of the study drug administration, the definition of "investigational material" should include marketed agents that may be undergoing Phase IV studies.

4. The patient's central record reflects the multiple study participation and adverse events or therapy experiences.

The enrollment and continuation decision processes are among the most important aspects of clinical research. Although the quality of a study can be enhanced by effective recruitment and documentation, the overall integrity of the study depends mostly upon a selection and retention process that satisfies the intent of the study design. An effective enrollment/continuation process will include a mechanism for self-evaluation to assess the extent to which the objectives of the study are being met.

Compliance of Patients Currently on Study

Compliance is an important issue in the conduct of research. The quality and eventual value in establishing a drug's efficacy and side effects depend upon the patient ingesting the medication and undertaking the scheduled evaluations. Bringing patients into the research process as participants in these goals is an excellent beginning. At the practical level, whether or not patients appear for visits, undertake necessary blood tests, or submit required diaries is an undeniable matter of record. Whether the medication dispensed is taken or used is not so easily established. This section considers ways of enhancing patients' medication taking and visit compliance.

DETERMINING MEDICATION COMPLIANCE

Some of the many ways of determining medication compliance in a research setting are listed in Table 23. In practice, in short-term protocols such as bioavailability involving only a few doses, actual observation of the ingestion and swallowing is used. In long-term studies, less certain and indirect methods are employed.

Observed ingestion is often used in short-term studies and is effective. Sometimes in a Phase I study searching for side effects, a subject may "cheek" the medication in order to avoid placing himself at risk of the side effects almost certain to occur as the dose increases. This can be minimized by a routine inspection of the mouth after ingestion and swallowing of the tablet. To a great extent it can be avoided if the dose is prepared in liquid form and is observed to be placed in the mouth

TABLE 23. Methods of Determining Medication Compliance in the
Research Setting

Observed ingestion with mouth inspection
Pill count
Diary of time of ingestion
Measuring blood or urine levels of agent
Measuring urine levels of inert marker placed in medication
Measuring a predictable pharmacodynamic response
Use of devices noting the time a pill is removed from package

---

followed by drinking of water. Blood levels can almost always reveal whether "cheeking" is being practiced. However, these are not available during the conduct of the study.

On rare occasions, vomiting occurs shortly after the ingestion of the dose. This may be deliberate, a side effect of the medicine, or unrelated to either. Vomiting as a side effect usually can be predicted with many medications. The vomiting usually occurs after absorption is complete, usually 30 to 120 minutes after ingestion. All subjects should be observed for about one hour after dosing, not only for safety but also to prevent induced vomiting of a dose. If an intact tablet or capsule is observed in the vomitus, another dose can be given safely. If it is partly destroyed, suggesting partial absorption, this should be recorded but the dose must not be repeated. Records should reflect which subjects are prone to vomiting to avoid their inclusion in future studies.

The pill count is the most common method of determining medication use in outpatient studies. A standard study usually provides medication sufficient for the planned interval (e.g., 14 days) plus a few extra days in case the follow-up is delayed (e.g., 3 or 4 days' extra medication for a 14-day interval). The initial bottle, sealed by the manufacturer, would contain 35 tablets when only 28 are needed for the twice-a-day schedule. The patient returns with medication bottle at each visit. In his presence it is determined that 9 tablets remain, indicating that 26 were taken in the 14 days. Thus, two doses were missed. This observation should then be discussed with the patient in a nonthreatening manner, encouraging him to do just a little better. Many sponsors will ask that a medication diary be kept detailing the date and time of administration of medication and other pertinent symptoms or events. At the time of the pill count, the diary can be compared with it and helpful hints provided. This pill count and diary review with the patient must be conducted in a matter-of-fact manner, with a warm, helpful, and grateful attitude toward the patient. Improvement, rather than the inconsistency between the protocol and the pill count, should be emphasized. Thus, complimenting the patient on his truthful reporting (e.g., "I forgot to take the medication with me on my overnight trip") rather than berating him is in order. Missed doses are a fact of life even in excellent studies. In fact, if all subjects are perfectly compliant, inspectors suspect that the data have been adjusted. Patients who persistently miss doses and cannot correct the problem should be discussed with the medical monitor to determine whether or not they should be continued.

The open discussion on the counting of the pills with the patient is highly valuable in increasing compliance. It also permits the investigative team to acquire specific information about barriers to the study ("If I take that medication on an empty stomach, I suffer cramps for several hours") that may be of interest to the manufacturer. When there are compliance problems, coordinating the ingestion of a dose with an event of the day (e.g., meals, regular TV program, or noon whistle) is helpful.

Various studies the authors have performed have used other devices or means to determine compliance. Most drugs, by the time they are under trial, have products known to appear in the urine and blood. The levels to be expected with the dosages given are known. If, for any reason, the study staff believes the patient is not taking the medication, it may be appropriate to take a blood sample or urine sample (the time of collection must be known) and request analysis by the sponsor. Prior discussion with the medical monitor will allow the team to obtain the correct specimen. The sponsor's laboratories can analyze this without informing the team which drug the patient is receiving. Their answer may indicate that there is clear evidence that the patient is not taking the medication or that there is no evidence to this effect. (A patient on placebo would not have blood levels of the drug.) Table 24 lists some reasons to suspect that a patient is failing to take his medication.

In one study in which the authors were involved, the referring physician insisted upon seeing all of his patients enrolled in a hypertension study in his office just before every study visit. This factor, combined with the nearly perfect pill counts, led to the checking of urine levels for the study agent. Obtaining urine levels enabled the research team to determine that none of the patients were on the active agent and that most were taking other agents to control their elevated blood pressure. This proved a collusion between the physician and his patients in which they received but did not ingest the new drug. Conducting these extra tests, which were not required by the protocol, enabled the team to learn of this problem and resolve it before the entire study was jeopardized.

When the likelihood of noncompliance is high, provisions can be

TABLE 24. *Reasons to Suspect Failure to Take Medication*

Precise diaries and exact pill counts by a patient who is casual about many other
    details of protocol compliance
A therapeutic response that varies from excellent to poor from visit to visit
Side effects of nausea or headaches that are intermittent
Inconsistent reporting of drug-taking behavior upon interview

---

made in the protocol design to confirm compliance. A very successful
study of disulfiram had special tablets manufactured that contained
both riboflavin and either the experimental dose or a placebo. All patients were checked for compliance by the identification of the high
levels of riboflavin in the urine.

There are also many special devices that can be employed when
compliance is an important issue. In a study of compliance in alcoholic
tuberculous patients, each dose of INH was sealed in foil and stacked
on top of another. This pile of doses was placed in a spring-loaded
device so that only the top one could be removed for ingestion. A weak
radiation source was present on one side of the device and a film strip
on the opposite side, so that the foil-covered tablets shielded the film as
long as they were present in the device. When the film was developed,
the scientists could determine within two hours as to when each dose
was removed. It was loaded each time with a one-month supply. Obviously, such devices can be costly and their use must be incorporated
into the protocol. However, their use should be considered and discussed with the sponsor in studies where a high level of noncompliance is a likely possibility, particularly when noncompliance could
jeopardize the study.

If any additional tests will be performed to determine compliance,
subjects must be informed of them when they sign the initial consent
document. If a decision is made to institute such monitoring procedures while the study is under way, the PI should consult with the
IRB to discuss whether an amendment to the consent document is in
order.

IMPROVING MEDICATION COMPLIANCE

A positive, pleasant, and thoughtful relationship between the patient and the research staff goes a long way toward ensuring compliance. Medication ingestion, whenever possible, should always be
tied to an event of the patient's day such as arising, lunchtime, or the

children's arrival home from school. In order to devise these mnemonic aids, the staff must use its knowledge of the specific patient's personal habits and life-style to formulate effective suggestions for enhancing compliance.

Medications may come in prepackaged bottles, unit dose strips, or blister packs in which each day's dose is clearly delineated. With either unit dose packaging or blister packs, the staff can facilitate compliance if necessary by marking days of the week or other useful information on the actual package. If the population under study is very forgetful or the regime is complex, plastic pill holders, in which each day of the week is marked and the time of ingestion is noted, may be obtained from health supply stores. These are useful with certain groups of subjects (e.g., in studies evaluating an agent for the elderly or severely depressed).

The staff can avoid many medication problems by a "dry run" exercise during which a staff member simulates a patient storing, opening, and ingesting the medication as required one to six times a day. The staff should be thoroughly versed in the special problems and side effects of the medicine before interacting with patients (e.g., requirement that the drug always be taken with food, anticipation of sleepiness as a side effect). Brief but clear medication instruction sheets are helpful. The staff should be aware of other household members, specifically addressing the hazard to children or pets should they get hold of the medication. A paste-on label listing the study clinic's phone number can be provided with the medicine so that the subject is encouraged to call about items about which doubt or uncertainty arises.

Instructions for patients who have unusual problems, such as working 11:00 p.m. to 7:00 a.m. or transcontinental drivers of trucks, should be clarified with the sponsor at the outset. Reminders in the form of bathroom mirror stickers, kitchen table calendars, alarm clocks, or family-initiated reminders are excellent devices for some patients. Occasionally, for a critical study, daily telephone call reminders from the staff may be necessary.

EXAMPLE 1. Penny-Wise, Pound-Foolish

An excellent investigator lost his research coordinator and did not replace her because the large study had only three months until completion. A secretary was trained to complete CRFs and the PI chose to complete the patient contact work himself. Errors in pill counts and major problems in compliance with medication appeared, such that four of the remaining six patients were dropped for noncompliance. Interviewing the patients provided some insight. The former research assistant had been so friendly and had called the patients frequently be-

tween visits. They really missed her presence and interest in them. In contrast, the physician was too rushed, could not spend time with them, and berated them for mistakes. They did not mean to harm the study but they had unintentionally lost interest in it when they were without an attentive and available caregiver. The value of a concerned assistant in enhancing compliance should never be underestimated.

ENHANCING PROCEDURE AND VISIT COMPLIANCE

Compliance with visits and procedures is readily assessed and is an important indicator of the caliber of a research team. The quality of the investigation and the reputation of its staff are judged in large part by how well they are able to motivate patients to comply with the protocol. Although compliance is easy to assess, good compliance is necessary to guarantee safety and the collection of valid data. An anticipatory approach is usually the best one and helps reduce the on-study hassles the staff and patient must face. All studies have an acceptable "window" for visits. If visits are at two-week intervals, usually it is acceptable for a patient to come in anywhere from 10 to 18 days after the previous visit (i.e., there is a 4-day window). The length of the window is largely determined by how much extra medication the patient has. Planning the study schedule with the patient's personal calendar and continually educating the patient as to why compliance is a benefit to safety and evaluation are useful.

Setting aside one or two hours of PI or staff time each week for patients to discuss issues of personal significance or concern goes a long way toward maintaining a positive relationship and reducing the likelihood that the patient will miss an appointment as a means of gaining attention. This offer of additional special time, to be used entirely at the patient's choice, is usually not needed but allows the patient to feel that the PI and staff are truly accessible should any circumstance arise. When the patient chooses to take advantage of this opportunity, an issue of deep personal significance is usually raised and thoroughly explored in an atmosphere that is less task-oriented and rushed. It is the authors' experience that very few patients use this time, even fewer abuse it, but that it is helpful to have it available.

EXAMPLE 2. Close Supervision

A group of alcoholic patients who had been dropped from a protocol studying daily disulfiram for reasons of noncompliance entered into a different type of protocol. They came to the hospital three times weekly to take their daily medication (disulfiram) in the presence of a study nurse and took it at home on the other four days. They were given two bus tokens for travel. Each week they were phoned once to remind them to collect and mail a urine sample in the next 12 hours. Containers with prepaid postage were provided. Twenty patients undertook this study. Eighteen continued for three months (the end of the study) with no missed appointments, and no urine results failing to show ingestion of disulfiram on the day sent. Only two patients were erratic in keeping appointments. Thus, a group of patients provided with reminders and convenient means of complying with the protocol adhered to a regimen that seemingly they could not accomplish on their own.

Holding group meetings of participants is another way of making patients feel special and part of the research process. These can be scheduled on a day when many subjects are attending to offer subjects the opportunity to take advantage of the social aspects of participation. Providing small thank-you's in the form of snacks in the morning, a cola or coffee if the protocol permits it, or a birthday cake for all participants to honor a subject whose birthday came on that particular day (or even week) is valuable.

The staff that helps the patient "map out" the study schedule on his own personal calendar can anticipate some of the common scheduling hassles, such as personal or staff vacations or conferences or holidays. These can then be dealt with without disrupting the protocol schedule or the patient's personal schedule too much. This planning will make it easier for the patient to be flexible in return without feeling resentful, hassled, or put upon. A patient's flexibility on scheduling matters should be amply noted, praised, and rewarded by the staff because so many scheduling problems can be quite difficult to solve. The staff may also show appreciation to the patient by making a special effort to coordinate multiple tests/procedures in a logical, efficient manner that minimizes consumption of the patient's time and efforts. The staff's thoughtful tips about a procedure also can preempt patient dissatisfaction. For example, the patient should be told beforehand that the eye doctor will dilate the pupils and that the patient may not be able to leave or drive right after the exam.

A particular quality that patients greatly appreciate is promptness. A clinic or office operation that minimizes waiting time, and that does what it says it will do promptly and courteously, builds the patient's confidence in those who care for him and enables him to plan his nonstudy time better. Patients who feel that the research staff respect their valuable time and involvement are far more likely to reciprocate by being prompt and courteous themselves. Simple amenities provided to the patient reinforce ther feelings as well. Coffee and Danish offered after an early-morning fasting procedure acknowledges the inconvenience the patient has borne and serves to ease the hassle somewhat. Such inexpensive but thoughtful gestures will not be forgotten by the patients or the staff, for that matter.

When the waiting time is expected to be longer than usual, most patients are very appreciative of being notified of the fact, of being told when the procedure can be expected to start, and of being offered an alternative of how to use their time effectively (e.g., drawing blood before the procedure rather than after, as is usually done).

For a variety of reasons, many patients enrolled in studies may be unable or unmotivated to comply with the medication or procedure requirements. A conscientious research team will make an effort to anticipate those problems that may be caused by a difficult protocol or an uncooperative subject. Where necessary, provisions should be made to monitor medication taking to preserve the validity of the study results.

Enhancing patient compliance requires the staff and PI to continue recruitment well after a patient has been enrolled in the study. Special attention to little reminders and rewards that may make it easier for a patient to comply with the rigors of the protocol go a long way toward making the on-study experience a positive one. Such efforts portray the team's attitude that the research patient is special and that his time and cooperation will not be taken for granted. The contribution of satisfied and enthusiastic subjects is essential to produce a study that favorably reflects the skills of the research team.

FURTHER READING

Eraker, S.A., Kirscht, J.P., and Becker, M.H., Understanding and improving patient compliance: A review, *Ann. Int. Med.* **100**:258–268, 1984.

Greenberg, R.N., Overview of patient compliance with medication dosing: A literature review, *Clin. Ther.* **6**:592–599, 1984.

Peto, P., Pike, M.C., Armitage, P., *et al.*, Design and analysis of randomized clinical trials requiring prolonged observation of each patient, *Br. J. Cancer* **34**:585–612, 1976.

CHAPTER 14

Adverse On-Therapy Experiences

Types of Reactions • *Necessary Data to Gather in Any Suspected Drug Reaction* • *To Break or Not to Break the Code* • *Reporting Substantive Reactions to Both the Sponsor and the IRB* • *Using Data to Evaluate an Adverse Experience* • *Documentation of Follow-Up*

When the status of health is examined minutely by periodic biochemical measurements, meticulously detailed investigations of the eye, heart, or kidney, and leisurely inquiry about symptoms, variations from the baseline or normal ranges are encountered 5 to 15% of the time. Should an intercurrent viral infection arise, extreme muscular exertion occur, or severe anxiety develop, biochemical and symptomatic abnormalities will concomitantly increase. Mild symptoms of anorexia, irritability, fatigue, altered sleep, and constipation are similarly variable and commonplace. The problem arising in any study is to ascertain which symptoms or laboratory variations may be caused by the agent under study and, therefore, may be classified as adverse drug reactions (ADRs), and which changes are from other causes. These symptoms or variations are commonly referred to as adverse on-therapy experiences (AOTEs). This chapter suggests an approach for managing adverse experiences in cases where the protocol does not provide guidelines for withdrawal of medication or evaluation of the events.

Careful clinical assessments must be supplemented with other activities essential to an effective system for managing adverse experiences. First, the research team must have a mechanism in place to collect accurate data on the adverse events. In addition, the team must report any significant adverse events promptly to the sponsor, whether or not they are thought to be drug-related. The team should also be prepared to follow subjects with adverse experiences until resolution or until a determination of etiology is made. Finally, the team should act to preserve the health and safety of the patient above all else in managing such events.

TABLE 25. *Levels of Implication of a Drug and an Adverse Event*

Level	Evidence
Almost certainly related	Rechallenge positive; typical timing and characteristics of onset and cessation
Probably related	Timing of onset and features typical; course not documented
Possibly related	Timing not typical, features suggestive of alternative diagnosis; documentation poor, history positive for similar occurrence in the past
Probably not related	Timing very atypical, behavior after drug withdrawal atypical, features without precedent for a well-studied drug
Not related	Established to be present before the study drug was given; clear alternative diagnosis established by a diagnostic test, a biopsy, or an assessment of extreme improbability

To this end, any change in symptoms or laboratory tests must be carefully correlated with an accurate history of onset of the new finding and with other symptoms and signs relating to the most likely organ and its possible diseases. The sequential course of the possible reaction over time with its relation to withdrawal or continuation of the drug is most important. If all of this is done meticulously and the randomization code to determine whether the patient was taking active agent or placebo is not broken, it is readily possible to assign the potential to five categories relating the agent to the adverse event (Table 25). These are as follows: certainly not related (unrelated), probably not related, possibly related, probably related, and almost certainly related. A possible adverse experience for which an unrelated cause is established is considered an intercurrent illness rather than an adverse experience. Finally, the real significance of the reaction can be established when the frequency of occurrence of the adverse experience is tabulated and the code is broken in order to compare the frequency of adverse experiences associated with placebo to those of the active agent.

EXAMPLE 1. *Drug Hepatitis*

A patient's blood sample in a steady state cross-over study of bioavailability indicated liver tests that were clearly elevated with AST 420 and ALT 305. Using only this information, it would be possible to conclude that a liver reaction to the drug had occurred. If the new agent were given second (in the cross-over design), it might well be implicated. Careful follow-up four days later indicated that the patient had reported a mild sore throat the day before the study ended, and on the fourth day poststudy had had mild tender lymphadenopathy. He subsequently showed a typical antibody response to the Epstein-Barr agent and had atypical monocytes on the smear of his peripheral blood, unnoticed at the termination blood but quite clear later. This episode was diagnosed as infectious mononucleosis. Follow-up indicated no relation to the drug.

TYPES OF REACTIONS

Table 26 lists representative reactions that may manifest themselves as symptoms, findings on examination, or findings in a laboratory test. Most of the time when these occur, it is initially unclear as to their severity and significance. An excellent fund of medical knowledge (or immediate access to knowledgeable consultants), which includes specific knowledge about the actual drug and similar molecules, and a constant awareness of what episodic infections are now prevalent in the community, all aid in making decisions regarding adverse experiences.

The overriding consideration in treating and evaluating an adverse event is the maintenance of the patient's health and safety. Thus, emergency reactions require prompt, appropriate therapy and usually require removal from a study. On the other hand, mild occurrences of highly significant symptoms, signs, or even laboratory tests may require further observation for clarification while the patient remains on the drug before a decision regarding continuation can be made.

EXAMPLE 2. Heart Block

A normal volunteer in a Phase I study seeking dose tolerance developed an arrhythmia that proved to be third-degree heart block. He was taken to the hospital under the care of a cardiologist with an interest in arrhythmia. Subsequent study, including bundle of His pacing, suggested that the event was clearly related to the drug under study. When approximately 100 patients had been studied, this patient proved to be the first of 3 who developed this adverse effect.

The key philosophy in evaluating any abnormality is to document its extent or magnitude, follow its course carefully over the next few days or hours, and utilize the new information gained by this addi-

TABLE 26. *Representative Types of Reactions to Assess*

Type	Classification	Examples
Emergent		Anaphylaxis, cardiopulmonary arrest, convulsion, severe bronchospasm, aspiration, syncope, serious pain, change in vision or mental state, speech change, tachyarrhythmia
New symptoms	High significance	Rashes, bleeding, severe pain, heart irregularity, inability to pass urine
	Intermediate significance	Headache, looseness of bowels, anxious feeling
	Often low significance	Constipation, mild loss of appetite, nocturia, insomnia
New signs	High significance	Arrhythmia, rash, severe agitation, lethargy, severe tenderness, fever, new tachycardia
	Intermediate significance	Mild changes in blood pressure, hepatomegaly, skin hemorrhage, syncope, mild tenderness
	Often low significance	Mild agitation, mild slowness of motion, possible hepatomegaly, possible heart murmur, apparently new
New lab test results or changes from baseline	High significance	Leukopenia, low platelets, elevated creatinine, twofold change in liver tests, hematuria, major change in coagulation
	Intermediate significance	Mid proteinuria, trivial changes in liver function tests, moderate changes in electrolytes or acid-base assessment
Changes from baseline diagnostic test results	High significance	ECG, tonometric pressure, ejection fraction of heart, electrical activity of brain
	Often low significance	Chest film, nerve conduction time, global evaluations of anxiety or restlessness

tional observation to make a decision on whether the medication should be withdrawn. Sometimes the abnormality is observed after the agent has been discontinued. Careful following of the subsequent course of the abnormality will usually permit an accurate decision as to whether or not it was related to the drug. When significant abnormalities appear, testing for organ damage in separate objective ways is beneficial for the evaluation. Thus, with new skin rashes, eosinophil counts may be helpful. With elevated urea, testing the creatinine and urinalysis are useful. With elevated alkaline phosphatase, testing the GGTP and the 5-nucleotidase is adjunctive.

EXAMPLE 3. Low Platelets

The final blood on a Phase I study of a new agent on a normal subject indicated a platelet count of 50,000. It was repeated 48 hours later and was 65,000. All other aspects of the CBC were normal but there was inadequate clot retraction. Reexamination of all previous studies on this man indicated that his entry platelets were slightly low at 140,000 and that 2 of 11 platelet counts in the past were under 100,000. Because he had been studied many times, this was attributed to poor technique, and he was allowed to enter studies. He was sent to a hematologist at the study's expense and was evaluated as an outpatient. The hematologist concluded that the patient had idiopathic thrombocytopenia, which likely bore no relation to the drug.

NECESSARY DATA TO GATHER IN ANY SUSPECTED DRUG REACTION

A meticulous history, dating by all possible means the onset of the new finding and providing all reasonably related information on other symptoms, signs, and pertinent laboratory findings, is of foremost importance. The authors have often encountered patients with recurrent skin rashes who suppress this information in order to qualify for a study and compound the difficulty of final evaluation by not promptly revealing the accurate history. Obtaining confirmation of the patient's history to evaluate a potential reaction may necessitate discussion with relatives.

When a reaction seems substantive, consultation with a colleague, if only by phone, will often alleviate the conflict of interest the investigator sometimes experiences in his desire to keep the patient under study, on the one hand, and his desire to minimize possible health risks to the patient, on the other. This consultation should be documented in the research chart. Usually someone experienced in evaluating adverse experiences can give advice on the magnitude of the risk and make the decision regarding continuation much easier. Sometimes a few additional days of observation can be safely obtained on the agent by making frequent clinical evaluations and, where appropriate, repeating the abnormal tests. Subsequent daily telephone calls to the subjects will reassure them that the PI is closely following the event.

It is important to observe what is happening to the abnormality over time, since this often will clarify the course. Usually the abnormalities are mild and the agent may be continued. If the problem clearly disappears while the agent is continued, then obviously it has no relation to the drug. Since sometimes the evaluation of a reaction is costly (e.g., a cardiologist's review is desired or a CT scan is needed), it is often possible to get the sponsoring company to agree to pay for whatever tests are needed to evaluate the reaction. Communication by telephone with the medical monitor will usually allow the investigator to secure this permission. Such a telephone call should be noted in the patient's research record, indicating the principals involved, the essential elements of the conversation, and the date.

TO BREAK OR NOT TO BREAK THE CODE

It is almost never necessary or appropriate to break the code indicating whether the patient is on placebo or active agent. The decision to discontinue an agent should be made without knowledge of whether or not the drug is active. This decision must be based upon the medical significance and severity of the abnormality. A patient with platelets of 10,000, many hemorrhages, a positive tourniquet test, and poor clot retraction needs prompt discontinuation of the agent. Although subsequent evaluation may reveal other causes, it is better to be safe than sorry when the risks are so great. On the other hand, a patient with doubling of the AST or ALT over a two-week period may be followed on the agent while additional observations are being made. Treatment of the adverse event can be undertaken in most cases without knowing the identity of the study drug. Breaking the code is necessary only when it serves a valid clinical purpose. The team's curiosity about the association of the drug with the reaction can be satisfied at a later time when their objectivity will not be affected by the information.

The only reason to break a code is when one of the agents being studied is commonly used and is needed in therapy for a life-threatening reaction for which there is no alternative drug (e.g., digoxin, phenytoin). On rare occasions, a child ingests a toxic dose of the drug and the code must be broken to identify an antidote. If the code is broken, and the agent is identified as active and available, a Med-Alert bracelet should be obtained simultaneously by the physician. These can be purchased at any pharmacy. In some 30 years of clinical investigation, the authors have broken codes for patient benefit only once or twice. It is almost always unnecessary.

EXAMPLE 4. Need to Break Code

A patient in a year-long placebo-controlled trial of a new antihypertensive agent found his three-year-old granddaughter sitting with the empty vial of experimental medicine. Though the substance was in a child-proof container, it was subsequently learned that the patient had not put the lid on tightly because he previously had difficulty in getting it open.

Within 20 minutes, the code (present in the PIs file) was broken. For-
tunately, the gentleman had been receiving the placebo. Later that day
all of the missing tablets were found alongside a chair cushion. The
patient continued in the study with the concurrence of the medical
monitor and his statistician even though the code had been broken. The
rationale for the decision was that BP readings were the only outcome
measures being utilized so the patient's knowledge that he was receiving
placebo would not significantly affect the data. Furthermore, the patient
had satisfactorily completed six months of the trial already. There can be
no question that the code needed to be broken in this circumstance.

REPORTING SUBSTANTIVE REACTIONS TO BOTH THE SPONSOR AND THE IRB

Reactions that are life-threatening or permanently disabling, or
ones that require hospitalization, prescription drug therapy, or a visit to
an emergency room are considered substantive reactions. Reactions
such as anaphylaxis, syncope with related findings of injury or prolonged unconsciousness, life-threatening changes in liver, kidney,
heart, or coagulation, convulsions, overdose, congenital anomaly, cancer, or death require a prompt telephone report to the sponsor, followed
up by a written report. Such reports are in order whether or not the
events are thought to be drug-related. To save time and effort, the same
report may be provided to the IRB. Data on any subsequent diagnostic
tests that are performed should be recorded and provided to the sponsor and the IRB to facilitate the eventual assignment of relation to the
drug.

The FDA requires a brief written report of all drug-related adverse
experiences (whether mild or major) and an assessment of their estimated relationship to the agent under study. (See FDA Form 1639,
which has been included in Appendix B.) Reports of minor adverse
experiences are taken from the CRFs when they are submitted from the
field. Reports of significant adverse events are required to be made
within 15 days of receipt of the information. These reports are usually
made by the sponsor, who has a mechanism in place for the medical
monitor's evaluation of the event and perspective on the overall incidence of the reaction.

USING DATA TO EVALUATE AN ADVERSE EXPERIENCE

The most urgent task is to assess the precise temporal relationship
between the abnormality and the adverse experience. This assumes

great importance when termination chemical examinations reveal abnormalities that were not suspected. The drug is no longer being administered, yet the creatinine, for example, rose from a baseline of 1.2 to 5.0 following the study. It is urgent to double-check this result to determine whether it is real and associated with other evidence of loss of glomerular function (BUN elevation, elevated uric acid, possible retention of phosphate, change in pH, or change in urinalysis). If confirmed to be abnormal, the reaction should be followed to resolution. This is part of the responsibility of the PI and is one of the factors that distinguishes a well-done study from a poorly done one. If other pertinent tests are needed (e.g., markers of lupus, glomerulonephritis), they should be carried out to assist in the evaluation.

EXAMPLE 5. Retinal Damage

A patient taking disulfiram for alcoholism was doing quite well in a multidisciplinary program. He sought a referral two months into disulfiram therapy to an ophthalmologist for a change in glasses and was pleased with the new lens. Three months later he sought another appointment. At this time, the ophthalmologist noted a substantial deterioration of vision from 20/40 corrected to 20/100 corrected and suggested a toxic reaction. Reluctantly, the responsible physician discontinued the disulfiram. In 60 days, the vision had returned to a level better than the baseline measurement and the patient no longer needed glasses. Neuritis, eye damage to optic nerve or cataracts, and behavior difficulties are frequently overlooked side effects of medications. These changes develop in prolonged protocols or are seen in Phase IV or postmarketing studies. This adverse experience was clearly related to the disulfiram.

EXAMPLE 6. Lab Problem

The bloods in 7 of 24 subjects in a Phase I open-label study showed an elevated creatinine immediately after the agent. Since the urea and other kidney studies were normal, an interference with the test for creatinine was suspected. The parent compound did not influence the colorimetric test but the principal metabolite did. The sponsor collaborated in showing this effect, which subsequently helped many investigators.

EXAMPLE 7. Heart Block

A patient with chronic diarrhea obtained unique and total relief with a new agent while participating in a protocol and was provided drug for the next two years in a compassionate protocol while the agent continued under evaluation. One of his six monthly ECGs showed first-degree heart block. Review of his entire file indicated at least one pre-

vious instance of prolonged P-R interval to 0.26 but this was not observed in the reading. Subsequently, the interval returned to 0.21. Evaluation by a cardiologist indicated an abnormality, probably of a long-standing nature. This abnormality was present on and off the drug. The patient was subsequently given permission to continue on the drug and chose to do so. The evaluation, in this instance, clarified a complex situation and allowed a solution that seemed both safe and appropriate.

The maintenance of the blind is of great value for it allows the sponsor to assess objectively whether or not the reaction occurred more frequently on the active agent than on the placebo. A PI should not hesitate to consult with the medical monitor, consultants, and the chairman of the responsible IRB to discuss some of these possible adverse reactions. The final assessment of the relationship of the adverse event to the study drug should be noted in the patient's record.

DOCUMENTATION OF FOLLOW-UP

Some subjects seem to disappear from the face of the earth after the study is over. This poses a problem because then laboratory studies collected at the final visit, which do not become available until one or two days later, cannot be discussed with them. When it is consistent with the protocol, these blood tests sometimes may be obtained 12 hours earlier so the results will be available at the final interview. The chapter on referral discusses other means of following up research subjects. There are many devices that can be used to encourage compliance with follow-up. For example, obtaining the name of the physician to whom results should be mailed, withholding a portion of payment until after the final test results are returned, or scheduling a final debriefing are all devices that improve the availability of follow-up of any abnormalities that may occur.

If there are substantial abnormalities, the research record should document all efforts made to phone or contact the subject. A letter should be written about the abnormality, including an offer to repeat the lab tests without charge or to send the results to another physician should the patient so desire. Should all of these fail, the PI may give up trying to locate the patient, but a clear record of this effort should be entered in the patient's research chart.

This chapter suggests a methodology for evaluating the severity of an adverse experience and assessing the need to discontinue study medication. This methodology is meant to be used as a tool to assist the investigator in cases where the protocol does not clearly specify the conditions under which the study drug must be withdrawn. Whatever the nature and cause of the event, it is essential to keep in mind that prompt treatment of the adverse experience must remain the first priority. Once the individual patient has been stabilized, the sponsor should be contacted immediately with a report of the event and the patient's status. The PI should continue to report follow-up information to the sponsor until the event has successfully been resolved. Rarely does this clinical treatment require knowledge of which study medication the subject was receiving. Furthermore, although an assessment of the relationship of the event to the study drug is of value in deciding whether the subject should continue therapy, it should not influence the investigator's decision to report the event. Adverse experiences that are serious and unexpected should be reported promptly to the sponsor regardless of their cause.

CHAPTER 15

The Referral Process

Types of Patients • Barriers to Referral • Ways of Lowering Barriers to an Effective Referral Process • Preparation • Completion Rituals

Referrals to other physicians or locations of care are an everyday and necessary occurrence in an active research practice. Some reasons necessitating these referrals are listed in Table 27 and, therefore, need to be discussed no further with the exception of the final item. Patients, regardless of the reason for referral, fall into five different groups. Each category listed in Table 28 is different in terms of the duration of the relationship with the research team, the patient's level of expectation, and the investigator's level of responsibility to the patient and the protocol. Regardless of which group the patient falls in, he needs to be aware of the differences between the private medical care and clinical research care relationships. The latter is highly structured by the protocol, is very selective, is limited in the scope of care provided, requires more documentation, and is finite. An adequate referral process takes these differences into account. The success of this process can be measured in terms of patient satisfaction, a good image projected in the medical and lay communities, increases in the number of word-of-mouth referrals from both rejected and completed study candidates, as well as good staff morale and self-esteem.

This chapter discusses each group, suggesting ways to enhance the success of the referral process and reduce barriers to effectiveness.

TYPES OF PATIENTS

GROUP 1: PATIENTS REJECTED AFTER MINIMAL SCREENING BECAUSE OF INELIGIBILITY. Patients referred by a physician or responding to advertisements will be screened for basic eligibility and many will be

TABLE 27. *Reasons That May Necessitate Referral of Subjects to Other Physicians, Clinics, or Sites of Care*

The principal mission of the research team is not general or private medical care. While the staff is prepared to deal with medical issues beyond the scope of a particular study, the staff's primary focus is the completion of high-quality research and its documentation. Matters not relevant to the study may require referral to outside providers when:
The investigator's capabilities, interests, and training are not suited to the particular needs of the patient's condition.
The capacity of the investigator's practice to take on new private patients is limited.
The financial viability of the investigator's practice to take on new private patients is limited.
"Arm's length" care is necessary to avoid the appearance of a conflict of interest or of an attempt to suppress or "cover up" untoward consequences of the investigator's decisions.

rejected after one or two critical facts have been elicited. The trained staff is prepared to deal with these patients who obviously have some problem and are expecting something from the investigator. The patients will react positively to the rejection if it is done with sensitivity, pleasantness, and a general referral back to the patient's private doctor or to any of the physicians or clinics approved by the investigator. Such a list should be prepared by an experienced staff member prior to initiation of recruitment, with careful review by the investigator. Because the investigator and staff have little or no involvement with the patient at this stage, the investigator's medicolegal and ethical responsibility is to provide the patient with a positive encounter, a general referral, and a brief explanation of why the patient's participation in the study is not possible. Some patients desire a little more and may feel the rejection is a personal one. A restatement by the staff or physician of the criteria for entry and its safety rationale will usually suffice. Rarely does this type of patient request to talk directly with the investigator. For this group of patients, elaborate follow-up systems to ensure compliance with follow-up are not necessary and usually are not feasible.

GROUP 2: PATIENTS FULLY SCREENED BUT REJECTED FOR PARTICIPATION. Problems uncovered as a result of the screening process may sometimes emerge. The investigator has the responsibility to each screened patient, regardless of the patient's potential as a future study candidate, to ensure continued care of chronic conditions and appropriate care of newly identified ones. The conscientious investigator

TABLE 28. Types of Patients Requiring Referral

Group	Description	Duration of relationship	Patient's expectations	Investigator's level of responsibility			Example
				To patient	To protocol	To referral physician	
1	Rejected after minimal screening	Very brief	Very low	General referral obligation	None	None	Exclusion due to age, sex, or use of prohibited medication
2	Fully screened but rejected	Short (days)	Low	Specific referral necessary	Maintenance of exclusion statistics; no follow-up documentation necessary	Letter or staff call	Patient found to have gastric cancer on screening endoscopy needs a specific referral for follow-up care
3	Dropped from study prior to completion	Short to long	High	Specific referral necessary; complex nature of relationship between study and referral physicians must be clarified	Follow-up documentation necessary; relationship between adverse event and study drug must be assessed	Telephone call to clarify who makes the decision regarding the relationship between the study drug and the adverse event	Adverse event necessitating discontinuation from the study

(continued)

TABLE 28 (Continued)

Group	Description	Duration of relationship	Patient's expectations	Investigator's level of responsibility			Example
				To patient	To protocol	To referral physician	
4	Requiring treatment for intercurrent illness	Long	High	Specific referral necessary; PI obliged to discuss financial issues	Follow-up documentation necessary	Telephone call to outline rationale for continuing study medication in light of adverse event	Patient with a skin rash determined to be related to study medication requiring care and follow-up
5	Completed	Long	High	Specific referral necessary	Follow-up documentation necessary	Letter with referral documents, including baseline and follow-up status	Patient completing a hypertension study requires a specific referral to an internist

will feel this responsibility, especially in regard to those patients with newly diagnosed problems, and will want to notify the primary physician of the findings directly by phone or by a standard letter. A standard letter stored on a word processor can greatly simplify the process and facilitate timely communication with the patient's physician.

EXAMPLE 1. Urgent Referral

A 44-year-old woman presented for endoscopic screening for an ulcer study. The endoscopist saw a cancer. Biopsies confirmed this disease, making her ineligible for study. She had no regular physician. After discussion with the PI, a surgeon at a hospital in which she had confidence was selected. An appointment was made. The biopsy and endoscopy reports were in the surgeon's hands at the time of the appointment and appropriate surgery was conducted within nine days of the initial endoscopy. The patient was pleased with the surgery and the prompt referral.

Permanently rejected patients who have a full screening done that produces much baseline information usually will be pleased when these results are offered to their regular physician. The disappointment of rejection from the study can be lessened by particular attention to this detail. This will cement the referral back to the patient's physician and will enhance the relationship involving the investigator, the patient, and the medical community at large.

The effective, efficient investigator will handle temporarily rejected, fully screened patients in a different manner. Patients with chronic or newly diagnosed medical problems should be cared for outside the context of the research team. The genuine referral of these patients to more appropriate caregivers who have been oriented to the study purpose and objective and who are on a good working basis with the investigator should be undertaken first. Once the problem has been clarified and stabilized, the team may reconsider the patient for participation in the study. This "holding" arrangement sometimes can be worked out with the patient's private physician if the investigator is careful to involve the private physician in the process.

EXAMPLE 2. Reasonable Action

A 38-year-old engineer with rheumatoid arthritis wished to join a study. At screening, his temperature was 101° F and there was a large boil in the right axilla unrelated to his arthritis. In all respects he qualified, but his WBC was 14,800 and his ESR was 44. He was referred to a local family

*medical office within the neighborhood and was accompanied there with
our records (after a phone call). The boil was incised, he was seen by that
office one week later, and he returned that same day for repeat WBC and
ESR. He qualified and entered the study a few days later.*

An effective recruitment process produces many candidates and
affords the luxury of choosing the best participants. Flexible referral
relationships that allow the temporary exclusion of "marginal" study
candidates with newly diagnosed or unstable medical problems will
enable the investigator to meet the study enrollment objectives without
compromising patient safety or overspending the budget allowance.

The patient's cooperation often is best obtained by telling him why
he is not quite suitable for the study, what is necessary to make him
suitable, and how the finances of the care will be handled. The patient's inability to pay is often the reason why this type of referral does
not succeed. The investigator is wise to acknowledge in advance to the
physician accepting the care of the patient that this is of concern and,
where feasible, to refer the patient to a facility prepared to provide
services to lower-income groups. Alternatively, recruitment of qualified patients is sufficiently valuable in some studies that payment for
the care is sometimes undertaken.

GROUP 3: PATIENTS DROPPED FROM THE STUDY PRIOR TO COMPLE-
TION. The informed consent process makes each patient entered into
the study aware of the permissibility and possibility of his dropping or
being dropped from the study prior to its completion. The investigator
must be actively involved in the referral and tracking of subsequent
care of these patients because they have received the investigational
therapy under his supervision. Referrals for dropouts with adverse
events require special attention and care for this reason. The investigator and the patient must have a clear understanding of the level of care
needed, the level of documentation needed, the manner in which the
care will be paid, as well as the time involved. The physician best
suited to provide care under these circumstances and how the control
of information flow will be managed are matters that require consideration at this point also. The patient experiencing an adverse event will
need to be provided with the rationale for choosing a specialist to care
for him (rather than his own physician if he has one). The investigator
must be prepared to go over this with the patient and to discuss with
the referral physician the special care and documentation requirements
as well as the financial arrangements for this care.

This type of difficult referral is made easier if the investigator has a

clear idea of the sponsor's policy regarding reimbursement for the treatment of drug-related adverse events and for the evaluation of events
possibly related to the treatment. The investigator must be careful not
to give the physician or the patient the impression that the sponsor's
reimbursement policy is open-ended, carefully explaining that it is
meant to provide the evaluation and short-term treatment of an adverse
event. The investigator is responsible for the control of this process and
must make the issues clear to both the patient and the referral physician. The determination of whether an adverse event is drug-related or
simply an intercurrent illness based on the referral physician's evaluation and studied opinion is for the investigator to make. This means
that the referral physician must communicate directly with the investigator regarding this matter and must understand that it is the investigator's responsibility to communicate these results or opinions to the
patient. If a suspected adverse event is determined to be an intercurrent
illness with no relation to the study, the investigator must inform both
the patient and the consultant that the patient should receive any further treatment required as a private patient. Thus, the patient may make
arrangements directly with the consulting physician to provide the
additional care.

As is evident from this discussion, the selection of a referral physician by the investigator is critical. Haphazard referral of this type of
complicated patient to physicians unfamiliar with research care problems will result in much worry and hassle for the investigator. A poor
choice also exposes the study to an increased risk of poor documentation, disgruntled patients, and a poor image in the medical community.

EXAMPLE 3. Itch and Rash

*A patient in a trial of a new cephalosporin for urinary tract infection
developed severe localized pruritis and rash during the second week of a
21-day study. The lesions seemed typical of pityriasis rosea but the patient was highly concerned about continuing the drug. A referral to a
dermatologist known to test drugs frequently confirmed this diagnosis
and reassured the patient to continue the antibiotic and complete the
study. A formal report, including the biopsy, was sent to the investigator.
The dermatologist's bill was paid by the sponsor.*

GROUP 4: PATIENTS WITH INTERCURRENT ILLNESS. This type of patient requires a referral process similar to that of the above group. The
additional feature is that the referral physician and the patient must
participate with the investigator regarding the decision to continue in
the study. The decision to continue in light of an unrelated illness is a

difficult one that must be made by the investigator and consented to by the patient in light of the consulting physician's findings. The referral physician and the investigator must have a clear understanding of their respective roles. The successful development of this complex relationship between the investigator and the referral physician requires direct and careful communication, most easily accomplished in person, but feasible by telephone. Follow-up of the referral by hand or mail delivery of key documents is needed. Because the initial decision to continue the patient in the study may be made with limited information, the referral physician must be sensitive to the need for timely evaluation and rendering of an opinion. Although continuing written documentation is essential for the research record, this usually is too slow for effective communication. Thus, it is customary for the consultant to communicate his opinion by telephone as promptly as possible. Referral physicians unable to offer these services in a timely or consistent manner should not be utilized.

The obligation to inform the patient of the determination regarding whether the adverse event is drug-related or an intercurrent illness is solely the investigator's. If the investigator feels that the adverse event is an unrelated illness, it is up to him to inform the patient that the subsequent care rendered by the referral physician is the patient's financial obligation. The investigator must inform the referral physician of this fact as well. The referral physician will then be aware that he should expect payment directly from the patient or a private insurer. An investigator who executes this function smoothly and matter-of-factly ensures that the relationship between the referral physician and the patient will be grounded in the usual assumptions and expectations of private medical care. If it is not done well, the misunderstanding between the patient and the referral physician will jeopardize the relationship and cause resentment toward the investigator by both the patient and the referral physician.

GROUP 5: PATIENTS COMPLETING THE STUDY. Since nearly all patients completing study will need referral, the remainder of the chapter will deal with some of the issues common to this group. These issues also may be relevant to the other categories of patients discussed previously. The reader should readily see the applicability of this section to all referrals despite its focus on patients completing the study.

BARRIERS TO REFERRAL

PATIENT KNOWLEDGE/AWARENESS. Often a patient is not aware of the limited context of the research care and may fail to see the rationale for the referral. With these patients, it is often helpful to review how clinical research and private medical care differ.

The purpose of the research team is to provide a limited part of the patient's care, the part related to the specific research protocol. The team's responsibilities require a different orientation, different record-keeping procedures, and perhaps even different facilities from those used for routine practice. Individualized care for conditions other than those of the research cannot be delivered by the research team. It is the investigator's job to ensure that the patient has access to physicians or clinics to provide the nonresearch-related care. There may be barriers to meeting this obligation. The patient may not understand the necessity of division of research and unrelated medical care for the following reasons:

1. It may not be made clear to him by the staff during the consent process.
2. The patient may feel he has a single problem that is cared for entirely within the protocol context.
3. The patient may see the difference but prefers to ignore it for financial reasons. The private medical care is an expense the patient may not want to face.
4. The PI and staff may have blurred the distinction during the study to simplify evaluations and retain the patient.

PATIENT FEELINGS ABOUT REFERRAL. Some study patients develop intense negative feelings at the prospect of having the investigator refer them to another physician at the end of the study. These may be expressed in various ways (Table 29). Each of these feelings can impede the effective transfer of care and may even interfere with compliance in the latter part of the study. Verbal patients will express these feelings directly, alerting the experienced staff to their existence. Other patients may be less in touch with their feelings. Clues to these feelings may be found in noncompliance at the end of the study or in the late appearance of vague new complaints about the study drug. Patients' inquiries about getting the study drug for long-term use just for themselves (e.g., compassionate use exemptions, requests for just one more visit, lab test, or procedure "just to make sure" or for "just one prescription to get started before I see my new doctor") may occur frequently. Such requests are good clues that the patient needs some time to discuss his feelings.

EXAMPLE 4. Confused and Inadequate Referral

An unemployed hypertensive subject was enrolled in a one-year study of efficacy of a new agent, was well controlled, kept his appointments regu-

TABLE 29. *Negative Feelings a Patient May Experience about the Prospect of Being Referred*

Dependency—separation anxiety

Abandonment—"My problem was so special that I was picked to be in the study. Now it's over and they aren't going to care for me."

Worthlessness—"Now that they have gotten what they wanted and the study is over, I'm being discarded. I'm not special anymore."

Grief—loss of significant support and nurturing by the staff

Financial anxiety—"How will I pay for a private doctor?"

Concern about long-term side effects—"Will they occur and how will my new doctor know anything about the study medication and its potential side effects if anything happens 20 years from now?"

Fear of disease recurrence or progression—"I'm sure the study drug helped me. What will I do without it?"

---

larly, and seemed compliant. He had a flare-up of psoriasis, was given samples of topical agents that helped the skin condition, and so did not see another physician. Later the patient came in for unscheduled visits for a severe chest cold and diarrhea. Each time he was very pleasant and wanted to be sure that he did nothing to interfere with the protocol study. Because he could not comfortably afford a private doctor, he received care on each of these occasions. As the end of his study approached, his visits for extra things increased more and more, for the study had made him very dependent. When his study ended, he did not cooperate at all in getting a new doctor to treat his hypertension and continued to come back to the clinic staff. The referral process for this patient was handled very poorly.

INVESTIGATOR/STAFF-RELATED ISSUES. Just as the patient has concerns that may block effective referral, so may the investigator or his staff. The research personnel may wish to provide ongoing care for patients who have been involved in studies in the hope that patients will enter future protocols. While the incentives are great to "recycle" patients or to maintain patients in a "pool" or "stable," the desire to do so must be tempered by several important concerns. Is the patient truly receiving optimal continuing care between studies? Experienced investigators not infrequently encounter sophisticated patients who through unsupervised, suboptimal self-medicated regimens maintain their disease condition to enhance the likelihood of their future participation. Chronic conditions like hypertension, arthritis, depression, and duodenal ulcer disease are subject to this kind of problem. These patients, although readily available to the clinical researcher, are often poorly compliant with the study medication because successful control of their disease leads to eventual termination. The investigator must guide and encourage patients to seek appropriate long-term care and control of their condition, rather than ignore or subtly encourage this dangerous practice.

The staff may avoid the patient's negative feelings for a variety of reasons. The most common is the staff's feeling of helplessness or anger in the face of the patient's anxieties. Staff members may feel that the patient's financial problems are unsolvable, that they cannot control whether or not long-term side effects occur or whether the new doctor will treat the patient as well as they did. The staff may feel guilty or ambivalent about using, hurting, or inconveniencing a research subject. This guilt makes it hard for the staff to face the patient's feelings of abandonment or worthlessness. Certain staff members may also enjoy feeling needed by a dependent patient. Each of these staff reactions is a liability for the referral process. Some investigators believe that only they can provide the appropriate care and attempt to continue treating the patient after his study participation has ended. If a patient has had an adverse reaction, the investigator may be reluctant to refer him to another physician's care because he does not want to have to answer the accepting physician's inquiries regarding the event.

Some experienced investigators assume the private medical care of their past research subjects. This produces many problems, though none are insurmountable. On the positive side, the investigator already knows the patient, the responsiveness of his disease to treatment, and his experience with at least one drug. Poststudy follow-up visits are often needed to evaluate any late side effects. These can be followed more easily if the subject is a patient in the PI's practice. On the negative side, the investigator who accepts the patient reluctantly because the patient cannot face the discontinuation of the relationship will be poorly motivated to provide the subject's long-term care. The transition from research to private patient status often requires the patient to be seen in a different location and with a different staff. Although such a change is evidence that the research care relationship has shifted to a private care one, confusion over billing and collections may occur, nevertheless. The investigator who does not refer patients back to their original providers may appear to be in competition with his colleagues in the community. Such a perception could have a negative impact on future referrals to the study, since it is difficult to sustain the view that the PI is not stealing patients. Finally, the influx of new study patients into the private practice subtly changes the character of the private practice in ways that may prove undesirable. These new patients may overload the investigator and staff to the point that they have no time to devote to research activities.

EXAMPLE 5. Smooth Referral

Ms. H answered a radio advertisement for patients with ulcers and healed her disease promptly while on the protocol. She had never had a
regular physician and asked if she could become a patient of the study
doctors. The endoscopist accepted private patients, but she needed a
more general doctor. After some discussion, she chose a female internist
with an office near her place of employment and was sent to her newly
chosen doctor with a letter of referral. Her endoscopy reports, laboratory
evaluation, and physical examinations were included. We talked with
her by phone about three weeks after the study with us had ended and
found that she had met with her new doctor and was delighted.

WAYS OF LOWERING BARRIERS TO AN EFFECTIVE REFERRAL PROCESS

Effective referral occurs daily despite the many barriers. Yet there
are a number of things that make the process easier, less hassle-prone,
and more beneficial for staff and patients. A clear understanding must
be reached between the PI and the patient as to what level of care is
needed and the role in the subsequent follow-up of the physician who
originally referred him to the study. Unless the PI has unique qualifications, recognized throughout his community for treatment of the patient's condition, referral should always be undertaken. Table 30 indicates some actions that can be taken to make this transition easier.

PREPARATION

The staff can be helped immeasurably by the preparation of the
investigator's acceptable referral list. A staff member can prepare for

TABLE 30. Ways of Reducing the Hassles of the Referral Process

---

Preparation
  Staff preparation
  Individual patient preparation
Completion rituals
  Certificate of participation
  Final payment
  Debriefing sessions
  Poststudy follow-up visit or call
  Referral papers
Formation of peer groups, buddy systems
Encouragement of friendly contacts, not medical ones

---

the PI's review a list of physicians and clinics and the types of patients they accept. Often consultants who have been recruited to perform routine study procedures can offer assistance in this regard. If the team expects to refer a large number of patients to particular physicians or clinics, the PI can contact those offices to describe the team's program before beginning to refer subjects. An uncomplicated referral then can be handled by the research secretary and the accepting physician's secretary with a form letter and a call indicating that the patient will be calling for an appointment. The patient must not be ignored in this process and should always make the call for the appointment himself. Patients are far less likely to honor appointments made by the staff on their behalf. "Paving the way" makes it easy for the patient to carry on for himself. The investigator must prepare the staff for the emotional reaction that they and their patients may experience. The investigator should also provide the staff with a rationale and an information base for the referral, so that the staff can pass it on to the patient.

Nowadays most practices or clinics have descriptive pamphlets that detail their fee schedules, hours, emergency coverage, hospital affiliation, and similar items. Having these on hand is a great help to a patient. The individual patient must be prepared for referral from the onset of the study. Patients with a regular doctor should be identified and approached with the thought that they will return to this doctor's care. The other patients, from the start of the study, should be asked to think about their referral preferences, and at each visit some attention should be paid to this process. For example, the staff could introduce the idea as follows: "I know that you have just entered the study and will be under our care for your study problem. However, for other problems that may occur which are unrelated to the study, you might think about whom you would like to care for your problems. We are familiar with many physicians and clinics in the area and can help you choose one after you have thought about your preferences." Statements like these prepare the patient for subsequent discussions at a later date. The patient's requests for appointments and prescriptions for unrelated illnesses are best addressed early on and prior to the end of the protocol.

COMPLETION RITUALS

The rituals that finalize a study, once established and practiced by the staff, give a sense of completion and worth to the patient as well as make it crystal clear that he must now get his care elsewhere. The rituals represent opportunities for the staff and patient to deal with the anxieties and feelings outlined already and greatly facilitate the referral process.

The final presentation of a certificate of participation is a way of showing finality, combined with appreciation, to the patient. It also gives the patient "something to show" for his effort and involvement. An investment of $2 to $5 for a nicely printed certificate is well worthwhile.

The manner in which the final study payment is paid can be important as well. Its prompt, personal, hand-to-hand presentation, with a few words about the payment process being only a token and a fraction of what the patient really deserves, helps bolster the patient's sense of worth in the special context of the research process. Emphasizing that this is the last payment helps set a tone of finality to the procedure.

Debriefing and poststudy follow-up evaluation visits or calls can be used quite effectively with a minimum of effort or time. Many patients may decline the offer of a brief visit "just to chat" but usually are genuinely surprised and quite talkative when they are called for a brief telephone follow-up. This telephone exchange gives the patient time to reflect on his feelings and to have any lingering concerns or questions answered. The call also serves as a way of checking if the patient did in fact keep his follow-up appointment with his new doctor. If not, further support and encouragement can be offered at this time.

Finally, there are referral papers. These may include a copy of a simple summary letter from the investigator sent to the accepting physician, a copy of lab or ECG reports, or patient education and self-care pamphlets. They serve to personalize the referral process and the staff's commitment to help the patient get good follow-up care. Once again, the patient is given something in black and white to show for his involvement.

SECTION VI
Data Management

This logical and simplified approach to research record keeping allows new investigators and their staffs to produce superior studies that surpass all regulatory requirements. Since proper documentation is essential to all aspects of the research enterprise, this section contains a special introduction to topics such as confidentiality and recording techniques applicable to all aspects of documentation.

CHAPTER 16

Principles of Data Management

Principles of Data Recording • *Planning for Confidentiality*

The decision to participate in pharmaceutical research imposes regulatory responsibilities to document all clinical and administrative activities pertaining to a study. Appropriate arrangements also must be made to ensure the confidentiality of records and their long-term availability to regulatory agencies. Although these record-keeping requirements are rather extensive, methods can easily be devised to streamline data collection and recording so these administrative activities do not prove burdensome. The chapters that follow describe efficient systems for documenting clinical activities and regulatory communication. These methods provide audit points and quality assurance controls that are essential in any research operation.

A research record system has four components. These are the scheduling logs, the research chart (as distinguished from the routine medical chart), the case report form (CRF), and the regulatory file. The completion of all of these records may be aided by using study checklists that offer reminders of protocol visit schedules and record-keeping requirements. Scheduling logs are similar to routine appointment books, which already are kept in most facilities. These meet the dual purpose of providing an outline of all patient activity and a mechanism for verifying timely receipt of study-related test results.

Patient-specific research records fall into two broad categories: the research chart, accompanied by any checklists used to facilitate data collection, and the CRF. Both are described by the proposed FDA regulations (21 CRF Part 54). The research chart constitutes a patient's medical record of the events leading to, during, and immediately following his participation in a protocol. Notes of visits, copies of consultants' reports, and notes of telephone conversations with the patient and the sponsor are retained in this record. It is from these documents that the CRF data are extracted. The research chart should always contain more information than is required on the CRF and should be re-tained at all times by the investigative team. Research charts should be generated for patients who are screened and disqualified from par-ticipating in a specific protocol as well as for those who actually are enrolled in a study. If a patient is involved in a study at the facility at which he receives his medical care, copies of clinically relevant re-search documents should be included in his medical chart.

The purpose of the CRF differs substantially from that of the re-search chart. The CRF, which is routinely developed by the study spon-sor, is designed to collect safety and efficacy data that the sponsor has deemed necessary to document the routine details of a subject's ex-posure to the test medication. It is not meant as a substitute for the more comprehensive research chart, which the sponsor expects to have available to provide any additional details needed to evaluate specific clinical events.

The administrative counterpart to the research chart is the reg-ulatory file, in which all general study correspondence with the spon-sor and the IRB is retained. This file provides a chronology of the course of the study and includes such documents as a list of the person-nel involved in the research and all versions of the protocol and amendments. FDA 1572/3 forms and related regulatory documents should be stored here, along with copies of all correspondence with the Institutional Review Board.

PRINCIPLES OF DATA RECORDING

All study records constitute regulatory documents that must be created according to established principles of data recording. The prin-ciples of data management dictate that any records created must be difficult to alter and easily verifiable by inspection of supporting docu-ments or, rarely, by subject interviews. The principles of data manage-ment have been outlined in Table 31.

PLANNING FOR CONFIDENTIALITY

CONFIDENTIALITY OF SUBJECTS' RECORDS. Subjects participating in a clinical investigation should be offered reasonable assurance of confi-dentiality appropriate to the sensitivity of the data being collected. It has long been customary to devote greater attention to the preservation of confidentiality of research data than to that of medical records or other charts developed in routine practice. This practice evolved

TABLE 31. Principles of Data Recording

Use black ink. All entries must be legible and in black ink to provide a permanent record of each transaction.

Sign every entry. All entries on a study document must be signed at the time that they are made.

Make no erasures. Erasures and correction fluid should not be used. The erroneous information must be crossed out, the new entry made, and the change initialed.

Resolve or explain all inconsistencies noted in the record. A note of explanation must be included before dismissing as inaccurate any clinically relevant information noted in a chart or log (e.g., a patient's poorly recalled history of previous surgery that is not substantiated in records obtained from the treating practitioner).

Note any omissions. Omitted data should be entered in the next available space with an explanation of the lateness of the entry. A comment is in order on very late entries (those discovered more than 1 to 2 weeks after the event) in the research chart as well.

Leave no blank spaces. All blank spaces or sections of a log should have a line drawn through them once the date passes. Weekend and holiday dates should be included on any calendars with a note as to whether any activities took place. At the close of the workday, record the next day's date on any log pages, leaving no blank spaces.

Sign documents cautiously. No research document should be signed unless it accurately reflects the clinical situation described. A blank CRF or chart document must never be signed. The date of the signature should reflect the date on which the record was reviewed.

Use bound logs wherever possible.

---

largely owing to the influence of IRBs, who express the view that patients participating in research activities are asked to accept many risks and inconveniences. Unnecessary dissemination of medical history or research data represents an inconvenience to which subjects need not be subjected. The extent to which access to the records can feasibly be limited must be discussed as part of the consent process, and any assurances provided during that negotiation must be honored by the research team.

Careful planning undertaken as the study is getting under way can reduce the risk of accidental or unnecessary disclosure of sensitive medical data. Possible methods of organizing and labeling research records to preserve the subjects' privacy are as follows:

1. Codes such as patients' initials or an abbreviated combination of their first and last names should be used when writing chart notes or CRF data. A key linking these codes to the patients' names and medical record numbers can then be maintained separately in the event that it is necessary to retrieve the patients' complete medical records in the future. A numerical

    code should also be established and used consistently with the initials, particularly if patients' initials are used to refer to them.

2. A research code number should be assigned in addition to initials as a means of identifying subjects. In most cases, sponsors provide CRFs that are prenumbered with codes that can be employed for this purpose. The drug code is not a sufficient numerical reference since some studies involve washout or other screening periods in which the patients are considered enrolled but have not yet received coded medication.

3. When appropriate, research records may be maintained separately from the subjects' medical records. These should contain source data for all evaluations required as part of the protocol and would be the only records to which regulatory agencies or sponsors would have access in the event of a routine inspection.

The use of codes on documents such as laboratory reports is not recommended as routine practice. Laboratory reports contain little subjective data and so closely resemble one another that they can easily be mislabeled or misfiled if too few identifiers are used. Since these reports are commonly screened independent of the subjects' complete charts, it is best to minimize possible errors of misinterpretation by leaving subjects' names on these documents. Laboratory reports also are routinely sent to other providers and will be accepted more readily with appropriate identifying information. Investigators desiring to preserve subjects' confidentiality in the event of an inspection may wish to consider providing copies of these reports labeled only with the patients' initials and code numbers.

    Although some CRFs request identifying information such as medical record numbers, the sponsor is not required to have access to these and should not, in fact be provided with them on the CRF. It is becoming increasingly common for sponsors to requires that a confidential follow-up form be completed on each of the subjects who enter the study in the event that new toxicity information becomes available at a later date, which necessitates notifying them. Before agreeing to such a request, however, the investigator should ascertain from the sponsor how these records will be stored so the subjects can be made aware of any potential risks posed by submission of these data. Sponsors who collect such data should have separate, locked storage facilities available with some standard operating procedure describing the corporate authorizations required to retrieve these and the circumstances under which such access would be required. These forms should be stored in sealed envelopes apart from the CRF files. If the data being collected are somewhat sensitive (e.g., a study of venereal disease), the investigator should perhaps confer with his IRB and sponsor regarding the extent of the risks posed by such a requirement. Alternative arrangements, such as storage of the envelopes with the IRB or the investigator, may be permitted in such circumstances.

Whatever the special precautions taken to preserve the subjects' confidentiality, it is customary to eliminate identifiers from all data used in reporting or presenting the results of an investigation. The term *identifier* refers not only to patients' names and addresses but also to medical record numbers, Social Security numbers, or other uniquely assigned codes that would allow the patients' names to be easily linked with their research records.

As in the medical practice setting, some caution should be employed in responding to telephone queries from the sponsor or subjects' relatives. In a pharmaceutical firm, procedures for collecting safety data by telephone are well established and usually involve only the medical monitor or the CRA. Calls from other employees with whom the team is not familiar should be screened carefully, both to preserve confidentiality and to guarantee that the information being provided will flow through the proper channels. When in doubt as to whether a request is appropriate, the employee to whom it was directed should take a message and check with the PI before releasing any information. A similar procedure is in order for responding to telephone requests from patients' or their families. In studies where sensitive data are involved, an employee can easily verify the patient's identity over the telephone by asking him study-specific questions, such as whom he saw at his last visit, or his drug code assignment. The appropriateness of a family member's request for routine information can best be judged from what is known about the patient and his personal situation. Sensitive data are best reported only to the patient unless he has specifically granted permission for a relative to obtain the results on his behalf. It is always desirable to call the inquiring party back with the information, since this offers an opportunity to verify his identity.

CONFIDENTIALITY OF PROTOCOL AND RELATED DOCUMENTS. The same planning undertaken for preservation of subjects' confidentiality also applies to the many reports and documents received from the sponsor. The protocols, CRFs, investigational use circulars, and other study-related materials distributed by the sponsor are considered trade secrets and should be stored in a way that does not permit access by competitive firms or unauthorized employees. Facilities at which multiple studies are being conducted should contain an area for sponsor use that is free of posted confidential materials such as protocols or study flow sheets. Drug supply cabinets or files containing records of studies conducted for other firms should be locked or arrangements must be made to supervise sponsor personnel during their visits. The considerable financial and administrative resources that sponsors devote to the development and monitoring of clinical investigations easily could be jeopardized if adequate precautions are not taken to preserve confidentiality of information meant only for the research team.

CHAPTER 17

Scheduling and Log Systems

Appointment Books • Alphabetical Card Index • Laboratory Specimen Log • Patient Sign-In Log • Diagnostic Medication Log • Record of Payments to Subjects • Study Medication Log • Record of Sponsor Visits

Medical facilities generate many records for purposes such as financial accounting, general administration, and supply dispensing that are needed to produce accurate reports on their business and medical activities. Records of transactions with research subjects, such as petty cash disbursements, appointment scheduling, and dispensation of medication for diagnostic procedures, serve a secondary function of corroborating data recorded on CRFs by reflecting the patient's progression through the facility. When presented as supporting documents, these records engender confidence that CRF data submitted to the sponsor and the FDA are both accurate and authentic. Although investigators are not specifically required to maintain scheduling logs, it is wise to establish some combination of the administrative systems described below to support CRF data and serve as backup sources that can be used to resolve possible transcription or other documentation errors.

Even in limited research operations, record-keeping systems should be developed for tracking laboratory specimens, diagnostic medication use, study medication use, and petty cash disbursements. In smaller facilities, combining several functions into a few logs may be appropriate. Specimen tracking may be recorded in the appointment book, for example, to minimize the inconvenience of working with many different log books.

In establishing these record-keeping systems, it is worthwhile for the research team to keep in mind that the principal investigator is responsible for the integrity of any system developed to provide supporting documentation of study events. Conflicting or poorly maintained records call into question the validity of data and can cause audits to be unnecessarily prolonged. While it is wise to develop administrative systems in which visit dates and other basic information can be independently recorded, these systems should involve only as much duplication as is needed to engender confidence in the study data and provide a confirming source of visit information. The team should devise only as many administrative systems as reasonably can be maintained and which serve to facilitate the conduct of the research.

APPOINTMENT BOOKS

Books for scheduling appointments are recognized by the offices of most physicians as essential organizing tools for a busy practice. Entries in the research appointment book should be made with attention to the principles of data recording listed above and should have the following minimum contents (also see Figure 9):

1. The name of the patient should be indicated with the date and time of the scheduled appointment. If the date the appointment was made is important, that, too, should be noted.
2. If the facility conducts a number of studies with the same personnel, the type of visit and study in which the patient is participating should be listed. A clear notation should be made to verify that the appointment was kept.
3. Any cancellations should be documented in the appointment book and rescheduled appointments noted as such. Erasures should not be permitted.
4. Every date, including weekends and holidays, should be recorded with a special notation if no contacts occurred. Appointment books that list only those dates on which patients' visits were scheduled do not provide a clear reference for resolving possible transcription errors or confirming that no pages have been misplaced.
5. In a facility involving multiple investigators, the name of the assigned physician should be noted.
6. If desired, the dates on which sponsor and FDA personnel visited the facility may be noted in the appointment book as well.
7. If a relationship has been established with a subspecialist to perform specific safety evaluations for the study, he should be advised of the need to maintain his usual records of the visit, including documentation of the visit in his office appointment

Monday, December 2			
9:00 Ida Smith	M-32—5th week	DH 11-1	Showed up
9:30 Art Holmes	M-32—24th week	DH 8-1	Rescheduled DH
10:00 Phil Marion	SK-7241 Inf. Consent Dr. Riley	AL Nov. 29	Showed up
Tuesday, December 3			
9:00 Marel Siltz	M-32 Screen blood here	DH 11-29	Here
10:15 Marel Siltz	M-32 Audiometry—Dr. Ohr	DH 1-29	Kept
11:00 Art Holmes	M-32 24th week	DH 12-1	Here
Wednesday, December 4			
9:00 BM Tanzy	Screen M-32	DH 12-2	Here
9:30 Oscar Lenz	Screen M-32	DH 12-2	Rescheduled DH
10:00 Tammy Ants	Screen M-32	DH 12-2	Here
11:00 Oralee Jones	Screen M-32	DH 12-2	Did not come DH
Thursday, December 5			
9:00 Oscar Lenz	Screen M-32	DH 12-4	Here
Friday, December 6			
No Clinic Activities			

FIGURE 9. Appointment book format (study use only).

book. The team may wish to note the dates of these visits to track receipt of consultants' reports.

The necessity of meticulously documenting and scheduling study visits in the appointment book must be stressed to all personnel checking in subjects or accepting cancellations.

ALPHABETICAL CARD INDEX

An alphabetical card index listing each of the studies in which a patient has participated should be maintained at any facility conducting or planning to conduct multiple studies. This index can include an abbreviated problem list, which will aid in recruiting prospective candidates for studies of other disease states. It is wise to prepare an index card for any patients examined at the facility even if they do not enter the current study, since they may prove suitable for later projects. Additionally, if separate research charts are generated for each study in which a patient participates, this index provides a mechanism to access

```
Semnelweiss, Marie                   Born 1-1-39
22 S. Squirrel Hill Drive            Primary Dx = Essential Hypertension
Wayland, MA 01778                    Secondary Dx = Osteoarthritis
Home (617) 348-7166   in Boston Thursdays
Spouse:  Harold                      Work (617) 602-4433
Protocol:  Searle Enovid             Start 3-3-81   Pt# 6038
Protocol:  MSD—3128                  Start 2-12-84 Pt# 16-8
```

FIGURE 10. Sample alphabetical card index.

a patient's complete file. A sample index card that is useful for this purpose is provided in Figure 10.

LABORATORY SPECIMEN LOG

It often proves a challenge for a busy research operation to monitor for the timely receipt of laboratory reports from the variety of laboratories it may use. The log book format presented in Figure 11 provides a convenient mechanism to document laboratory transactions and highlight those reports not yet received. This log should be reviewed daily by a staff member and any reporting delays investigated promptly.

Developing a method to verify that consultant, laboratory, and special test results, such as ECG reports, have been seen by the physician is essential. Methods that have been successfully employed for this purpose all require notations of such reviews on the lab slips or reports. These methods are discussed in Chapter 18.

PATIENT SIGN-IN LOG

In very active facilities, a simple log book in which the patient can sign his name under the date of each visit is an excellent supporting document. This is best developed using a bound log book. This log provides a record in the patient's own handwriting documenting his visit. If desired, this log can be used to document sponsor visits as well. If a patient neglects to sign in, a staff member may enter the patient's name with his or her own initials and a note as to why the log was not signed. At the end of the day, the next day's date should be enterd with no free space.

Who	What	When	Study #	Time picked up	Report received
Monday, April 7, 1986					
Mary Jones	Blood	9:15 a.m.	L-3106	Noon	4-9-86 AR
Phil Manson	Blood Urine	9:18 a.m.	Screen MN-20	Noon	4-8 AR
Tessa Plow	Blood Urine	9:45 a.m.	Screen MN-20	Noon	4-11 AR
Marion Mann	Urine	11:30 a.m.	Repeat	Noon	4-7 AR
Tuesday, April 8, 1986					
NO SPECIMENS					
Wednesday, April 9, 1986					
Mary Jones	Blood	9:00 a.m.	L-3106	11:30 a.m.	4-11-86 AR
Frank Jones	Blood Urine	9:10 a.m.	L-3106	11:30 a.m.	4-11-86 SN
Ann Canne	Blood Urine	9:45 a.m.	Screen MN-20	11:30 a.m.	4-11-86 AR
Thursday, April 10					
NO SPECIMENS					

FIGURE 11. Laboratory specimen log.

DIAGNOSTIC MEDICATION LOG

Physicians who administer medication such as analgesic agents as a part of diagnostic procedures related to a study (e.g., endoscopies, catheterizations, uterine or sinus cultures) are required to maintain separate chronological inventories documenting their dispensation. These chronological records are required so the supplies that have been documented as used can be compared at any time with the actual supplies on hand. A sample log of this type is included in Figure 12.

These logs are meant as inventory records and are not required if individual prescriptions are written and supplies purchased separately for each patient. In a hospital setting, these records are retained by the pharmacy and need not be duplicated.

Controlled substances or other medications requiring special han-

| DRUG NAME: | Sterile Valium | | | | | | |

DRUG NAME: Sterile Valium

DOSAGE STRENGTH: 25 mg/ml   DOSAGE FORM: i.v. liquid

UNITS RECEIVED: 25 amps   LOT/SERIAL NO.:   R-6130628

STAFF MEMBER ACKNOWLEDGING RECEIPT: P. J. Murray   2/4/86
                                                      (Signature)   Date

Patient	Date	Procedure	Quantity Received	Used	Discarded	Signature
Anne Jane	2/11/86	Gastroscopy	25 mg	15 mg	10	Selma/RN
Mary Thomas	2/11/86	Gastroscopy	25 mg	7 mg	18	Selma/RN
Andy Marino	2/11/86	Gastroscopy	25 mg	25 mg	—	Selma/RN
Horace Philben	2/13/86	Gastroscopy	25 mg	10 mg	15	Selma/RN
	2/13/86	21 amps in medicine cabinet				IBER/MD

FIGURE 12. Procedure medication inventory log.

dling must be inventoried frequently to confirm that no supplies have been lost or stolen. Any discrepancies noted should be documented with a witnessed signature. Any disposal of supplies also should be recorded with a witnessed signature. The regulations governing the storage and use of controlled substances are discussed in the section on drug accountability.

RECORD OF PAYMENTS TO SUBJECTS

A petty cash receipt book or office checking account must be maintained for accounting purposes to document transactions with patients. This record offers confirmation of the patient's visit. If a petty cash receipt book is maintained (which is signed and dated by the patient *at each visit*), the separate sign-in book referred to above may not be required. Standard petty cash slips found in office supply stores should prove adequate for this purpose. Facilities presenting checks rather than cash to patients should make a notation of this transaction in files that are easily accessible, since inquiry regarding payment status occurs frequently.

STUDY MEDICATION LOG

A chronological inventory of supply dispensation and return must be maintained by all facilities conducting pharmaceutical research. Its purpose is to indicate when and to whom medication is dispensed and returned. The maintenance of these records is required per the proposed regulations and should be part of any log system employed at the facility. A sample log format and detailed discussion of drug accountability are contained in Section VII.

RECORD OF SPONSOR VISITS

In an audit, investigators may be asked to provide documentation of the dates on which sponsor personnel visited the facility. The appointment book and sign-in log described above and the CRF tracking log described in a later section offer alternative sites for recording the essentials of such visits. Sponsors also may have their own log formats, which they will present at the initiation of the study. If any of these methods prove inconvenient, the research team may wish to consider documenting sponsor visits by noting on the CRF copies the initials of the sponsor personnel reviewing or retrieving them and the date. This latter method offers confirmation of what was actually accomplished at the visit.

Some of the administrative records described above are of value to the research effort purely as accurate scheduling methods. Others are required to comply with regulation or accepted accounting practices. Combined, they all contribute to research record keeping in three important ways: (1) They serve to corroborate that the visits described on the CRF did, in fact, occur since the records are generated by multiple parties; (2) they provide a means of resolving the inevitable transcription errors that will occur in a system involving such extensive record keeping; and (3) they offer a convenient mechanism for tracking the paper flow of study-related documents. It is to the research team's advantage to establish administrative systems that further these three objectives with the least duplication.

CHAPTER 18

The Research Chart

Format of the Research Chart • *Content of the Research Chart*
• *Research Chart Entry and Review* • *Integration with Facility's*
Medical Chart

The purpose of the research chart has expanded considerably in the past decade due to advances in data-processing technology and the regulatory agencies' desire for extensive documentation of subjects' eligibility and clinical course in a study. The data that sponsors are collecting now on all patients with exposure to a study drug require highly standardized record keeping compatible with sophisticated computer technology. The advent of this standardized computer-compatible CRF has ruled out using the CRF as a comprehensive record of a patient's course of study. The research chart has evolved as a separate record that contains all of the details of adherence to the protocol. It also links patients to the previous care they received prior to the study and their later reentry into the medical care system following the study. This record assumes increasing importance in supporting the authenticity of the research data now that subjects have begun to take part in studies at facilities at which they have no history of previous treatment. In fact, the proposed FDA regulations governing the obligations of clinical investigators (21 CRF Part 54) require that case histories of a patient's eligibility and course of therapy be developed independent of the CRF to support the integrity of the data-collection process. Thus, the research chart has become perhaps the single most useful research document generated on a patient's clinical course of study. Table 32 lists the materials that are included in such a chart.

The research record is the property and responsibility of the research team and should be retained in the study area at all times to ensure its availability and confidential use. It can be stored separately or kept as a part of the patient's office medical record, particularly if the office records do not circulate. The research chart, combined with the

TABLE 32. Typical Reference Documents in a Research Chart

Informed consent
Copies of key reports documenting eligibility (e.g., old X-ray report showing arthritis
  of knees, hospital discharge indicating heart condition)
Patient's release of information form for old records
Doctor's correspondence referring patient
Patient correspondence
Old medical records
Raw eligibility documents
Eligibility checklist once enrollment occurs
Locator sheet, address, phone numbers, emergency contact

study checklists discussed later in this section, constitutes the essential
raw data needed to complete the study case report forms.

FORMAT OF THE RESEARCH CHART

The information included in a research chart is of two types: (1)
essential reference documents that are developed but used only infrequently, and (2) chronological reports of study-related contacts and
research interventions that are referred to quite frequently. The first
category consists of a copy of the informed consent document, referral
letters to and from the patient's private physician, and administrative
correspondence with the patient. The second category includes all progress notes made at the time of the patient's visit, the results of laboratory evaluations or other study procedures, and notes of significant
telephone communication with the patient, his family, the sponsor, the
IRB, or any consultants involved in his research care. The problem-
oriented medical record is an ideal format for recording this second
category of data and structuring progress notes. The research chart
must be designed to accommodate the variety of test report formats and
reference documents that will be placed in it.

All useful systems should include a mechanism for securing loose
documents as soon as they have been reviewed. Systems that the authors have employed for various studies are listed in Table 33. Chart
documents should not be filed until they have been reviewed and
signed appropriately by a study physician.

Research facilities conducting multiple studies should prominently list on the front or inside cover of the chart the names of the
studies in which the patient has participated previously. While research charts can be developed as either patient-specific (covering a
patient's involvement in all studies) or study-specific (covering a pa-

TABLE 33. Developing a Research Chart Format

A manila folder can be used. The top sections can be modified with two-pronged
metal clips to attach progress notes. Reference documents and correspondence can
be placed on the left, with all notes placed on the right side of the folder. Lab work
can be attached chronologically on lab pages toward the back of this section with
transparent adhesive tape to facilitate photocopying for referrals.

A clipboard can be used for each patient. Chronological progress notes can be kept on
the front, with reference documents stored at the rear of the clipboard in a large
mailing envelope. This system is best suited to short-term studies involving few
documents and is not useful for long-term record storage.

A study notebook can be established for each subject. Pocket folders can be used to
retain loose documents, with reference ones filed in one pocket and diagnostic and
laboratory tests filed in the other. Progress notes can be filed in the binder
chronologically.

Bulky, extensive interview records or long copies of CRFs are best kept in a separate
folder in a filing cabinet.

Full- or half-page-size envelopes can be attached to the research record to retain loose
reports.

All types of records must prominently display the subject's name or initials and
patient number or drug code. If the study medicine has been color-coded, it is
advantageous to prominently use the same color consistently on the research record
for easy reference. Each chart page should have identifying information such as
initials and patient number or drug code.

For long or complex studies, a summary page noting key qualifying diagnoses,
hospitalizations, and study information can be placed on the front of the chart.

tient's involvement in one study only) documents, the latter approach
requires a cross-reference system so records of previous studies can be
retrieved. The alphabetical card file described in an earlier chapter is
ideally suited to this purpose.

CONTENT OF THE RESEARCH CHART

All data that are pertinent to the suitability of the patient for study
and all information that is needed to judge the quality of the team's
conduct of the research must be documented in the research chart. The
research chart is the source document from which all CRF data will be
extracted and should contain a complete chronology of the screening
process, study participation, and referral for routine care following the
study. In simple studies, the research chart need not be much more
extensive than the CRF. For example, in a study of headaches in which
subjects are monitored for a few hours following receipt of an analgesic
or a placebo, the chart may consist only of the screening evaluation,
outcome assessments (likely to be simply photocopies of the CRF

TABLE 34. *Standard Elements of a Research Chart*

Information required to contact patient or responsible family member in an
  emergency
Documentation of patient's appropriateness for entry into study[a]
Documentation that patient has disease state under study as defined by the protocol
  and good medical practice[a]
Baseline safety measurements (e.g., laboratory test results)[a]
Appropriate informed consent, oral and written, prior to the performance of any
  study-related procedures[a]
Documentation of dosing decision (Note in chart and on lab reports that clinical and
  lab data have been reviewed and are considered acceptable for entry. Telephone
  discussions between investigator and staff on special problem issues should be
  documented as such and subsequently countersigned by the investigator.)
Medical release form
General health status of patient, noting any adverse experiences in detail with
  medical management plan (required each visit)[a]
Changes in concomitant medication noted since previous visit, with reason
  (required each visit)[a]
Comments on study medication compliance, both observations and actions taken to
  counsel patients about compliance if appropriate (required each visit)[a]
Physician's documentation that it was appropriate for patient to continue in study
  (required each visit)[a]
Patient diary records with comments in progress note or on card itself, if permitted
  by client, of potential inaccuracies
Communication with client regarding eligibility or continuation decisions
Documentation of all visits or telephone contacts of medical or scheduling import
Reasons for any unscheduled visits
Calls by patient to report adverse events with action taken by center and physician
  to arrange proper follow-up (The outcome of any adverse events, even those
  occurring at the final visit that are followed up after the patient has completed
  the study, should be noted in the record and on the CRF.)
Calls to sponsor and IRB to report serious adverse events with documentation from
  sponsor of FDA reporting (if provided by client)[a]
Calls to patient to remind him of appointment
Summary statement of patient's participation
  Status of disease under study, comparing initial and final diagnoses
  Response to medication
  Adverse events noted during the study
  Suitability for future protocols
Final disposition of patient
  Debriefing at end of study or at the conclusion of screening if patient is deemed
    ineligible
  Referral to local medical community if active disease remains present or patient
    wishes general care referral

---

[a]These items are required specifically by the proposed FDA regulations 21 CFR Part 54.

sheets), and the signed informed consent form. Table 34 lists the categories of information contained in a research chart and a description of those standard categories. Whatever the study's complexity, the research chart must be sufficiently detailed to establish the subject's identity and eligibility, exposure to the test medication, and final disposition.

RESEARCH CHART ENTRY AND REVIEW

Any staff member gaining information about the patient or having contact with him for purposes of study should document the encounter in the chart, dating and signing the entry. Scheduled and unscheduled visits, all issuances of medication, all telephone calls with sponsor concerning the individual subject, and evidence of review of the laboratory work or special tests should be included. Figure 13 is a sample page from such a chart.

If a reaction occurs, all actions taken in relation to it and all follow-up contacts, including referrals, results of the referrals, and eventual outcome of the possible adverse event should be noted in the research chart. Excellent charts will contain thoroughly documented follow-ups of abnormalities found in laboratory evaluations, particularly those noted at the final visit. For example, abnormal liver function tests noted at the exit evaluation may be associated with a delayed hepatotoxicity from the drug or may be an unrelated hepatitis. The events of the ensuing few days or weeks that clarify whether the abnormalities represent an adverse reaction should be noted in the chart and communicated to the sponsor.

All clinical documents should be reviewed and signed by a study physician before being filed in the subject's records. To best utilize the investigator's time, staff members may be asked to scan all reports, highlighting abnormalities and significant changes from baseline for physician review. Investigators at high-volume facilities usually provide the staff with guidelines for reviewing lab work that specify ranges not considered clinically significant, those meriting observation or repeat, and those requiring immediate medical review. Such a standard operating procedure should be in place at any facility in which review of lab data is delegated. The incoming data should be reviewed daily by the staff so any clinically relevant findings can be acted and commented upon promptly. Medical personnel can then make themselves available for routine signatures two to three times per week as volume requires. Following medical review, the signed documents may be filed in the subject's charts. Any other phone calls to the sponsor, the FDA,

Antonia Jones   (AJ, Subject 17 in Robbins Study 136-85-3) Sept. 3, 1985. Enrolled by Dr. Riley. First medication and diary given. AST

Sept. 5 Phoned for clarification on diary. Seemed confused so plans to stop by in a day or two. AST

Sept. 7   Confused on diary so we took her info. and transcribed it into a new document starting 9-3 (old in data pocket). She seems to understand clearly now. Did not have medications with her. AST

Sept. 15   Retn visit 1. BP 120/80, wt. 121. No complaints volunteered. Diary and pill counts reconciled. Returned bottle with 7 tablets; diary excellent (in data pocket). New medications issued. AST

Oct. 14   Second visit. BP 120/80, wt. 116. No attempts at dieting. Diary and pill counts perfect. Bottle returned and diary in folder. Issued new medication. JN/tech. To see Dr. Riley.

Oct. 14   Unexplained 5 lb. weight loss. Nice weather and more frequent excursions with dog, only changes. Does not have signs of hyperthyroidism to my exam. Pulse 72. Delighted with wt. loss. Will follow and see next month. WAR/md.

Oct. 24   Changed appointment to Nov. 12. FLI/MD

Nov. 12   Third visit. Diary very poorly kept and patient upset. Wt. 116, BP 120/70. No complaints but clearly is miserable. Pill counts off by 3 and cannot remember when they were not taken. Pt. wants to continue study. Thinks she can do better. Did not wish to see Dr. Riley and did not want to discuss the problem. Promised to phone. AST

Nov. 15   I called her at work. She called back later. Things much better. Invited me to lunch next week for discussion. AST

Nov. 23   Lunch. Discussed unexpected death of her neighbor's daughter and how upset she was but could not talk to anyone about it. Just talking seemed a great relief. Reports study fine. AST

Dec. 18   Fourth visit. Wt. 119, pulse 72, BP 110/80. Looks great in new outfit and no complaints. Pill counts and diary exact. New bottle given; old bottle returned. Routine safety blood taken today. AST

Dec. 19   Blood returned, all normal. Called to tell her that this OK. AST

FIGURE 13. Page from a research chart.

or staff about an individual patient should be documented in the research record. Results of audits of the record should be kept as a part of the overall study, or the auditor may note them as a progress note.

It deserves emphasis that these documents should include information that may not be required on the CRF but does reflect the process by which the data were gathered. If, for example, a patient interviewed informed the first interviewer that he had taken a specific medication

for hypertension until the previous month and, upon subsequent questioning, revealed that he actually had stopped the medication two
months previously, the raw data should reflect both the patient's first
response and the resolution of the inconsistency by the investigator. In
contrast, the CRF will reflect only that response which the investigator
has concluded is accurate.

INTEGRATION WITH FACILITY'S MEDICAL CHART

Investigators in a hospital or private office setting who are conducting outpatient studies must also consider whether they wish to
establish a research chart apart from the medical record. Such a practice is nearly always essential in outpatient work if the protocol requires multiple visits or if study patients can be expected to receive
medical care for other conditions at the facility. Medical records containing research charts that circulate within a facility often are not
accessible for research visits and so cannot be used as the only records
of the patient's course of study. Some IRBs recommend maintaining
separate research charts to preserve the confidentiality of aspects of a
patient's medical history that are not relevant to the study (e.g., a previous psychiatric history for a hypertension study). Since it remains the
research team's obligation to retain documentation of the subject's
course of study, medical records available for general use rarely suffice.
In outpatient studies where separate research charts are maintained, a
list of all patients' medical record numbers should be kept in the event
that their medical charts are needed. A note and copy of the informed
consent form should be placed in each subject's medical record to
indicate that he is involved in a research protocol with the name of the
research team member who can be contacted for further details. In
some institutions, it may be appropriate to include copies of all clinically relevant study documents in the subject's record and retain the
originals in the research chart. Research manipulations on hospitalized
patients should be recorded in their medical charts with copies retained for research records.

CHAPTER 19

Study Checklists

Checklists for collecting the data required for a protocol and a patient's medical care can prove quite useful in structuring the research staff's interactions with subjects. The staff can use the development of these checklists as an opportunity to consider the sequence in which patients will be scheduled for the various study procedures. These same check-lists can be provided to research subjects for their study planning. Table 35 summarizes the many types of reminder documents that can be developed.

There are several types of checklists that can be used quite effec-tively to facilitate data collection and remind the team of important eligibility requirements. The first of these is the eligibility checklist, which has been presented in Figure 14. Many CRFs include checklists that outline the basic eligibility requirements. These can easily be amended to include items of particular interest to the team (e.g., a signed consent document or scheduling availability). Eligibility check-lists should summarize baseline screening requirements such as age, weight, and sex, and important admonitions such as specific medica-tions prohibited during a study or requiring a washout. Since the study physician performs only some of the eligibility checks, such as the physical exam or the ECG, and the research staff performs others, such as drug history, age, or weight, this checklist can be used to ensure that a comprehensive baseline review occurs before the patient is entered. The checklist can be initialed by the responsible staff member as each requirement is met.

Visit flow sheets are useful for complex studies to provide a chronological summary of the visit requirements and each patient's status in the study. These flow sheets can be placed on the front of the subject's chart for easy reference and completion at each visit. The flow sheet will then be accessible if subjects telephone to reschedule ap-pointments or request the dates of any they have forgotten. Figures 15 and 16 offer alternative flow sheet formats.

Disease-specific history forms are useful for studies involving high screening volume in which much of the initial eligibility data can be

TABLE 35. *Useful and Necessary Study Checklists*

Necessary
  Eligibility checklist (Figure 14)
  Flow sheet to track schedule of visits (Figures 15 and 16)
Useful in special circumstances
  Checklist for complex visit (Figure 17)
  Standardized questionnaire (taken from CRF)
  Global mental state questionnaires
  Symptom checklist
  Disease-specific history to aid recruitment
  Telephone "interview" sheets

NAME: Thomas Harry

DATE: 3/7/86

Any single "no" renders patient ineligible

	Yes	No
Eligibility criteria	(Initials of tester)	
Between ages of 21 and 60	TB	
Does not now take any meds regularly*	TB	
Is nonsmoker (no cigs for 1 month)	TB	
Normal to screening physical exam	WAR/MD	
(except arthritis)	3/5	
Has at least two major joints involved	FLI/MD	
on X ray by arthritis	3/7	
Chest X ray in last 6 months (Nov. 1985)	TB	
Some incapacity on timed walking test	TB	
Screening CBC and labs normal	TB	
Ophthalmological exam normal	TB Raft	
	3/6	
Judged compliant by staff	TB	
Signed informed consent	TB	
Patient *told* no alcohol and no		
OTC medicines without permission	TB	
	3/7	

*Defined as daily at any time since February 1, 1986.
PI Signature _____ Date _____

FIGURE 14. Eligibility checklist.

SANDOZ 362

Patient: P.J.

Subject: 5014

	1	2	3	4	5	6	7	8	9	10	11	12
Week	1	2	3	4	5	6	7	8	9	10	11	12
Visit	1	2		3		4			5			6
Date	3/6	3/14		3/20		4/4			5/2			
Interview	X	X		X		X			X			X
BP check	X	X		X		X			X			X
Detailed form 3	X			X					X			
Dose change				X					X			X
MD physical	X											X
ECG	X											X
Eye MD	X											
Pill count	X	X		X		X			X			X
Chems	X			X								X
Urine	X			X								X
Give meds	X	X		X		X			X			X

FIGURE 15. Study flow sheet.

collected by telephone or by the staff in preliminary interviews. These can be developed jointly by the investigators and staff and be updated during the study as the team's screening techniques are increasingly refined.

The many details of a research protocol must be available at a glance to research team members scheduling and caring for subjects. If designed to facilitate protocol adherence and communication with subjects, study checklists serve as convenient references for frequently used study information.

Patient _____ Drug Code _____ Patient/CRF No. _____			
Procedure	Baseline exam	Visit 1	Visit 2	Visit 3 (Final)
Visit window	Day −7−0	Day 12−16	Day 26−30	Day 40−44
H&P/Symp. Rev.	6-1-86	6-12-86	6-29-86	7-10-86
Cardiologist	6-2-86			7-12-86
Initial when completed				
Supine BP readings				
Concomitant meds				
Adverse events				
CBC/DIFF/ SMA-12				
Urinalysis				
Medication check				
Honorarium				

FIGURE 16. Visit flow sheet.

PATIENT NAME: _____ VISIT DATE: _____

PATIENT/CRF NO.: _____

PROCEDURE   *STAFF INITIALS*

Height and weight.   _____

Pulse, BP, and respiration.   _____

Collect blood for SMA-12, CBC with differential.   _____

Collect urine specimen.   _____

Obtain 3 blood pressure measurements after patient has   _____
   been supine for 10 minutes and average.

Evaluate whether patient's diastolic blood pressure has   _____
   increased greater than 10 mm Hg. If yes, discontinue
   patient from study—see discontinuation
   requirements.

Question patient regarding any adverse experiences   _____
   occurring since the previous visit. (Refer to notes of
   previous visit for continuing adverse events.) Note
   follow-up plan if required.

Question patient regarding changes in concomitant   _____
   medication (explore changes for possible adverse
   events). Note name, dosage, frequency, and indication
   for medication.

Collect used medication supplies and pill counts, and   _____
   note whether patient was compliant.

Dispense next set of supplies if appropriate.   _____

Schedule next visit.   _____

Provide honorarium.   _____

FIGURE 17. Visit checklist, Protocol XX-9999, Visit 3.

CHAPTER 20

The Case Report Form

Case Report Form Completion • *CRF Tracking* • *Circumstances under Which a CRF Must Be Submitted* • *Corrections or Additions to CRFs* • *Frequency of Submission*

CASE REPORT FORM COMPLETION

Since sponsors ordinarily provide extensive guidelines concerning the details of completing their CRFs, these will not be covered in depth here. It is important to note that each sponsor has specific requirements as to how the company wishes specific data elements recorded. Sponsors may be willing to provide a sample completed CRF that can be used as a training document for the staff. Feedback as to the staff's success in complying with the completion guidelines will be provided in the form of written requests for additional data or on-site reviews with the CRA staff. It is the investigator's obligation to ensure that any valid errors noted in these reviews do not recur. The team's response to any deficiencies in CRF completion will be a factor in judging its suitability for additional studies. Since most pharmaceutical companies evaluate their field forces' performance partly by the quality of the CRFs submitted from their assigned sites, satisfied monitors are more likely to recommend a facility for placement of future projects. As a result, the CRAs will make fewer demands of the investigator's time during the study.

Because CRAs are the primary reviewers of the clinical data generated for the study, most sponsors do not permit them to record data on the CRF during site visits. The CRA's role is to provide clarification as to how the facts were gathered and to orient the team as to any additional information the sponsor may require for safety or regulatory reporting. He or she should not prohibit medical personnel from recording data on the CRF that is felt to be medically relevant in evaluating the case. Any concerns regarding an individual CRA's practices of CRF review should be directed to the medical monitor of the project.

Protocol: _____
X = Visit Collected by Sponsor

CRF no.	Patient initials	Baseline evaluation (pp. 1–6)	Visit 2 (pp. 7–11)	Visit 3 (pp. 12–16)	Comments
0001	JC	6/10/83X	6/20/83X	6/30/83X	Completed
0002	DM	7/5/83X	7/15/83X	Discontinued. Developed rash. CRF collected 8/10 by JL of Lederle	
0003	CC	8/3/86X	8/13/86X	8/23/83X	Completed
0004	DDX	CRF begun in error. Patient declined at initial visit. CRF returned to sponsor.			
0005 ⎫ 0006 ⎭		Blank CRFs destroyed 12/10/84 at study conclusion. ADM/Study Coordinator			

FIGURE 18. CRF/visit flow sheet.

CRF TRACKING

CRFs vary considerably in length and may be collected by sponsors either in sections or as complete records. Having the staff maintain a flow sheet (see Figure 18) that lists visit dates and CRF submission dates will permit close monitoring of these documents. All CRF numbers that have been assigned by the sponsor should be listed on such a log and their status noted. This log should also include a record of any blank CRFs returned to the client or destroyed at the conclusion of the study. A tracking system for CRF submission is a necessity at high-volume facilities where CRFs for patients who discontinued early in the study can easily be misfiled in a drawer, only to be discovered well after the conclusion of the study. It is the team's obligation to see that any CRFs that contain data are given promptly to the sponsor. It may be helpful for investigators considering developing such a log to ascertain whether their CRA routinely keeps one. If the CRA provides the team with a copy of his log at the conclusion of each visit, the team could be spared having to keep this additional record.

CIRCUMSTANCES UNDER WHICH A CRF MUST BE SUBMITTED

A CRF must be completed on any subject who receives even one dose of study medication, whether or not that subject is to be considered evaluable. The research team should also consult with the CRA concerning any more stringent requirements that may apply to specific studies (e.g., studies involving defined screening periods that must be completed before subjects are assigned coded medication). In institutional settings in which residents or fellows may be motivated to participate primarily for financial reasons, they will not likely be anxious to complete CRFs on early discontinuations for whom they will receive no remuneration. It is important to review this point to ensure that CRFs for unevaluable patients are submitted in a timely manner.

CORRECTIONS OR ADDITIONS TO CRFS

Companies also have very specialized mechanisms for recording corrections to data or requesting additional information once the CRF has been submitted to their headquarters. Some sponsors require that the CRF needing correction be returned to the investigator. Others provide a separate form on which any missing information or clarification will be requested. Clarifications may be requested by telephone if the case in question involves a significant adverse event. Written confirmation should be provided of all such telephone requests. The research team should also note in the subject's file that the conversation occurred. In processing these requests, the team should keep in mind that the CRF that the sponsor has on file *must be identical* to that which is in the site's records, since it is the sponsor's copy that would be included in a regulatory submission to FDA. If any relevant information on a patient's case is learned after the original CRF has been submitted, it is the team's responsibility to see that it is included in the sponsor's records as well. In the absence of a specific mechanism for adding to a subject's CRF once submitted, the investigator may simply send a letter to the CRA or the department that processes these documents detailing the new information and requesting that it be added to the subject's file.

FREQUENCY OF SUBMISSION

It is desirable that CRFs be completed immediately after the patients' visits and be available for CRA review within one or two weeks of the visits. Postponing completion or review and signing of these documents will quickly cause a backlog that will prove difficult to eliminate as enrollment increases. If such a backlog appears to be developing, it is best to reduce or discontinue enrollment immediately until the backlog is resolved. Should the problem become severe, sponsors themselves may insist that enrollment be discontinued until the administrative problems are rectified and may view the team's performance unfavorably as a result. The flow sheet described above offers a convenient mechanism for the staff to monitor CRF submissions and to identify any such delays before the sponsor feels obliged to resolve the matter.

Sponsors with field monitoring forces require that they visit every one to three months, depending on the site's enrollment volume and CRF submission status. Data should not be allowed to remain in the field for greater than three months under routine circumstances, since such a delay does not permit sufficiently prompt review for adverse experiences or recovery of missing data. The staff should be oriented to the need to contact the CRA to request a visit if data submission is delayed. Since investigators' grant installments are based on the number of CRFs on file with the sponsor, prompt submission of data has financial advantages. The staff must prioritize for the monitor's review CRFs for patients who have had significant adverse experiences that have been reported to the sponsor by telephone.

Sponsors have the legal responsibility to tabulate and report adverse experience data to the FDA. The primary document on which these reports are based is the CRF. The promptness with which investigators submit these records to the sponsor will greatly enhance this important safety monitoring and reporting mechanism.

CHAPTER 21

Records of Excluded Patients

RATIONALE FOR RETAINING RECORDS OF EXCLUDED PATIENTS

A well-designed enrollment process ensures appropriate selectivity of subjects from within the population responding to recruitment efforts. The quality of this process can be documented only by careful recording of interactions with patients who were ineligible or who refused to join the study. Detailed documentation of these encounters serves medical-legal purposes as well since the majority of interactions with patients reveal some findings of medical import. These records further serve as a source of potential subjects for studies that the team may choose to undertake at a later date. This chapter will outline methods of storing records of excluded study candidates that permit these objectives to be achieved most expeditiously.

CONSIDERATIONS IN ORGANIZING THE RECORDS

Individual records must be generated for each patient who visits the facility and is seen by a staff member for screening. These records should contain reports of all tests or evaluations performed and a clear indication of the basis of ineligibility. These records are a valuable source of prospective subjects for future studies and should be prepared as carefully as is feasible with the staff resources available. Subjects considered unsuitable for one type of study but who express an interest in future participation should be clearly identified with a brief statement of their preferences. If he is eligible, the reason (if known) that the patient did not participate should be listed along with the patient's final disposition. Guidelines for organizing these records are as follows:

1. A complete, physically separate file should be established for each candidate. This file can be as simple as a stapled set of the documents generated during screening.
2. Many sponsors require that exclusion logs be maintained of patients who were not considered appropriate for entry. If the sponsor does require that such a log be maintained, the desired format should be presented at the initiation visit.
3. Many IRBs require a log of patients who refused to participate.

These records can be filed either alphabetically by study or in a general screening file. However, the filing system should allow the team to retrieve promptly the records of all subjects who were excluded from a specific study as well as to locate the record of an individual subject who cannot recall for which study he was considered. Systems in which records are stored in a general screening file must include exclusion logs for each study. The exclusion log is a chronological list of all subjects considered for a particular study and the reason(s) they were excluded. Chart systems organized by study should employ the alphabetical card index to retrieve patients' charts using their names only.

One of the potential benefits being offered to all patients who express a desire to participate in the study is the access to any medical information acquired during the screening process. Prompt responses to requests for these records constitute positive publicity with prospective candidates and local practitioners. These records should be organized in such a way that requests can be honored promptly and with minimal inconvenience to the staff.

CHAPTER 22

Regulatory Document Files

THE IMPORTANCE OF REGULATORY DOCUMENTS

While clinical records provide a chronology of an individual patient's course of study, regulatory document files may be thought of as the administrative counterparts to the clinical records. These records should reflect the sequence in which employees and physicians joined and left the research team and the timing in which protocol changes or updated safety information on the medication was received and acted upon by the team. Documentation of compliance with IRB requirements should also be retained in these records. Since pharmaceutical firms and the FDA have well-established mechanisms for documenting changes to the investigative team (i.e., submission of revised FDA 1572/3 forms) or receipt of amended protocols (i.e., return of signed and dated copies of the protocol to the sponsor), these regulatory files will largely consist of copies of documents submitted to the sponsor and the IRB. A checklist of the required elements is included as Table 36.

One of the criteria that outside auditors employ to judge the quality of a research operation is the timeliness with which the research team reviewed and took action on any materials received from the sponsor. It is wise to date the receipt on all study-related correspondence and to establish a system for the team's prompt review of these. Judgments made as to the necessity of taking action (e.g., reporting new safety information to the IRB) should be documented by the responsible staff member so the review process will be clear to any auditor examining the files. Investigators should keep in mind that regulatory inspections

TABLE 36. Checklist
Regulatory and Administrative Files

Patient exclusion log   —
Patient assignment sheet   —
Patient visit/CRF submission flow sheet   —
Protocol signed and dated by the principal investigator   —
Amendments or revised protocols signed and dated by PI   —
Consent document(s) approved by the IRB   —
Sample CRF annotated with instructions for completion   —
Investigational use circular (all versions)   —
Copy of signed FD 1572/3 form and any updates   —
C.V.'s of principal investigator and collaborators   —
Correspondence with IRB:
  List of IRB members and copy of bylaws   —
  Initial submission and letter of approval   —
  Submission and approval of amendments   —
  Submission of safety updates on new drug   —
  Submission of annual and final reports   —
  Reports to the IRB concerning significant AOTEs   —
Normal laboratory values (including revisions with dates these became effective)   —
Laboratory accreditation number and effective date   —
General correspondence to and from the sponsor   —
Documentation of general telephone contacts with sponsor   —
List of study personnel and employment dates   —
Sponsor site visit log   —
Drug accountability records (transferred from medication area at the study's   —
  conclusion
Grant agreement and financial correspondence (these may be removed in the   —
  event of an inspection)

---

are often conducted well after a study has been concluded. Recording administrative information such as the names of study personnel may seem superfluous as the study is proceeding but will be of great use subsequently in interviews with inspectors.

FDA 1572/3 FORM AND CURRICULUM VITAE

An FDA 1572 or 1573 form must be submitted for any trial that involves testing a new drug or new use of an available drug. FDA 1572 forms are to be used for earlier phase studies (Phase I or II) in which the pharmacology of the test agent is still under investigation. FDA 1573 forms should be filed for Phase III and IV studies that primarily involve expanded safety and effectiveness testing. Sponsors will inform investigators as to which of these is the correct document to file for a particular investigation. These forms were developed by the agency to secure the investigator's commitment to conduct a clinical trial in accordance with applicable U.S. regulations. These forms request information on the training and experience of the study principal investigator, the names of the individuals who will be functioning as collaborators under his direction, and the study locations. A sample completed FDA 1573 form has been included in Appendix C. The form is presented to the sponsor prior to study initiation and is then forwarded to the FDA to be added to the test product's IND. The form may be updated during the study should any staff or facility change occur. Instructions for completing either form are as follows:

1. The principal investigator (PI) is considered the primary medical administrator of the study and is responsible for both protocol execution and regulatory compliance. He and any colleagues wishing to share this responsibility as coprincipal investigators must list their training and experience and sign the form on page 2.

2. Many sponsors have begun to limit the choices of PIs to physicians (including osteopathic physicians) for clinical trials. Doctors of Pharmacy are permitted to serve as PIs for pharmacology studies. These are company-specific requirements that should be clarified with the sponsor. Only licensed M.D.'s and D.O.'s should be listed as PIs.

3. The selection of a PI is significant not only for professional purposes such as publication and funding but also for administrative purposes. The PI alone must sign many of the case report form pages or regulatory documents issued during the study. Where feasible, assigning a co-PI facilitates timely document processing. Listing a second physician as either a PI or a collaborator (see below) will assure the necessary coverage should the PI be unavailable.

4. A *curriculum vitae* (C.V.) is routinely attached in place of completing the sections concerning the PI's background and experience. Many sponsors collect the *curricula vitae* of collaborators (see below) as well, although they are not required to do so. The content of a *curriculum vitae* suitable for regulatory submission is specified in Table 37.

5. The term *coinvestigator* is often used in general discussions to refer to physicians participating on the research team. This term has no significance for regulatory purposes. A physician serving on the research team must be either a PI or a collaborator.

TABLE 37. The Curriculum Vitae

  I. Personal data
     A. Name   Social Security #
     B. Birthdate   Citizenship
     C. Office address and telephone
     D. Home address and telephone

 II. Education and degrees
     A. Undergraduate
     B. Medical school
     C. Internship
     D. Residency
     E. Fellowship/other professional training

III. Professional experience
     A. Academic appointments and/or general clinical responsibilities
     B. Research experience
     C. Administrative responsibilities
     D. Special talents or experience—languages, editorial boards, civic activities

 IV. Board certification or eligibility (list dates)
  V. Current licensure (list states, numbers, and expiration dates)
 VI. Hospital affiliations (list years only)
VII. Membership in professional societies
VIII. Publications

---

6. Collaborators are the research team members who prescribe the study medication under the PI's direction. Sponsors usually restrict the listing of collaborators to physicians involved in conducting the protocol or performing invasive study-related procedures. Thus, endoscopists, for example, are routinely listed as study collaborators, whereas ophthalmologists performing routine baseline safety tests are not. Collaborators need not sign the FDA form.

7. The requirement of listing a colleague who covers for the investigator in an emergency will vary with the sponsor. If an investigator is to be absent and he has oriented a colleague who will conduct the study in his absence, this individual should be listed on the form before he takes part in the study. Physicians who cover for the PI in an emergency usually need not be listed on the form, provided that no new subjects are enrolled during that period. In such circumstances, the PI must countersign all reports prepared by the covering physician in his absence.

8. The FDA form should include a listing of all sites at which supplies will be stored or patients will routinely be seen for the purposes of the study. The primary site is defined as the site from which the majority of supplies will be dispensed and

stored. Facilities such as clinics used on a limited basis, those at which invasive study-related procedures are performed, or any facilities at which supplies will be stored are ordinarily listed as secondary sites. Sites of noninvasive tests, such as ophthalmology or audiometry, need not be listed on the form.

REVISIONS TO FDA 1572/3 FORMS

The FDA form must be modified to reflect any changes in medical staff or facilities used for the study. Revisions should be submitted to the sponsor when possible before the new physician begins seeing patients or the new facility is used as a study site. The preferred method of processing amendments to the form is to prepare a new form, revised and dated appropriately, for the PI's signature. This provides clear documentation that the PI has authorized the revision. The addition of a co-PI must be documented in this manner. However, the PI may add collaborators or study sites with a letter written to the sponsor, including the C.V.'s of any collaborators, should the sponsor require them.

PROTOCOL AMENDMENTS/INVESTIGATIONAL USE CIRCULAR

Any new safety or protocol information received from the sponsor should be dated and reviewed promptly to identify precisely how it differs from the previous version and influences performance and regulatory requirements. The PI must determine whether or not to revise the consent document and submit the change for IRB approval. Those changes or updates not requiring approval should, nevertheless, be forwarded to the IRB for its records. Protocol amendments in particular should be signed and dated by all principal investigators and a copy returned to the sponsor upon request. Implementation of amendments that affect the patients but are not new safety measures should be delayed until they have been authorized by the IRB.

NORMAL LABORATORY VALUES AND LABORATORY ACCREDITATION

Any changes in the normal laboratory ranges for study-required tests should be provided to the sponsor with the date on which they occurred. Copies of current laboratory certifications should be retained on file and provided to the sponsor upon request. State certifications or accreditation by the College of American Pathologists are the documents that sponsors most commonly request.

LIST OF STUDY PERSONNEL AND EMPLOYMENT DATES

A simple list of the staff's dates of employment, job titles, and handwritten initials will be of great value for inspections. It is advisable for the team to develop and maintain such a record for each study by having new personnel record their names on a staff list when they join the team. If such a list is not maintained, the investigator might ask his personnel department to produce the necessary information since the study records are being placed in long-term storage.

CHAPTER 23

Record Storage and Access

RECORD RETENTION AND STORAGE

The principal investigator of an FDA-regulated clinical trial must retain the administrative and clinical records pertaining to the study for one of the following periods, whichever is shortest: (1) a period of two years following the date on which the test article is approved by the FDA for marketing for the purposes that were the subject of the investigation; (2) a period of five years following the date on which the results of the investigation are submitted to the FDA in support of, or as part of, an application for a research or marketing permit for the test article for the purposes studied in the investigation; (3) in other situations (e.g., where the investigation does not result in the submission of the data from the investigation in support of, or as part of, an application for a research or marketing permit), a period of two years following the date on which the entire clinical investigation (not merely the investigator's portion of an investigation involving more than one investigator) is completed, terminated, or discontinued, or the exemption (IND) under which the investigation is being conducted is terminated or withdrawn by the FDA.[1]

These requirements are specified in the proposed FDA regulations cited below and are currently being followed by much of the research community. In signing the FDA 1572/3 form, the investigator agrees to abide by a more limited version of these regulations. Sponsors generally advise that investigators plan to retain their records for a period of at least five years following the completion of the study as a whole. They also wish to be notified before an investigator destroys any records so they can have an opportunity to verify that no inspections or

```
┌─────────────────────────────────────────────────────────────┐
│ LONG-TERM STORAGE              Box __ of __                   │
│                                                               │
│              John J. Smith, M.D., Jane C. Doe, M.D.           │
│                    Principal Investigators                    │
│               Scientific Drug Company, Protocol XX-901        │
│                        Completed 6-1-86                       │
│                Records can be destroyed in June, 1991         │
│            DO NOT DESTROY WITHOUT CONTACTING PRINCIPAL        │
│                         INVESTIGATORS                         │
└─────────────────────────────────────────────────────────────┘
```

FIGURE 19. Storage label.

resubmissions of the data are planned. These record retention requirements apply to subjects' clinical records, records of correspondence
with the sponsor and the IRB, and any supporting materials such as
petty cash logs or appointment books.

Following the completion of all IRB and sponsor reporting requirements, provisions can be made for long-term storage of the study records. Each subject's CRF can be placed in his research record for storage
with the study regulatory file in a labeled box. If the records of excluded patients have been filed by study, these can be added to the
long-term storage container as well. Appointment books or logs developed for one specific study should be included in this long-term file. If
appointment books or other scheduling logs were used for multiple
studies, these can be placed in a long-term file storage at the end of the
calendar year. All such boxes should be labeled as in Figure 19.

Chapter 22 on regulatory files lists the items that should be retained in preparation for an FDA or sponsor audit. Regulatory documents, combined with the CRFs, research charts, and all logs in which
study data were recorded, should be retained consistent with the record-retention requirements listed above. As is discussed in the chapter on FDA inspections, study records are best reviewed for completeness before they are placed in storage. Copies of any documents
that have been lost can then be obtained from the sponsor or the appropriate hospital department prior to storing the files.

EXAMPLE 1

*The institutional review board chairman for a company undertaking
extensive numbers of contract investigations moved to another city. His
records were moved to the office of his successor, who maintained them
while the studies were current, then moved them to dead storage maintained by the company.*

Another institutional review board ceased operation as a planned portion of incorporating its activities into a single national committee. All of their records were moved to permanent storage by the contract company. Both of these moves solved a complex problem.

EXAMPLE 2

An active investigator evaluating drugs for hypertension retired from practice and closed out his office records. His office records and research records were intermingled because many of his office patients were research subjects. He was informed that his office records should be maintained for six years after their last entry. Since this requirement met the storage requirement for his drug studies, he kept all of his records intact.

TRANSFER OF RECORDS IN THE EVENT OF RELOCATION

Research records themselves should be stored in a secure location with access limited to the research team. Often they are stored in a locked cabinet or room near the study supplies. In studies on hospitalized patients, research data are ordinarily recorded in the medical record, which must be stored in a manner compatible with hospital policy. Research records remain the responsibility of the principal investigator both during and following a study's completion. If an investigator relocates to a new facility or finds himself unable to maintain study records for the required time period, it is his obligation to see that these are transferred to another party able to assume responsibility for complying with these requirements. Sponsors, IRBs, or coprincipal investigators may be called upon to fulfill this responsibility in those rare cases where the investigator is unable to store them himself. The sponsor must be notified of any such arrangements that are made so the FDA can be advised of the new location of these files.

EXAMPLE 3

An investigator evaluating many office preparations for gynecological use died suddenly. All of his research records were meticulously kept in separate files. His office assistant made prompt arrangements for a new investigator in the same building to complete the several patients under observation. Each set of records was prepared for sending to its sponsor. Approximately one-half of the sponsors accepted them. The remainder were put into storage with his office records. The practice was subsequently sold to another physician. A request for research records after one year indicated that they had been discarded by the new owner. Clearly the sponsors who did not choose to move the records to their

control were lax. The majority of physicians in practice are unaware of
the record-retention responsibilities. When research-related records are
intermingled with office records, it is very difficult for a new owner to
provide needed information.

ACCESS TO RECORDS BY REGULATORY AGENCIES, SPONSORS, AND OTHERS

The FDA requires access to investigators' records as a condition of accepting studies in support of a regulatory submission. This encompasses CRFs, clinical records pertaining to the period of study and establishing the patient's eligibility, appointment books and other supporting documents, drug accountability records, and administrative files of contact with the sponsor and the IRB. It also includes any certifications that the facility meets current standards to conduct procedures required by the protocol. It does not encompass records of financial negotiations between the sponsor and the investigator except in unusual cases where unorthodox practices are suspected. In routine inspections the FDA representative may also copy relevant sections of a CRF or source document *once the identifiers have been removed.* Copies of records that include identifying information should be requested only in the context of a "for-cause" audit in which the agency has reason to believe that the subject's consent was not obtained or that the data themselves are fraudulent in some way. In the latter circumstance, investigators ordinarily seek legal counsel before releasing any such documents.

Under the proposed regulations for sponsors, companies are required to ensure that a research team being considered for participation in a clinical trial has adequate medical and staff resources and an adequate patient population to conduct the study. Thus, sponsors may request a summary of the types of studies being conducted at the facility, with the number of patients and specific disease states involved. They should not be provided with the names of studies or sponsors, however. It is also the sponsor's obligation to conduct reviews of the research data at appropriate intervals during the study to compare research records and other source data with the CRFs. Thus, the sponsor must have access to all records available to the FDA as described above. In its on-site inspections, the sponsor must also verify that any recording of data on the CRFs by personnel other than the investigator is supervised and its accuracy appropriately checked. Such an assessment requires that the monitor observe the study in progress to establish how this review process occurs. The sponsor is also required to determine the adequacy of the facility being considered as a study site and, therefore, should be provided with any special certifications applicable to the type of study being conducted. Arrangements should also be made for the sponsor to visit any satellite facilities. The confidentiality issues discussed above apply to any such visits.

The subject's research chart constitutes his medical record of study care. This chart should be disseminated to providers and third-party payors under the same confidentiality provisions that apply to other health care records developed at the facility. That is, any such requests should be made in writing, accompanied by the patient's written authorization, and should involve only those records needed for the purposes specified in the request. Telephone requests from nonsponsor personnel should be verified with the subject before any data are released. Providers requesting a subject's study record are routinely provided with a copy of his research chart rather than the CRF, since the former is more comprehensive. The original research chart is the property of the investigative team and should not be released.

The chapter on the IRB process includes a discussion of records to which IRBs may have access.

REFERENCES

1. 21 CFR Part 54, Obligations of Clinical Investigators of Regulated Articles, Proposed Regulations, August 8, 1978.

FURTHER READING

American Medical Record Association, *Confidentiality of Patient Health Information: A Position Statement of the American Medical Record Association*, December 1977, 875 North Michigan Avenue, Suite 1850, John Hancock Center, Chicago, IL 60611 (312) 787-2672.

CHAPTER 24

Computer Technology in Data Management

Hardware Requirements • Software Requirements • Scientific Considerations • Operational Issues

As has been discussed in earlier sections, sponsors and PIs face continuing pressure to increase the speed with which they collect and evaluate clinical trials data. The many technological advances that have been made in data processing and telephone transmission in the past several years now offer attractive alternatives to traditional on-site data review methods. Sponsors are continuing to investigate both remote data entry and facsimile transmission as cost-effective methods of speeding the tabulation and analysis of research data. Increasingly, sponsors are approaching investigators to take part in clinical trials in which they will be provided with terminals, PCs, or facsimile machines to transmit study data and secure access to numerous useful reports. Investigators at active research facilities are also exploring the advantages of independently performing on-site data entry to improve protocol execution and permit faster publication of study results. Although the utilization of this automated data collection and reporting has numerous advantages, particularly when the hardware can be used for the investigator's nonresearch activities, it also has some drawbacks. This chapter will outline some of the issues a team should consider before agreeing to take part in such a project.

HARDWARE REQUIREMENTS

An investigator most commonly enters data using either a microcomputer or a terminal that can communicate with the sponsor's computer, often a mainframe. One accesses the sponsor's host computer with a modem that allows the user to execute programs on the remote mainframe. When a microcomputer is used, an investigator can independently store the data at the study site and upload the data to the sponsor's host computer via modem. Removable storage media, such as diskettes or tape cartridges, can also be employed and forwarded by mail to the sponsor at the end of each day. The batched transmission of data is more cost-effective than on-line data entry but does require special communications software that the sponsor must be willing to develop. Terminals are used when a site does not require independent storage and processing capability. The site enters all data directly into the sponsor's computer and must gain access to it whenever any study-related data are needed. Although in the past some of these systems could not function without dedicated telephone lines, dial-up lines now work quite effectively and have further reduced the cost of remote transmissions.

If appropriate software is available, the microcomputer is clearly a superior choice for remote data entry. Aside from its adaptability for other aspects of the investigator's practice, the PC is versatile in allowing investigators to communicate with one another and with a number of drug firms using the same equipment. With this technology, information concerning side effects or new recruitment techniques can be transmitted easily and rapidly to all study sites. Since terminals are more limited than microcomputers in the types of host computers with which they can communicate, investigators using them may encounter physical space problems if they decide to work with more than one firm, each of which finds it necessary to install its own equipment.

The task of transferring data between sites has been greatly simplified with the availability of mass data storage systems for the PC. Several companies now manufacture cassette and aluminum cartridge tape backup systems that allow up to 60 megabytes of data to be stored on a single four- by six-inch cartridge. Another innovative company, Iomega, has developed a disk drive that combines the portability characteristics of a floppy disk with the capacity and speed advantages of a hard disk. Twenty megabytes of data can be stored on a single eight-inch cartridge specially constructed to protect data from contamination and the disk "crashes" that can occur with hard disks. These mass storage systems permit efficient and cost-effective transfer of data between investigative sites or between a site and the sponsor.

A number of pharmaceutical firms also have investigated the use of facsimile transmission equipment and have been enthusiastic about its potential for speeding up submission and review of clinical data. This equipment requires a minimal investment and a modest operating budget now that desktop facsimile equipment is available that can be programmed to transmit data unattended during evening hours when telephone rates are cheapest. Although facsimile technology does not offer data-processing capability, it does provide a mechanism for sponsors to issue immediate feedback on CRF data. In-house review by the sponsor can also eliminate the need for some CRA visits. This technology is useful to the investigator in that it allows immediate written communication with the sponsor on complex cases.

SOFTWARE REQUIREMENTS

The larger pharmaceutical firms hire permanent staff and in-house consultants to create programs tailored to their specific needs. Others procure the services of independent contract firms who specialize in clinical trials software. Whatever its source, software developed for use in a clinical setting must meet several important criteria. First, it must be sufficiently flexible to accommodate cultural and linguistic differences in the usage of medical terminology. Second, the software must allow the team to create an audit trail of all transactions. If any revisions or corrections are made to study data, the original entries must be retained and the new data labeled with the date of the correction, its originator, and, where required, the reason for the change. The software should include prompts to remind the team of procedures that must be performed at certain visits. It should also be programmed with the numerical ranges that are acceptable in fields containing laboratory or other quantifiable data. Sophisticated packages allow the investigator to initial and comment on significant abnormalities directly into the database. Many also include "dictionaries" of terms that are acceptable responses in text fields. Software or SOPs that provide for all data to be entered a second time by a verifying staff member can be useful in assuring that error rates are kept to a minimum. If the system is designed for direct data entry during the patients' visits, it must allow the team to override fields for which data are not available so the interviews with the patients are not interrupted unnecessarily. Finally, the software must offer reasonable security, limiting access to the system to the research team only.

SCIENTIFIC CONSIDERATIONS

The capability for on-line reporting of eligibility and safety data has numerous scientific advantages. First, it would allow the sponsor to randomize new subjects on the basis of the characteristics of the current population, so the comparability of the test and control groups would be ensured. Subjects could also be more easily stratified in the randomization on the basis of the severity of their disease. In addition, remote data entry could effectively reduce the time required to gather and evaluate adverse events, thereby enabling the sponsor to identify serious safety issues more quickly. This capability would also permit immediate review of eligibility data, allowing the sponsor to confirm that subjects are not being selected inappropriately for participation. By its very nature, remote data entry requires high standardized data collection and, if used properly, can reduce the frequency with which missing data, illegible entries, or ambiguous comments are encountered on a CRF. Facsimile technology offers many of these advantages without requiring the burden of data entry functions to be shifted to the investigator.

OPERATIONAL ISSUES

Incorporation of computer technology into an office routine will require some resources in the form of personnel and training. The investigator considering such a venture should be certain that he has a staff member with time available to devote to the task. Since it is unlikely that remote data entry will eliminate the need for paper recording of study transactions, data entry tasks can be expected to add to, rather than replace, conventional documentation functions. This added responsibility can pose many problems for an employee if the data entry function conflicts with other tasks, such as insurance billing and appointment scheduling, that are vital to the PI's practice. The PI must also ensure that the sponsor can provide or finance comprehensive training for the chosen employee, particularly if he has had no previous experience with the equipment. If customized software is being used, this training support should include telephone access to technical personnel who can answer questions about any problems that may arise.

There are also many physical space and technical issues to be considered in performing on-site data entry. Adequate and secure space must be available to store the equipment, a requirement that can pose some hardship if the equipment will be used exclusively for the study. If the team were to become highly dependent upon the system, the local equipment or host computer's "down time" could prove quite inconvenient. The PI should ascertain whether replacement equipment would be provided if any repairs were required on the site's own equipment. Some consideration should also be given to the method by which data will be transferred to the sponsor. If data will be transmitted over telephone lines, the availability of the line and the necessity of being present while these transmissions are being made should be investigated and considered in the budget.

If the equipment will be used for general office purposes as well as for the study, some restructuring of the office routine may be required to guarantee that it is available for both sets of functions. Some offices recruit part-time data entry personnel who work in the evening when the equipment is not required for the research. The investigator and his staff must also make a firm commitment to timely data entry, particularly if the computer will be the source of much of the data relating to subjects' care. If properly used, remote data entry can improve data collection and protocol compliance. The technology is also ideally suited to many of the rote tasks, such as drug accountability checks and appointment scheduling, that are important to the research endeavor.

If the equipment will be used for on-line reporting during subjects' interviews, the PI must assess whether the data entry will adversely affect communication with subjects. If the limitations of the software force subjects to delay responses to questions or to answer them in a limited, highly structured way, the quality of the information elicited during the interviews may deteriorate. In the clinical setting, the PI must also ensure that he will have quick access to drug codes and medical data in the event of an emergency.

Investigators considering on-site data entry as either an individual project or a sponsor-funded activity will be required to support the undertaking with both personnel and office space. If the PI is willing to provide these, he should expect to receive some direct benefits in the form of equipment and timely access to reports of the study data. While remote data entry can produce many improvements in the quality of protocol execution and data collection, its success is highly dependent on the technical support available to support the project. In joining such a project, the PI should be certain his individual interests can be met and that the activity does not merely represent an attempt to shift the burden of data entry from the sponsor to the research team.

FURTHER READING

Houston, D.S., Plotting scientific data, *Lotus* **2**:57–60 (March), 1986.
Javitt, J., Computerizing a medical office, *Byte* **9**:171–182 (May), 1984.
Rosch, W.L., Hard disks and beyond, *PC* **3**:116–147 (September), 1984.
Zucconi, G., A computer in the doctor's waiting room, *Byte* **9**:108–118 (May), 1984.

Drug Accountability

Proper storage and dispensation of study supplies are essential regulatory requirements that can serve to prevent medication errors and produce high-quality studies.

CHAPTER 25

Drug Accountability

Storage and Labeling of Supplies • Supply Dispensation Procedures
• Drug Accountability and Record Keeping • Satellite Facilities
• Supply Transfers • Special Considerations with Controlled Sub-
stances

Research on pharmaceutical products imposes special obligations for their proper storage and dispensation consistent with FDA regulations (21 CFR Part 312). The PI has the obligation to maintain an inventory of the receipt and disposition of the products under study, including documentation of any returns to the sponsor, or destruction of supplies at a study's conclusion. The PI also is expected to assume responsibility for the activities of any of the physicians listed as collaborators on the FDA 1572/3 form who will be dispensing study medication under his direction. It is the PI's responsibility to assure that staff members are thoroughly oriented to the importance of documenting drug-related transactions and to the protocol criteria for dosing eligibility. This section will address the regulatory requirements governing supply disposition and describe mechanisms that can be employed to eliminate many common dispensing errors.

STORAGE AND LABELING OF SUPPLIES

Investigational drugs should be stored in a locked cabinet or closet so access can be restricted to designated members of the research staff. This area should be near the staff's office so a log of supply-related activities can be maintained easily. It is also wise to check with one's hospital pharmacy as to whether the institution requires that the pharmacy store and dispense all medications provided to patients. (If the pharmacy is staffed to provide these services, the staff need not assume this function.) The sections that follow will provide some suggestions for streamlining the dispensation process when a pharmacy is involved. Controlled substances (defined below) must be stored in a locked cabinet or other sturdy enclosure within a locked room for proper security.

Investigators conducting multiple studies must develop systems to prevent errors such as selecting an incorrect drug code or drug kit for a second study of the same medication. Simple coding mechanisms that are clearly posted and known to the patients and research staff greatly facilitate dosing activities.

1. Facilities conducting multiple studies with the same sponsor should store supplies for the different studies in separate locations within the facility. (These are often packaged similarly and could easily be mistaken for one another on a busy clinic day.)

2. Decals can be purchased at office supply stores quite inexpensively to color-code supplies. These can be placed on each bottle or box of medication for easy identification. Marking all boxes and bottles with a red sticker for one study and a blue sticker for another prevents errors.

3. As soon as a patient has been assigned a medication code, it is worthwhile to record his initials in bold ink on each box of medication included in that kit. If the study design is such that it is particularly important that the boxes be dispensed in a certain order, it may be appropriate to highlight the visit numbers as well. The highlighting system should be explained to the patient also.

4. A receptionist or second staff member may be enlisted to double-check the supplies being given to a patient, verifying that the latter has received the correct set.

5. The study subjects can offer valuable assistance in monitoring the dispensation process. If properly oriented, they can verify that they have received the medication that lists their correct initials and study color code. The subjects' involvement will assist the research staff and reinforce their critical role in the study's execution.

Once a study has been concluded, the supplies should be collected by the sponsor or arrangements made for destruction as soon as possible. If multiple studies are being conducted at the facility, the retention of unnecessary supplies does increase the risk of dispensation errors and should be discouraged. Many sponsors can arrange to return partial shipments of used supplies during the study if retention of large quantities poses storage problems. If no arrangements can be made for early return of the supplies, however, they should be packed up and stored away from the medication cabinet containing supplies for active studies.

SUPPLY DISPENSATION PROCEDURES

The PI should expect to receive an initial shipment of study supplies shortly after having submitted all regulatory and budgetary documents to the sponsor. Prior to receiving this shipment, the team should be instructed by the CRA as to whether the staff may open and inventory the supplies and begin enrollment. Some sponsors request that the supplies not be opened until the CRA has met with the team at the initiation visit. If the staff is permitted to examine the supplies and initiate enrollment, it is wise to have two employees perform this function jointly. If any supplies are found missing or damaged, then the sponsor must be notified immediately. Most sponsors allow interim supply shipments to be opened immediately and do not plan a special visit to examine these.

The decision to prescribe study medication rests with the PI and the collaborating physicians listed on the FDA 1572/3 form who are functioning under his direction. Once the medical decision to enroll a subject has been made and documented, the act of dispensing supplies to study subjects is best delegated to a trained member of the staff who can assume administrative responsibility for the day-to-day dispensation activity. The type of documentation needed to verify that a medical entry decision was made is described in the chapter on the research chart. Since continuation of a patient who is already on study often occurs presumptively pending laboratory results, additional medication is routinely provided to patients without obvious safety problems with the understanding that the continuation decision will be reassessed if significant abnormal laboratory results are reported. If abnormalities are reported that necessitate discontinuation of medication, arrangements should be made to collect the supplies as soon as possible so the subject is not unnecessarily exposed to investigational therapy. Coded drug supplies should not be used for the compassionate treatment of a patient who may benefit from known active drug.

If medication is being dispensed by the pharmacy, arrangements can usually be made to call in study medication orders on the day of the patient's visit and to accord the study patients priority in picking up these supplies. Alternatively, some pharmacists will permit the medications to be signed out to a member of the staff on the day of the patient's visit to eliminate unnecessary delays. Since most investigators set aside specific days on which to see study patients, this advance preparation can greatly streamline clinic visits.

DRUG ACCOUNTABILITY AND RECORD KEEPING

An investigator who dispenses supplies from his own facility is considered to be performing a pharmacy function and, therefore, must maintain a comprehensive drug accountability record that has the following three components: (1) an initial inventory of supplies received with identifying information such as lot number, dosage form, expiration date, and drug codes; (2) a chronological record of supply dispensation and returns by patients with a notation by the responsible staff member handling medication (this record should be maintained apart from the CRF and be organized for simple comparison at any time with the actual supplies on hand); (3) a final inventory of supplies returned to the sponsor or destroyed at the conclusion of the study.

Figure 20 offers a sample format suitable for the chronological log to which the inventory forms easily can be attached. The use of a bound log with prenumbered pages is necessary only if supplies will be received in an unspecified number of shipments and if the supplies have not been coded in a manner that would allow an auditor to confirm that all shipments have been accounted for in the log. For most studies, investigators are provided with one shipment of supplies listing all of the drug codes assigned to the site. If a pharmacy will be dispensing the medication, it is best to continue with that pharmacy's own system provided that it is compatible with the sponsor's requirements and records all of the information listed in Figure 20. The company CRA can assist the team in discussing with the pharmacy staff any modifications that may be required to meet the sponsor's needs.

Any shipments received from a sponsor should be accompanied by some documentation listing the package contents, which can be reviewed and initialed as an acknowledgment that the supplies have been examined. Supply returns must also be accompanied by a list of the specific bottles and codes being returned. Ordinarily, the sponsor's on-site documentation of supplies being returned is limited to a count of the number of partial and unopened bottles of each drug code that are being returned. A chronological inventory, which includes a count of the medication remaining in individual bottles, would serve as a reference for any detailed accountability information required at a later date. This inventory is routinely checked against the supplies on hand by the CRA during the study.

Received 10/31/84—15 sets of study medication (coded 333-1 to 333-15) Each set of coded supplies contains 2 bottles of 35 capsules each. See shipping label #1. 1/24/85 Received 15 sets of drug (coded 333-16 to 333-30). See shipping label #2.

			Dispensing record			
Pt # initials	Bottle #	Date given	By whom	# Returned	By whom	When
333-1 FT	1	11-3-84	TS	6 caps	TS	12-5-84
333-2 AL	1	11-4-84	FI	5 caps	TS	12-5-84
-3 TNT	1	11-16-84	FI	9 caps	TS	12-15-84
-4 AM	1	11-24-84	FI	7 caps	TS	12-22-84
-5 BS	1	11-24-84	FI	7 caps	TS	12-23-84
-6 SN	1	11-29-84	FI	6 caps	TS	12-29-84
333-1 FT	2	12-5-84	FI	4 caps	TS	1-7-85
2 AL	2	12-5-84	FI	11 caps	TS	1-7-85
3 TNT	2	12-15-84	FI	4 caps	TS	1-17-85
4 AM	2	12-22-84	WAR	3 caps	TS	1-24-85
5 BS	2	12-23-84	WAR	7 caps	TS	1-24-85
6 SN	2	12-29-84	WAR	8 caps	TS	1-30-85

6/6/85 All used supplies (bottles and pills) listed above from subjects 1 through 6 taken back by CRA, Elisha Marian (see signed inventory #3).

FIGURE 20. Protocol Bristol—333, drug accountability record.

In rare instances, a sponsor may permit a staff member to destroy outstanding supplies of medication and then simply to provide a document confirming this action. This can involve some inconvenience, however, and is a responsibility one should not routinely accept, since it involves arranging for the witnessed physical destruction of the supplies. Mechanisms that are appropriate for this purpose are incineration or dissolving the medication in water. Intact supplies should not be discarded in a refuse container, where they could perhaps be retrieved.

SATELLITE FACILITIES

The involvement of satellite facilities must be coordinated by the primary site so the study randomization scheme is not compromised. A satellite or secondary site is defined as a second facility at which subjects will be seen and/or supplies will be stored for the purposes of the study. Establishing a facility as a satellite rather than a second primary site (which has its own record-keeping systems and supplies) is desirable and appropriate if three conditions are satisfied: (1) The activities at the satellite can easily be coordinated by or with the staff through the primary site office, (2) the satellite can be expected to contribute only moderately to recruitment efforts, and (3) the subjects will be recruited from the same population base and will be seen by the same group of physicians covering the primary site.

The satellite structure imposes obligations regarding randomization, since the patients must be assigned study medication in the order in which they present for dosing from all of the participating facilities. A subgroup of supplies *cannot* be transferred to a satellite and dispensed independently. Study medication kits must be used in sequence so as not to compromise the randomization scheme. For example, Ms. Jones, a patient at Facility X, visits the facility on January 2, 1986, to receive her initial set of study supplies and is assigned Drug Code #001. Thirty minutes later, Mr. Smith, a patient at Facility Y, a satellite of Facility X, visits the satellite to receive his initial medication kit. He will receive Drug Code #002. A third patient, Ms. Reed, who visits Facility X for dosing later that afternoon should be assigned Drug Code #003. Research teams seeing patients at multiple sites routinely schedule clinics at only one facility per day so the next sequence of kits can be brought to the designated facility and assigned chronologically from that site. Unassigned supplies can then be returned to the primary site for the next screening session. Once a medication kit has been assigned, it can be stored at the satellite facility for the remainder of the subject's participation.

If the volume of activity at a primary site will not permit alternating its clinic days with those of satellites or involves separate staff, it is best to plan to maintain a separate inventory of supply dispensation and return at each site. Each site can then record supply transactions in its own log at the time of the patients' visits. The records at the primary site should reflect the date on which each set of supplies was transferred to the satellite. If patients are being seen by one group of staff members who travel to the satellite and maintain their offices at the primary site, the log at the primary site should prove adequate for both sites, provided it is either brought to the satellite on screening days or completed as soon as the staff members return to the primary site office. In such cases, a notation should be made in the log as to where the transactions took place.

SUPPLY TRANSFERS

On rare occasions, sponsors may request that supplies be transferred to another investigator participating in the program. In such cases, a specific listing of the supplies sent, signed by the principal investigator, with a space for the receiving investigator's signature, should accompany the shipment. The signed form should be returned to the originating PI and a copy forwarded to the sponsor.

SPECIAL CONSIDERATIONS WITH CONTROLLED SUBSTANCES

Investigators conducting research on controlled substances listed in any of the Schedules I–V must obtain a DEA registration number, which covers research activities involving the schedule of drugs into which the test product falls. Research involving controlled substances may also be regulated by state and local law. IRBs should be able to provide the address of the state Bureau of Drugs for obtaining information on any state registration requirements.

Under DEA regulation, some research activities may need to be approved separately from practice activities. Authorization is granted separately for approval of research on Schedule I substances and research on Schedule II–V substances. Investigators considering these types of research should check with their local DEA office to discuss whether a separate registration is needed. DEA licensees must reregister annually. A separate registration is required for each site at which the substances routinely will be stored.

The person holding the DEA registration must ensure that those employees or associates who will have access to controlled substances in his facility have been appropriately selected. Specifically, an individual who has had his DEA license revoked or denied at any time should not be allowed access to these medications. Additionally, provisions should be made when hiring new employees to screen for past convictions or narcotic use. It is advisable for employers to inquire of all candidates who may have access to these substances whether they have been convicted of a crime within the past five years or have used narcotics, amphetamines, or barbiturates other than for prescribed uses within the past three years. Furthermore, employers may wish to obtain the job candidates' written permission to verify the accuracy of their responses with the local courts, law enforcement agencies, and DEA, if required. Employers are also expected to apprise employees of their obligation to report any theft or diversion of controlled substances by other employees and to provide a mechanism for confidential reporting of such incidents.

Controlled substances listed in Schedules I–V must be stored in a securely locked, well-constructed cabinet within a locked room. Further precautions should be taken as necessary to guard against theft of these substances. Weekly inventories of controlled substances are scheduled at many institutions to monitor dispensation of these supplies.

Accountability records of controlled substance use should be maintained in a format similar to the investigational drug records discussed above. As an additional precaution, any disposing of controlled substances should be witnessed, with the names of the employees performing the activity listed on the log. These records should be compared at least weekly with the actual inventories on hand and any discrepancies noted with a witnessed signature.

Enhancing Credibility

Inspections and self-evaluations measure the quality of the team's performance and, when used for educational purposes, serve to motivate its members to produce and publicize work of high quality.

CHAPTER 26

Publications and Presentations

Deciding Whether or Not to Publish • *What Can Be Published* • *Ideas for Publishing* • *Steps in Preparing a Publication* • *Common Pitfalls in Writing Scientific Papers* • *Presentations at Meetings*

The publication of a paper, be it in a trade journal, in a peer-edited journal, or by verbal presentation, is of great value to a PI's personal reputation and that of his organization. Such a presentation enhances the recognition of the PI and should be structured to appeal to the desired target audience or readership. This chapter explores the methods of planning a paper, the process by which it is completed and submitted to an editor or a meeting chairman, and techniques for gaining exposure from such a presentation.

DECIDING WHETHER OR NOT TO PUBLISH

Considerations in deciding whether or not to publish are listed in Table 38. By publishing, a PI is accorded not only universal prestige but also the acceptance of his colleagues in practice and the industry. It requires a lot of time and may involve some expense. Companies that prepare publications for physicians usually charge $1000 for this service.

WHAT CAN BE PUBLISHED

Journals accept articles dealing with a variety of research topics, ranging from articles on the characteristics of a particular drug to broader review articles or "how to" papers. Since journals vary widely in content and intended audience, producing a publishable article is

TABLE 38. *Considerations in Undertaking Publications or Presentations*

Reasons for considering publication
  Enhancing personal and company prestige
  Gaining the recognition of sponsors and employers
  Encouraging improvement in the quality of the team's work
  Increasing business
  Establishing to others that the team supports quality research
  Gaining editorial scrutiny of the PI's work

Reasons against publication
  Contribution of an inordinate amount of time and resources
  Revelation of trade secrets
  Belief that one's paper adds almost nothing of value
  Modest value of data

largely a matter of selecting a journal with the reputation and audience best suited to the type of article the PI is able to produce.

Trade journals, particularly those with three-color advertisements, are widely read and usually feature "how to" papers. Peer-reviewed journals are more scholarly, are less well read, and feature high-quality original research. The publication of an article in a journal read by a limited but accomplished professional group is considered most prestigious. If a PI has a solid, unique, and outstandingly newsworthy paper, a prestigious journal, such as the *New England Journal of Medicine*, may be an appropriate vehicle. Otherwise he might consider a journal such as *Drugs*, which has wide readership. The publications with the largest readership are those that contain the greatest numbers of advertisements. This fact may be used to estimate the size and buying power of the readership.

IDEAS FOR PUBLISHING

Any results or techniques that are new and different or save time and money are highly publishable. The basis for the publication may be research experience with a particular drug or class of drugs, experience with a unique study population (e.g., elderly males), or a novel method of addressing a procedural problem encountered in conducting research. Examples of possible topics in these categories are discussed below.

If a team has performed several diuretic studies, for example, some possibilities for publications include age effects (or lack of an age effect) on the metabolic clearance of furosemide, racial differences in the excretion of furosemide, variability in absorption of furosemide in normal subjects, influence of meals on the absorption of furosemide, or effect of posture on the excretion of furosemide. An investigator may also wish to publish an improved method of laboratory analysis that he has developed for a drug, a new interference he has identified, or an unsuspected toxicity he has discovered.

An interesting aspect of a routine study may also be written up as a case report if it involves only a few subjects. For example, a new side effect observed in a small number of patients participating in a sponsored study is often reported in this fashion. The interested PI need merely advise the sponsor of his intent and proceed.

A scientifically interesting side study often can be added to a drug study at little expense. Although an independent ancillary project must be cleared with the statistician designing the study to assure that it will in no way weaken the design (e.g., break the blind), such studies usually are readily accepted. Thus, a series of blood samples could be collected from the well-characterized study population and sent to a collaborator for the determination of atrial naturetic factor.

An investigator in a multicenter controlled trial may gain an opportunity to publish data simply by indicating his interest in doing so. Sponsors usually are anxious to have reports on their data reach the academic community. If an investigator who would like to publish his part of the investigation should find that the sponsor is unwilling, he should persist in discussing his request until an amiable solution can be reached. Whatever the reasons for their reluctance, sponsors do not routinely prohibit an investigator from publishing if he so desires. The investigator need merely assure that he will not upset the sponsor with his action.

Long experience also may qualify a PI to prepare a paper on how to accomplish something that is problematic for less experienced investigators. A PI may have discovered a novel way to recruit patients (direct advertising), a way to predict compliance at one month (use of All-Bran for breakfast), a simple way to verify fasting for taking of blood samples (breath acetone), or a way to verify nonsmoking (urine cotinine). Each of these is of great interest to colleagues performing similar work.

STEPS IN PREPARING A PUBLICATION

Table 39 lists the steps to be considered in preparing a publication. Scientific writing, even for the greatly gifted, is no easy task and requires preparing endless drafts of the rewritten article in an effort to achieve greater clarify of expression. The task is such an arduous one,

TABLE 39. Steps in Publication

1. Identifying a message or question to be answered
2. Setting forth supporting data in a preliminary form
3. Reviewing the work with associates for constructive criticism
4. Exhaustively reviewing the literature to determine novelty[a]
5. Setting forth data in charts or tables[a]
6. Discussing readership and choosing a journal suitable for the type of article being prepared
7. Preparing manuscript in the style of the chosen journal[a]

[a]Services that can be purchased.

demanding self-discipline and patience, that the limitations of time often call for engaging professional assistance in both the writing and the editing. Although ghost writers are sometimes recruited to produce an entire publication, the author faces the risk of being presented with a finished product that does not accurately express his views.

COMMON PITFALLS IN WRITING SCIENTIFIC PAPERS

A common problem with scientific writing is often the very length of the article. Brevity of expression with utmost clarity should be foremost in the writer's mind because it is attractive to the busy reader. The length of the article should also be commensurate with the novelty of the data being presented. Publication costs more than $1 per word published. Thus, the more concise the message, the more it is appreciated. Classic articles often are models of simple communication and should be emulated. The minimal accomplishment is that the reader understand the message.

There are several techniques that can be employed to prepare a publication that is both succinct and of high quality. First, only the data and methods that illustrate the point should be included. Although a PI may have studied 500 hypertensive patients, if only 20 subjects provided the data that are important to establish the thesis, the publication should be limited to discussing those 20.

A tight outline, indicating the question being answered and the flow of the logic, should be made before beginning the writing. It makes the writing and organization easier. Reviewing other articles similar to the one the PI hopes to produce will give the potential writer an estimate of the size of his project. The approximate length of each subsection should be indicated in the outline. It is much easier to limit oneself at the outset to a particular length than to decrease by half a much too wordy effort.

Two weeks should be allowed to pass after each draft. If the draft is reviewed too soon after it is written, the author may be tempted to skim certain sections that are, in fact, in need of revision. Multiple reviews are so necessary to effective writing that sufficient time should be allotted for thorough editing. Colleagues should also be asked to read the work. Even though their views may not seem informed, a PI must consider that they represent readers and, whenever possible, should accommodate their views.

The manuscript that is sent to the editor should be proofread meticulously. References, in particular, should be checked multiple times. The PI should be quite confident that the authors who are referred to have their names spelled properly. Carelessness in manuscript preparation is usually construed as sloppiness in the performance of the work.

PRESENTATIONS AT MEETINGS

Professional meetings or conferences usually contain three types of presentations. First, there are general interest or plenary sessions at which prominent speakers or those with items of great current interest are invited to speak. If a PI has something of general value to say or show, he should not hesitate to communicate directly with the committee officers of the society responsible for the program. Such meetings are usually planned about four to six months in advance. The second type of presentation is the paper or posterboard of general interest that is selected from abstracts submitted for evaluation. The third type is an exhibit prepared for a rented space.

PREPARATION OF AN ABSTRACT. Newsworthiness or excitement should come forth in the text of an abstract. The title should accurately represent the content. However, if the conclusion is not overly exciting, perhaps the title should pose a question (e.g., Do Men over 80 Years Metabolize Estrogens Normally?). Although the answer is yes, the abstract need not reveal this until the end. The first sentence or two should summarize the PI's overall study plan. He should then present precise methods, numbers of study subjects, and results. The conclusions should be presented in such a way that the abstract is like a clash of cymbals with a tremendous crescendo to the final thought.

The author should be certain that the directions are followed meticulously in the preparation (e.g., margin settings or use of a specific form). Many times the abstracts are reproduced by photo offset and all must be uniform.

After submission, the abstracts are reviewed and the ones chosen for presentation are grouped together into similar topics. The PI will be informed of his abstract's acceptance and the format in which it is to be presented.

PREPARATION OF A TALK FOR A MEETING. Preparing a talk for a meeting requires similar attention to the theme and organization of the session. A PI should endeavor to learn as rapidly as possible how much time he has been allotted and exactly what other presentations will be included in his portion of the meeting. If there are several related items on the same subject, the investigator may need to know what the other speakers plan to present. If this is necessary, the PI can develop an outline of what he plans to present and send it at an early stage to the other speakers, asking them to indicate what topics they will cover.

The PI should also ascertain what the expected format will be. Are slides, chalkboard, magic markers, or overhead projectors to be used? The presentation should be organized so that the PI makes about one point each minute, with a clear illustration for each point. The text of the presentation should be written out and read a few times in front of a mirror, with the illustrations, to get relaxed. The presentation can be enhanced by doing dry runs with colleagues, checking the time carefully and arranging to finish with about 10% of the time to spare. Colleagues can critique the delivery and suggest how it can be improved.

PRESENTING A POSTER EXHIBIT. Preparation of a poster exhibit is a great challenge, for the PI must present written data in a small space, usually three by four or three by five feet, and make it self-explanatory. There are usually restrictions on what can be used. In preparing a poster, it is highly worthwhile to list the title and authors as well as the site at which the work was performed. Specifying the exact question that the study addresses also is of value. For the text of the poster, the abstract is generally reproduced and several illustrations of the significant data and the conclusions are presented. A PI may have a detailed handout of the study for the more interested person to take with him. A photographer or illustrator is usually employed to prepare some of the tables, graphs, and illustrations or, rarely, the entire poster.

PLANNING AN EXHIBIT SPACE. Paid exhibit space is a form of advertisement that is designed to attract the interest of potential customers and to enhance the reputation of the PI and the people he represents. The planning for an exhibit starts with an analysis of the cost versus expected gain. The cost of a suitable exhibit is $3000 to $5000. The expected gains are possible research grant offers, contracts, and new customers for services. The likelihood of achieving these goals can be estimated from talking with members of other research operations that have used this device. An advertising consultant is usually employed to put forward the unique features of the PI's operation. These may include a high acceptability of studies by the FDA, rapid recruitment, or early completion of contracts.

The willingness to submit one's work to the scrutiny of colleagues is an important step in establishing the credibility of a research operation as well as enhancing its prestige. Although an investigator may be involved with comparatively few projects that produce major findings, many seemingly routine endeavors have components that are noteworthy and deserving of publication. The PI who is keen enough to identify results and insights worthy of publication will find that these opportunities may serve to motivate his staff and associates to produce high-caliber research.

FURTHER READING

AMA Medical Association Manual for Authors and Editors: Editorial Style and Manuscript Preparation (7th ed.), Lange, Los Angeles, 1981.

Chen, C., Biomedical, Scientific and Technical Book Reviewing, Scarecrow Press, Inc., Metuchen, NJ, 1976.

Huth, E.J., How to Write and Publish Papers in the Medical Sciences, ISI Press, Philadelphia, 1982.

Style Book and Editorial Manual of the American Medical Association, Chicago, 1985.

CHAPTER 27

Preventing Fraud

Origins of Fraud • *Settings of Fraud and How to Avoid Them* • *Suspicion of Fraud* • *Methodologies for Determining Whether Fraud Has Occurred* • *Guidelines for Notifying Sponsor If Irregularities Are Discovered*

The field of clinical research offers numerous rewards to investigators who conduct successful studies of drug safety and efficacy. The most obvious of these are financial remuneration, subsidized business trips, and lecturing engagements that pharmaceutical sponsors offer to their investigators. If the research has significant academic merit, professional recognition also becomes an important motivation for conducting research on new drugs. These professional motivations can extend to the administrative and technical staff as well. In an environment of proper checks and balances, these motivations provide the inspiration for a team to conduct successfully recruited and well-documented clinical investigations. In an environment that is without the necessary resources or medical supervision, these motivations become the ingredients of research fraud. This chapter outlines the characteristics of work environments that can lead to research fraud and discusses how these occurrences can be detected when they occur and, what is more important, prevented.

ORIGINS OF FRAUD

It is the authors' contention that a properly designed system of data management and quality assurance will go a long way toward preventing substantial fraud. The orientation of patients and all staff on the uncertainties of the research process and the desire of the sponsor and the investigator to identify the truth about the agent under study must be continually repeated. Errors, omissions, missed observations or medication, and unkept appointments are constant aggravations in the research setting. These events are to be taken as indications to try a little harder and to educate a little more intensely those involved, rather than as items for pointed reprimand or beratement. The climate for fraud is one in which unreasonable expectations are set in both recruitment and adherence to protocols and minor errors are not tolerated. Although high standards and goals are of great value and must be shared, pursuit of these goals should never be considered more important than the truth.

While this chapter will deal primarily with fraudulent practices perpetrated by employees, it is worth noting that sponsor representatives, principal investigators, or even patients may be tempted to commit fraud for the same reasons that motivate employees to do so. The motivation to do well and be perceived by one's supervisors as a superior performer affects all employees of both the PI and the sponsor and, to some extent, trickles down to the patients. Although the PI may gain more than most by increased recruitment, the research assistant working with the PI and the CRA supervising the PI also profit if the study is completed rapidly and is found to be nearly error-free. Sponsor personnel who falsify records or encourage tampering with research data are most likely acting independently out of fear that they will be penalized if they have not motivated investigators to conduct a successful clinical trial. Sponsors recognize that the liability costs of introducing an unsafe product are much higher than those associated with a slower R&D process. Management is intolerant of employees who give tacit approval to fraudulent practices or suggest that the company encourages these. A principal investigator who fabricates research data, or tolerates or encourages low standards of data collection, may be responding to recruitment pressure from the sponsor, concern about financial security, or a desire to fulfill specific professional goals. Patients provide false history or wrong data on compliance only if they see that their responses earn them the approval of the staff.

Although fraud theoretically can be instigated by multiple sources, there are many ways of reducing the pressures that might lead to this behavior or identifying fraudulent practices once initiated. For example, some sponsor representatives who are pressuring the team to meet unreasonable recruitment objectives may simply require reassurance from their medical monitor that they are being judged on the quality of a study as well as enrollment statistics. Any investigator who perpetrates research fraud cannot likely continue such a practice for any length of time without arousing the suspicion of the staff. Pressure placed on patients to falsify research data largely can be eliminated if staff members are encouraged by their PI to approach compliance problems from an educational perspective, offering guidance as to how

TABLE 40. Methods for Discouraging Fraud

Select staff members carefully, using an interview process that emphasizes personal integrity as a selection criterion.

Orient staff members extensively on the need for truthful reporting of data, and repeat this orientation.

Establish a simple, confidential means of reporting suspected fraud by employees, sponsors, or patients. Evaluate any complaints in a thorough and confidential manner that protects the "whistle-blower" and offers the accused employee an objective review of the suspicions.

Establish expected averages for screening/enrollment and dropout/enrollment ratios and data errors. Conduct audits of each employee's performance at least every 2 months and scrutinize carefully any deviations from these averages.

Periodically spot-check each employee's performance in conducting every aspect of the study. Effective QA programs and CRA reviews all complement one another.

Reward examples of honesty and accuracy in reporting even if the finding caused a subject's data to be disqualified. An "Employee of the Month" award can be established to provide a bonus to employees who demonstrate initiative in the areas of truthful reporting or preserving patient safety.

In evaluating deficiencies in an employee's performance, focus on steps the employee took to rectify an error once discovered. For example, if a staff member forgot to order a particular laboratory test, did he ignore the error or take steps to procure the required sample so the patient's safety would not be jeopardized?

Meet with QA teams and other inspectors from the sponsoring company to learn any new techniques for improving data collection or auditing processes.

If feasible, establish a quality assurance program to evaluate adherence to standard operating procedures. Take advantage of resources available from the sponsor or facility QA team to request more frequent audits.

If more than three persons are involved in the research team, have leisurely open meetings (such as luncheons) to discuss quality, general study problems, or outstanding performance.

---

patients can improve adherence to protocol requirements. There are many checks and balances such as these that can be introduced to reinforce the ethical behavior most employees are anxious to display (see Table 40).

Research fraud usually manifests itself in two forms (see Table 41). The most common type consists of a minor alteration of a patient's medical history or compliance record to cover up an error, omission, or new disclosure that was made by either the staff or the patient in executing some protocol requirement. Staff members, anxious to please their supervisors or unwilling to undertake the cumbersome process of notifying the sponsor of the error, may be tempted to omit the discordant information from the record. For example, a staff member may suppress his discovery that a patient failed to report the use of prohibited medication since he does not want the patient or the study team to

TABLE 41. *Data Points That Are Commonly Chosen for Fabrication*

Entry criteria
  Known disqualifying factors suppressed
  Birthdate altered to meet eligible age range; weight or height altered
  Dates of prohibited medication use altered or suppressed
  History of drug or alcohol abuse or mental illness suppressed
Safety checks
  Procedure reports of previous visits or other patients' visits (e.g., electrocardiograms)
    used for current visit
  Blood and urine samples substituted from other patients
Visit data
  Visit dates altered to fit permitted windows
  Visits fabricated
  Medication counts falsified, with tablets discarded so inventories would corroborate
    false reports
  Diaries fabricated

---

be penalized for the error. Similarly, he may alter the dates of a patient's visit on the center logs and records if he discovers that a scheduling error has occurred or that the patient did not return within the allowable visit window. These omissions are difficult to detect unless the patient is questioned by the investigator on specific data that already were collected by the staff. A good internal QA program or an exceptional CRA may also detect this. Staff members who omit new findings do so largely out of a misconception that any deviations from a protocol, even those unforeseen circumstances that could not be prevented by the most experienced investigator, will result in the imposition of financial penalties on the patient and the facility. (In practice, sponsors rarely penalize investigators for an error or a patient's failure to comply with the protocol unless the deviations reach a threshold that suggests a deficiency in the recruitment process.) The investigator who sets reasonable performance standards and delineates the courses of action available to employees who encounter protocol violations can largely eliminate this problem. A data-management system that provides for a systematic review of CRFs with laboratory slips, petty cash logs, or other records of patient contact is also essential to ensure that more significant fraudulent practices do not develop. A satisfactory QA system also discloses such rigid attitudes and can identify the need for more on-the-job education.

EXAMPLE 1. Prohibited Medication Use

A young woman with an endoscopically proven duodenal ulcer had taken ibuprofen until one month before randomization into an ulcer study. The use of any regular NSAID in the 21 days before entry was a clear exclusion. After one week of treatment, the patient identified a prescription bottle that indicated she had taken ibuprofen regularly until 13 days prior to the entry endoscopy and, therefore, was clearly ineligible. The medical monitor of the sponsoring firm was promptly contacted with these new findings, and the investigator made a request that the patient be allowed to remain in the study because it seemed, in his opinion, an error and not a deception. The medical monitor concurred and the patient was allowed to continue. These data were entered into the medical record, and a letter was sent to the medical monitor verifying permission for this exception. We have encountered a few examples of this sort of information being suppressed to avoid disqualification of the patient.

EXAMPLE 2. Sloppy Entry Review

A protocol investigating an antipsychotic drug required a diagnosis of schizophrenia and two years off certain designated medications for entry. The study continued for one year. A QA auditor reviewing charts found that a patient four months into the trial had been on amitriptyline until six weeks before the trial began. This information had been recorded in the research record and in an abstract from the patient's physician that was also in the research record. This information seemed to have been ignored or suppressed in the eligibility screening of the patient. The PI denied knowledge of this disqualifying factor, as did the recruiting and treatment staff, yet the record was clear. The sponsor was notified and the patient was discontinued from the study.

All other patients in this study were closely monitored for eligibility and no other ineligible patients were identified. One-fourth of the patients were interviewed to verify their attendance at specific visits, lab work done, and their compliance with medication. The records were verifiable and were good. After this additional verification, it was concluded that this error resulted from sloppiness and was not part of a deliberate fraud.

The second form of fraud arises when the research team emphasizes recruitment and compliance as its primary goals and offers actual or implied rewards to the team members who reach these objectives. Investigators or research employees who may feel pressure to increase their enrollment statistics can respond to this stress by falsifying significant medical history data so patients will be considered eligible for a study. Left undetected, this practice can easily lead to complete fabrication of research records. This significant falsification can go unnoticed only in small research facilities, in which the investigator and/or staff members can easily enter into collusion, or in facilities without active medical supervision, in which there are no incentives to report un-

ethical behavior. These major violations can have adverse consequences not only for the subjects whose data are involved but for the
entire study. The investigator has an ethical obligation to provide the
visible leadership needed to prevent such violations. The chapters on
data management and employee training contain many techniques that
lessen the incentives for fraudulent research practices.

EXAMPLE 3. Falsified Eligibility

*An investigator permitted the entry of multiple patients into a study of
NSAID in arthritis who had mild elevation of the transaminase enzymes,
a clear protocol violation, by marking on each record that the very modest elevation was of no clinical significance. The frequency of this deliberate but minor protocol violation was impressive, and a sample of about
10% of the randomized patients was closely reviewed for other criteria of
eligibility. Active arthritis was required on the basis of laboratory findings, examination, X rays, or previous laboratory tests. Of the sample
tested, 3 of 15 patients were clearly ineligible. The research records clearly indicated that the PI had checked the same sources as our auditor but
had systematically recorded the findings incorrectly. Suspicion of fabrication was high, and confrontation with the PI on the matter was most
unsatisfactory. The records of all patients were subsequently reviewed
for eligibility and about 30% were found ineligible. After the first 3 ineligible patients were discovered, the sponsor was notified and the PI was
dismissed for failing to cooperate. The remainder of the staff stayed on
with the study, which was promptly transferred to another PI. The sponsor's representative participated in the subsequent review. Some 65% of
the patients remained in the study as fully eligible. The FDA was notified
and separately audited all of the clinical data and accepted the smaller
group of patients.*

*There can be little doubt that the PI, eager to fill the study, listed
eligibility data that were incorrect. There was no evidence of collusion of
the staff in this activity, because the false data were almost always those
gathered from other physicians by phone, from the reading of X rays that
did not have an original report, or from interactions with subjects.*

EXAMPLE 4. Too Good to Be True

*A blinded study of aspirin tablets versus rub-on salicylate ointment was
conducted in patients with athletic sprains. The end point of the study
was an in-depth interview in which the symptom and medication diary
covering the previous seven days was reviewed. Only one of the research
technicians conducting the study reported that no patients assigned to
her had failed to return for the follow-up and that all had completed their
diaries flawlessly. As some degree of noncompliance is expected in a*

study of this type, suspicions were aroused. Arrangements were made for seven of the technician's patients to meet with an independent auditor. Three of these patients readily admitted that they had requested to discontinue participation but were promised the full honorarium if they agreed to sign the diary prepared by the technician and claim compliance with the medication. Subsequent interviews with the remaining patients assigned to this staff member suggested that the fabrication involved only these three patients.

After confrontation, the technician involved left the facility and secured a new position outside of the drug-testing industry. The results of the audit of these three patients' data were noted on the CRFs so their data could be disqualified. The findings were shared with the sponsor's staff and employees of the facility. The remaining data were included in the submission to the FDA and were subsequently published.

SETTINGS OF FRAUD AND HOW TO AVOID THEM

The leadership of any organization is responsible for articulating the values and standards of performance for which the members should strive. In a research setting, the principal investigator is the health professional from whom the staff will seek direction regarding the ethical standards applicable to clinical and administrative research practices. An investigator who is absent from the scene, or who does not provide the supervision needed to reinforce the values he has articulated, contributes to a work environment that permits fraud. Any employees who are experiencing concern about the ethical conduct of peers, patients, or even sponsor representatives will choose to reveal these suspicions only to a responsible professional whose judgment they trust and who has the authority to investigate the matter immediately. However, in an environment in which the responsible leader is not present with any regularity, employees may become apathetic and lack the motivation to identify, much less report, any such ethical concerns.

The investigator who wishes to establish a strong working relationship with employees must arrange to be accessible for any questions they may have about individual patients or the general conduct of the protocol. While much of the routine communication can be accomplished efficiently in weekly team meetings, the PI would do well to speak individually with team members periodically in order to discuss possible methods of improving performance and problems of special interest. A routine of consistent communication of study information to the team is essential in establishing the PI as the primary administrative authority by ensuring uniform and timely information flow

necessary for employees to perform successfully. When the PI is unavailable by telephone for any protocol-related questions, he should
arrange for a coinvestigator familiar with the study to be available for
any questions employees might have and to notify employees of the
coverage arrangements. Upon his return, the PI should review the actions taken in his absence to ensure that misinterpretations or over-
sights did not occur.

The PI should also be certain to meet with the staff prior to the
sponsor's site visit to verify that CRFs have been completed and signed
for all subjects whose clinical and laboratory reports are available. He
should verify that drug accountability and other facility logs are being
maintained. He also should review the team's recruitment efforts with
the staff prior to the sponsor's arrival and devise a plan of action for
improving recruitment if necessary. Should the team identify any deficiencies in these critical areas, the PI should meet with the sponsor
representative (before the sponsor meets with the staff) to discuss the
corrective action being planned. These efforts should relieve some of
the anxiety staff members may experience when they feel that they
alone are expected to resolve the sponsor's concerns.

The PI who fails to orient new employees thoroughly also exposes
the team to the risk that day-to-day pressures may cause team members
to compromise their personal standards in the interest of expediency.
While experienced research professionals usually recognize that
clinical investigation serves a worthwhile purpose only if it produces
complete and accurate data to determine the value of a particular
modality, new employees just learning the basic research tasks do not
have such insight. In presenting the importance of a role in the clinical
trials process, the authors have had great success in reminding employees that the results of their research efforts potentially will be
reported in the PDR and academic publications for use by the medical
community in prescribing the drug. An appreciation of the fundamental purpose of research is essential in motivating employees to maintain
high standards. Research involves so much detail that the significance
of individual data measurements may easily be lost in the context of the
record-keeping system as a whole. Poorly oriented employees, particularly those who are sensitive to the financial pressures facing industry
R&D and the research facility, may be inclined to view their responsibilities as providing data to support a predetermined outcome. With
such an outlook, fabrication may seem a feasible means of meeting the
study objectives.

In contrast, employees who are strongly committed to the greater
societal and medical benefits of clinical research efforts frequently display the ingenuity and initiative needed to prevent potential violations

or disqualifications. For example, some staff members employed by the authors in the past have been so concerned about patients who have missed visits that they have traveled to patients' homes to collect laboratory samples and to interview them. This ingenuity has spared many absentminded subjects from having their case reports disqualified for noncompliance and has also assured timely identification of clinically significant adverse experiences. These employees clearly understood that test results that were delayed or visits that were missed were of concern not because they represented a blemish on an otherwise flawless case record, but rather because they constituted important monitoring of patients who were receiving therapy of unknown safety and efficacy. In the pressure to meet enrollment and CRF submission deadlines, the medical and scientific rationale for various study procedures can be forgotten rather easily. An investigator who takes the time to remind his staff of the fundamental purposes of the research effort can foster an environment in which these important goals remain the basis for all actions taken by the research staff.

PIs who aspire to have their employees meet ambitious recruitment objectives without sacrificing quality must carefully define their expectations. The investigator who expects perfection from either his employees or his patients delivers a clear message that he does not wish to learn of any incidents that may cause their performance to fall short of the stated goals. While subordinates may have great respect for a leader who is demanding and zealous in pursuit of worthwhile objectives, this admiration will be sustained only if they have confidence that his standards take into account the complexity of the task. The real world of drug testing includes patients who do not qualify for particular protocols, patients who choose not to participate, patients who do not comply with medication schedules, and even patients who suppress facts of their history and compliance to secure the approval of the research team. Employees who are not provided with the guidance and encouragement to report errors of enrollment or protocol execution may be tempted to cover up such transgressions, particularly if the breaches are discovered after a subject has been enrolled in the study. A reasonable attitude toward the inevitable scheduling mix-ups, lost laboratory results, and inaccurately reported histories encourages patients and employees to bring these matters to the investigator's attention without fear. In any complex drug study, the principal investigator is usually presented with protocol dilemmas that are totally new to him. When unique situations do not arise during the course of a project, it is very likely that staff members are failing to report these problems because they feel the investigator really does not want to hear about them.

EXAMPLE 5. Patient–Staff Collusion

An unemployed man was noted to have participated in three placebo-controlled studies of new agents for the treatment of duodenal ulcer. Each of these studies involved an initial endoscopy to verify the presence of an ulcer and follow-up endoscopies performed at two-, four-, or six-week intervals during treatment. One of the employees on the research team became suspicious because the patient's ulcer had not healed after participation in three studies and because he had had all of his appointments scheduled with the same research assistant. A detailed audit of the patient's records was initiated.

This audit revealed that a single endoscopy report had been duplicated and altered to provide documentation of the patient's eligibility for the second and third studies. Patient logs maintained at the facility failed to corroborate at least five visits for which data had been recorded on CRFs. Medication counts and diaries were completed almost without error, although the patient had been erratic in keeping appointments. An interview with the patient was arranged. He praised the person who had conducted his visits but could recall few details of the dates and appointments themselves. The staff person in question denied any knowledge of the irregularities.

These suspicions were followed up with an extensive audit of all records generated by the facility. Further concerns were raised and the research team chose to withdraw from analysis all data for which the facility had been responsible. The sponsors involved and the FDA were notified.

An appreciation of the complexities of the clinical trials process should not preclude a careful evaluation of errors that do occur. This is to ascertain whether mistakes stem from morale problems or an excessive work load. These errors can be evaluated with several considerations in mind: (1) Did the occurrence affect a patient's safety so significantly that disciplinary action should be taken regardless of the employee's explanation? (2) Did the employee openly acknowledge the mistake when discovered and take some action to rectify the problem? (3) How many times in the past have similar errors been made by the same employee or any other members of the staff? The answers to these questions can serve as valuable teaching tools in subsequent training sessions. For example, the employee who forgot to order a pregnancy test on a female patient but went to her house to collect a second specimen should be recognized for his quick thinking. In contrast, an investigator's observation that several employees forgot to order pregnancy tests may suggest the need for the group to implement suitable reminder mechanisms. This constructive problem-solving action will encourage employees to be open in identifying weaknesses in the current data-management system and recommending suitable solutions.

This same openness should be encouraged in any interactions between the staff and patients. Patients who do not fear that they will be penalized for forgetting to take their medication or not completing their diary cards will not likely be tempted to be dishonest in reporting. While noncompliant patients should be instructed as to the importance of medication compliance, safety reporting, and other protocol procedures, they should never feel that they will incur the wrath of the staff for having failed to comply with these requirements perfectly. Some protocols are not designed with patients' medication habits at all in mind. Patients who cannot meet the sponsor's ambitious standards are not necessarily less cooperative than those who have proven able to do so. It is preferable that the sponsor learn of any such weaknesses in the study design so future studies can be modified accordingly.

Recruiting and documentation methods that do not include multiple sources from which to verify visit dates and other important protocol information may also promote fraudulent practices. Employees who may be behind schedule in interviewing patients or completing research paper work will undoubtedly be more tempted to record fraudulent information on a record as a means of "catching up" on overdue paper work if fabrication proves much easier than actually conducting the visits. In contrast, clinic procedures that require patients to sign in at each visit and employees to keep various logs of clinic activity involve such detail that fraudulent documentation would not be a feasible means of escaping their administrative burdens. Medical histories generated in the patients' own handwriting, the logs and appointment books discussed in earlier sections, plus medical and laboratory reports offer valuable information that can be used to corroborate visit dates, enrollment qualifications, and other important protocol data. The principal investigator who combines spot checks of these records with confirming patient interviews encourages truthful reporting.

SUSPICION OF FRAUD

In spite of a PI's best efforts to create a supportive yet challenging work environment for research employees, a rare individual may, nevertheless, find fraud an acceptable tool to further his ambitions or resolve an unmanageable work load. The consequences of these actions can be so detrimental to patients that the PI must always be ready to

TABLE 42. Circumstances Suggesting Fraud

Unrealistically high performance in recruiting and retaining patients in a study, as
   well as an unusually low screening/entry ratio combined with poor and late
   documentation on the CRF
Sloppy and casual attention to logs, medication records, and clinical records,
   combined with a meticulously completed CRF
Error-free patient adherence to visit windows, with no requests for variances made by
   the staff
Absence of original raw documents
Discrepancies between logs and visit dates recorded on the CRF
Complaints issued by patients that they have not received the promised number of
   payments, with petty cash records listing payments that patients claim not to have
   received
Frequent scheduling of visits on evenings and weekends when no other staff members
   or physicians are present
Observations by quality assurance or medical personnel of major discrepancies
   between data produced at the time of patients' visits and that reported on the CRF
An employee wishing to work alone with one patient
Allegations or innuendos by employees about their peers
An employee expressing reluctance to have his colleagues cover his assigned patients

---

face the possibility of fabrication, no matter how unpleasant the prospect might be. Such suspicions will be aroused most often when the PI or a staff member observes a combination of irregularities in data recording and an employee's growing unwillingness to have any of his or her work reviewed by a staff member. Table 42 contains a list of circumstances that, when observed in combination, may suggest some irregularities. Several examples of research involving fabricated data are presented throughout this chapter.

A PI who learns that a sponsor representative is suggesting that employees falsify data should instruct them to respond that such conduct is not compatible with the team's ethical standards and that in the future such suggestions will be reported. The PI should then arrange to be present at future meetings with the representative. A request that the sponsor's CRA initial the stated change in the research record or verify the request in writing will eliminate this behavior. When the behavior is clearly fraudulent, the medical monitor should be notified.

EXAMPLE 6. Dates That Are Not Data

A CRA of many years' employment with the same pioneer drug firm regularly encouraged that visits outside of suggested windows be "adjusted" to fit the window on the CRF so it would pass muster and the case would be accepted. This repeated insistence was brought to the PI's attention and evidence was provided that the request had been complied with on several occasions. The CRFs were altered to show incorrect dates, while the research records were accurate. The medical monitor of the company cooperated in sending a company QA person to the scene, all of the known incorrect CRFs were corrected, and a new company CRA was assigned to the site. Within a year, the original CRA had left this line of work.

In the event that an employee is asked by the PI to falsify data or learns that such practices are occurring in the facility, he should contact a person in authority whom he trusts to report his suspicions. If he cannot identify an administrator or a physician with whom he feels he can discuss his concerns, he should contact the chairman or a member of the IRB. The circumstances that aroused these suspicions should preferably be documented in the employee's personal records so he will be prepared in the event of any future litigation. The understandable fear that such disclosure could result in dismissal should not motivate an employee to withhold any knowledge he may have of unethical conduct. Employees who participate in fraud or remain silent while the unacceptable practices are occurring will undoubtedly face a loss of credibility that will prevent them from being employed in research in the future. While it is highly likely that studies whose data are considered fraudulent will be discontinued, sponsors and institutional authorities will be inclined to protect the employees who have refused to compromise their personal ethics. These employees could then be placed elsewhere in the institution even though they had been recruited exclusively for that clinical investigation.

EXAMPLE 7. Grammar Lesson

Some 10% of the patients entered into a study with duodenal ulcer were found ineligible upon review by the company monitoring staff. An eligibility check sheet was used and was clearly ticked off for each critical item. However, upon review with the recorded research data clear exclusions were recorded that had not led to exclusion. A quality assurance visit quickly revealed the nature of the problem. The PI was a capable, highly overworked physician who neither understood nor communicated well in English, the language of the staff. All questions addressed to him led to a response: "Put them in" (the study) and any effort to communicate the lack of eligibility led to a great deal of noisy words about "that's your job," with no genuine discussion on the matter. A doctor-to-doctor discussion of the problem led the PI to pay major attention to his employee running the study and to employ a partner who communicated clearly and took on the responsibilities of the study. The problem disap-

*peared. The risk to these ineligible patients could have been avoided had
the undersupported, harassed, and intimidated employee sought advice
promptly from the medical monitor.*

METHODOLOGIES FOR DETERMINING WHETHER FRAUD HAS OCCURRED

If an employee, sponsor representative, or patient reports any observations of concern, the PI should document the conversation immediately. Any material that includes the name of the "whistle-blower"
should be retained in a file that is not accessible to any member of the
staff. The PI, the quality assurance staff, or an outside auditor must then
undertake a careful, systematic investigation to determine whether
fraud has occurred. If feasible, the PI most often conducts the initial
inspection to determine the extent of any irregularities. If the scope of
the task prohibits him from conducting the inspection personally, the
inspection can be conducted by a QA auditor or an IRB member not
involved with the day-to-day operations of the facility. The purpose of
this initial audit is to determine the extent of the irregularities and
decide on a course of action appropriate to the findings. The outside
auditor or the PI should follow a written plan listing the critical data
points that will be verified in each subject's chart and record which
patients were audited. Patient interviews by phone or in person may be
necessary if phantom patients are suspected. To further ensure the
objectivity of the process, these audits should be conducted routinely
and should not be limited to circumstances in which fraud is suspected. All employees should already be aware that their work will be
subjected to periodic inspection and that the findings of these audits
will be shared with the staff for educational purposes. If the inspection
is undertaken following a report of suspect behavior, it should be initiated within three working days of the report to the PI.

EXAMPLE 8. Ignored Whistle-Blower

*A long-term protocol required that patients take 80% of their assigned
medication to be allowed to remain in the study. Visits were scheduled at
one-month intervals. At each visit medication counts were undertaken
and diaries reviewed to determine compliance. The facility conducting
the study had enrollment and compliance rates that were significantly
above average. The supervisor of the facility was awarded several bonuses for superior recruitment efforts.*

During this time of heavy patient activity, a new employee who was involved with the study was dismissed after one month for failing to meet minimum standards of performance. Soon afterward, this former employee notified management that she had been dismissed for refusing to discard medication so compliance reports could be falsified. No action was taken to investigate the complaint. Several months later, other irregularities were noted that led to a comprehensive audit of the facility's operations. This audit revealed a number of clear inconsistencies between the facility's records and patients' recollection of their compliance with the medication schedule. These findings confirmed the former employee's report that data were being falsified.

Data involving more than 50 subjects recruited by this team were considered suspect as a result of the audit. The sponsors involved and the FDA were notified and arrangements were made to discontinue clinical trials research at the facility. The data were excluded from any regulatory submissions.

EXAMPLE 9. *The Patient Who Wasn't There*

An undercover narcotics agent entered a study of duodenal ulcer disease but insisted on maintaining anonymity, using a false identity and visiting the clinic when personnel other than one particular research assistant were not present. All of this patient's transactions were conducted by this same assistant, usually in the evenings or on weekends. When a QA auditor called the contact number, he could not identify anyone who knew anything about the patient. The physical examination described a voluptuous young woman of memorable physical features. The overworked middle-aged physician who signed the typed physical exam report verified the signature but pronounced with certainty that he had not examined such a woman. Further investigation revealed that two large panels of screening biochemical and hematology tests on Ms. X and another patient seen the same day were essentially identical. The evidence was clear that this patient was a total fabrication. A PI who provided little or no guidance and a doctor who signed a pile of papers without knowing their content and allowed many visits to occur after hours without investigating them enabled this fabrication to occur.

To conduct such an inspection, a review of CRFs and supporting data should be performed on a percentage of the patients to determine whether any irregularities are present. In most research settings, the records of at least 5% of the participants should be reviewed in their entirety along with the records of any subjects whose data have been reported suspect. CRF and research records should be compared with all available logs to confirm visit dates, procedures performed, and medication compliance. Reports of test results should be reviewed to determine whether these were altered or if original documents were replaced with falsified photocopies. If irregularities are noted, the audit should be extended to all patients' records. Further suspicions of irregularities require interviews with patients. At these sessions the patients' recollection should be tested on major aspects of the protocol, such as the number of diagnostic procedures performed, medication habits, payments received, and the number of appointments kept. These audits are best conducted by an outside professional, such as an IRB member or a consulting physician, since some patients or employees may prove reluctant to speak openly with the PI if in the past they had felt unable to approach him with any suspicions. The details of the audit process should be recorded meticulously in case any documentation is required to support the auditor's conclusions.

This audit should provide sufficient data to establish one of the following: (1) altered data are certainly present; (2) suspicious signs of alteration exist, though no clear inconsistencies were noted; (3) no evidence of fabrication exists, in spite of sloppy data recording; or (4) the study has been documented thoroughly and accurately. A summary of the findings of the audit should be shared with both the employees and the physicians. A review that is thorough and passes muster confirms that the facility is conducting the study in a highly ethical manner and offers a means of recognizing the achievements of employees.

If the audit reveals some uncertainty about the authenticity of the data, the employee involved must be questioned about the suspicious behavior and be reminded of the proper procedures for recording data. The incident should be recorded in the employee's file with a clear statement of actions to be taken if any irregularities are noted in the future. Provisions should be made promptly to observe the employee interacting with patients and recording data, so that deficient practices can be corrected.

If any clearly altered data are discovered, they should be presented to the sponsor with an explanation of how the conclusion was reached as to their fabrication. Employees who have participated in fraudulent practices must be removed quickly from any role involving data collection since their credibility will have been compromised. Employees who have been involved in any fabrication that has jeopardized patient safety must be released expeditiously. Whatever disciplinary action is taken, the employee's personnel record should contain a summary of the initial suspicions, the action taken to investigate them, the findings of the investigation, and the discussion with the employee and its outcome. With some effort, a detailed description of the circumstances can be presented without violating the confidentiality of the individual reporting the concerns.

EXAMPLE 10. *The Drug That Wasn't There*

Patients with mild hypertension (defined as blood pressure ranging from 140/90 to 150/105 mm Hg) were needed for a long-term study of a new antihypertensive agent. Following a placebo washout period to establish that stable hypertension was present, subjects were administered active medication in increasing doses for two to four weeks until the hypertension was controlled or a preset maximum dose was reached. One of the participating physicians referred many patients over the course of a few months, most of whom had to be discontinued because the maximum allowable dose of medication failed to control their blood pressure. When this phenomenon was first observed, diaries and compliance records were reviewed and the patients reported to have taken appropriate quantities of medication. All subsequent patients this physician had referred had urine specimens collected and analyzed by the sponsor for the presence of active drug. None of the patients remaining on active medication at the time of the analysis had the experimental drug in their urine despite their assurances of compliance. Collusion between the referring physician and the patients was suspected and confirmed by seven of the patients.

All patients supplied by this physician were excluded from the regulatory submission. The sponsor was notified of the findings and supported the investigator's decision.

GUIDELINES FOR NOTIFYING SPONSORS IF IRREGULARITIES ARE DISCOVERED

Once it has been established that any CRF data are of questionable authenticity, the sponsor must be notified so these data are not included in any efficacy analyses. Since the sponsor must avoid the appearance of selecting data to include in its FDA submission, the company will likely be reluctant to exclude a patient without clear documentation of the reasons for the decision. If data on a group of patients cannot be supported because the investigations indicate that some of the observations were fraudulently reported, a clear notation on the CRF to this effect with a cover letter detailing the findings constitutes sufficient notification. These CRFs must be submitted to the sponsor even if they will not be included in any efficacy analyses so the necessary safety reporting and accountability for the study medication can be performed. Although a minority of sponsor personnel may discourage reporting potentially disqualifying events, it is the principal investigator's prerogative to sign only those CRFs representing cases with which he is satisfied. While auditors and FDA personnel may ask to review the documents that led to this decision, they will usually accept the investigator's assessment of the findings.

When fraudulent data are discovered in more than one CRF, the sponsor and the FDA should be made aware of the problem as early as possible. Although financially costly (in more than 75% of reported cases, sponsors make no payments for such patients), these occurrences should be uncovered and reported openly so the investigator can preserve his integrity and professional reputation. Although a PI may fear that evidence of fraud will jeopardize his professional standing as a responsible investigator, sponsors and regulatory agencies customarily have exhibited greater understanding toward PIs who report such findings than toward physicians who depend on outside auditors to unearth serious irregularities.

Clinical research serves a worthwhile purpose for both society and the sponsors only if it produces accurate conclusions about the safety and effectiveness of agents under study. Any research participant or employee who distorts data jeopardizes the interests of both the study population as a whole and the sponsor, the two parties who will bear the most significant costs should any inaccurate conclusions be drawn from the study. The PI has the difficult role of providing active, concerned leadership that constantly highlights standards of performance that are compatible with both productivity and personal integrity. He must steadfastly provide the assurance that systems to monitor the quality and authenticity of the data collection process are established, maintained, and used for educational purposes to reinforce the importance of truthful reporting. In creating a supportive yet challenging environment, the PI must also be prepared to face the fact that individuals unable to meet these standards may resort to fraud to achieve their perceived goals. The PI who is keenly attentive to the pressures employees, patients, and sponsors face in fulfilling their study responsibilities and who thoughtfully assists them in overcoming these frustrations will likely produce a truly superior research effort.

CHAPTER 28

Quality Assurance

Types of QA Activities • QA for a Simple Study • QA in Larger Operations • QA and SOPs • What QA Must Accomplish • Criteria for a Successful QA, PI, and Administrative Relationship

Quality assurance, henceforth referred to as QA, is a monitoring process within an investigative group, be it large or small, that measures and documents how well the PI and his staff are doing what they wish to accomplish. A QA program is structured to allow an independent observer the opportunity to evaluate how well the team is conducting the study—specifically, its level of compliance with current regulations and the team's own standard operating procedures. Quality assurance usually includes some scrutiny of the actual data-collection process as well. Larger research organizations have a person or even a department devoted to QA functions. In smaller facilities, each person on the research team may be given a small assignment to observe and report on a section of the operation in which he is not directly involved. Alternatively, a person working in the field who understands the nature of the work can be engaged to provide part-time QA services at an affordable price. Whatever the arrangement, QA is usually conducted on about 5 to 10% of all activities at most facilities.

TYPES OF QA ACTIVITIES

QA activities should have a measurable outcome. To that end various data-collection activities are selected and compared with the standard operating procedures or protocols that outline how the activities must be carried out. Table 43 provides some examples of QA.

It is to be expected that the majority of these comparisons will indicate that the PI and staff are fully compliant with regulations. How-

TABLE 43. *Quality Assurance Activities to Conduct and Report*

Observation of data collection compared to protocol
  Timing of samples, drug ingestion, meals
Comparing various clinical procedures with SOPs
  Techniques of collecting, separating, and storing blood
  Laboratory procedures
  Adherence to procedure for repeat abnormal tests
  Presence and functioning of safety equipment
Comparing various protocol procedures with SOPs
  The informed consent process
  Review of laboratory reports
Comparison of CRFs with raw data
Comparison of research records with logs, appointment books, and records of drug
  dispensation
Comparison of research records with patients' accounts of visits, payments, blood
  samples, etc.

---

ever, it is surprising that even in the best-run outfits occasional lapses do occur. These deviations may suggest the need for more training, more diligence, and, occasionally, changes in work assignments or loads. Sometimes the QA process reveals that an SOP is obsolete.

QA FOR A SIMPLE STUDY

A gynecologist is undertaking a study of a new formulation of two standard and proven ingredients for the treatment of monilia vaginitis. The new formulation used as a vaginal suppository is being compared with a marketed product in a blinded fashion. Patients are identified in the doctor's office, smears are made for monilia, and the patients are recruited at that point. Patients currently on systemic and antifungal drugs, using intravaginal medication, or allergic to either of the two test ingredients are the only ones excluded. The office nurse administers the informed consent and the questionnaire of symptoms. Each patient is given sufficient medication for eight days from manufacturer-prepared kits that appear identical and have identical directions, though, in fact, only one of the two preparations is given. The patient returns in six to eight days for a repeat examination, including smear by the doctor and a repeat interview by the nurse.

A satisfactory QA program would include a review of the recruitment qualifications, the informed consent process, the compliance with medications, and the CRFs. A sample of the smears that the doctor looked at verifying the monilia could be reviewed in pathology. A

Conducted in office of Dr. John Phillips 6/18/86: Six of 84 completed patients had charts reviewed, specifically, subjects #4, 14, 24, 34, 54, and 74. All charts documented that the patients had been in the study and contained signed informed consent forms. Subjects 24 and 34 were reached by phone and confirmed participation in the trial and the informed consent process. Both improved; neither had unpleasant side effects. During the audit, patient 87 was entered. The patient's slide was separately reviewed in pathology and diagnosis confirmed. The informed consent and review of exclusions were witnessed by observer. It was noted that Katherine Sampler, R.N., performed all tasks according to protocol. Patients 85 and 86 returned with pills and diaries. Both were reviewed and were confirmed by observer to be in order. The observer had no suggestions for improvement.

Marie Reed, R.N.

FIGURE 20. QA report on treatment of monilia vaginitis 6/20/86.

separate person (a technician or another nurse) could review a small sample of the charts to verify that the charts fully document that the patients are qualified and that they participated in the study. A few of the patients could be telephoned to confirm that they were in the study and asked details about the informed consent. A good QA program would include an examination of 5 to 10% of the transactions. The methods of QA should be documented in a report indicating what was done and what was found.

A satisfactory QA report might well be the report of the sponsor's CRA. An example of a QA report on the above study is shown in Table 44.

QA IN LARGER OPERATIONS

Regular, planned QA assignments by an outside scientist must be carried out in order to avoid neglecting this important function. QA should investigate every substantial portion of the data-gathering operation. All of the items in Table 43 should be observed at one time or another. The adherence to the entry requirements and exclusions and the observations demonstrating efficacy should be meticulously observed. Safety features and compliance to the treatment also require observation. When a single full- or part-time QA person cannot be hired, it is possible to assign five or six different employees so each observes one function for about one hour per week and writes a report. This usually will provide all needed information. An outsider or a separate employee usually can perform better than regular employees, who may be intimidated about auditing their co-workers.

QA AND SOPS

All research facilities conducting multiple studies must develop some standard operating procedures (SOPs). The methods of separating and preserving bloods until analysis, the choice of laboratories to conduct the analysis, the postural position of patients after single-dose bioavailability, and the relationship of dosing to meals are all examples of items that may be important to a study. Thus, some procedures should be established as to how they should be carried out. SOPs are also useful for record storage, specimen pickup, and lab slip review. QA has a specific responsibility to see that SOPs are being followed and, indeed, that pertinent SOPs are available for use in staff instruction. Safety SOPs are essential for such things as how to get a patient with serious side effects to the hospital, how to choose the hospital, and how to inspect or replace the research facility's own resuscitative equipment so it will be available for an emergency.

SOPs are usually resisted in small operations, but they are valuable in the training and protection of employees, in allowing the PI to set the standards by which he wishes to be judged, and in clarifying aspects of the study that are confusing. Examples of three SOPs follow:

· EXAMPLE 1. SOP When PI Is Unavailable

All medical matters are referred to the doctor covering my on-call schedule. 301-243-1771 will reach a physician. All administrative matters should be taken up with Mrs. Anne Wolper, who can be reached at 246-8910 work hours or 247-8910 at home. If hospitalization is necessary, refer patients if possible to Mercy Hospital. We have an account with Speedy Ambulance Service (242-7221) to transport these patients.

Signed: Philip Dartmouth, M.D.

EXAMPLE 2. SOP on Responsibilities of Mrs. Anne Wolper

Mrs. Wolper acts as research assistant to me on SKF study 312469. She screens patients, administers the informed consent, reviews diaries, can provide patient medication except for the first visit, arranges appointments, and contacts patients frequently with the results of their tests. She does not conduct physical examinations, evaluation of reactions, or review of laboratory work.

Signed: Philip Dartmouth, M.D.

EXAMPLE 3. CPR Requirements

All physicians, nurses, phlebotomists, and research assistants with any patient contact must have a current American Heart Association basic

TABLE 45. *Useful Areas for Creating SOPs*

Delegation of staff responsibility
  Delegated duties of each staff person
  Arrangements when PI is absent
  Responsibility for medication release
Protocol clarification
  Separation and storage of specimens if not in protocol
  Pickup procedure for specimens
  Review of returned laboratory tests, procedures, and consultations
  Dosing procedure, mouth inspection, position after dosing, and timing in relation to
    food and drink if not part of protocol
Operations
  Watch and clock synchronization when several clocks are used
  Storage of research records and CRFs
  Checking of safety kit equipment and supplies

CPR card. *Employees must obtain this as a condition of employment within six weeks of being hired. Employees whose cards expire after six months or more with us are to arrange for renewal but will be paid three hours' salary upon showing an updated card. Dr. Riley will maintain records of the date of each employee's most recent certification. A photocopy of the updated card should be submitted to receive the salary payment.*

CPR equipment will be checked weekly by Sally Morgan, R.N. Ms. Morgan also will orient all new employees to the location of the equipment and procedures for notifying her if it is used so it may be promptly checked and any missing materials replaced.

Signed: *Philip Dartmouth, M.D.*

Table 45 provides a listing of functions for which SOPs are valuable.

WHAT QA MUST ACCOMPLISH

QA produces documentation that both the staff and PI are following protocols and SOPs, are recruiting appropriate patients, are administering appropriate informed consent, and are following up the patients according to the dictates of the protocol. In fact, QA, particularly when unannounced observations or audits are conducted, exposes inadvertent errors in performance or other omissions, unallowable shortcuts, and slight protocol deviations that can become the basis for education and future improvements in performance. A recent QA audit in the authors' organization showed that the nurses were *not* questioning all subjects about allergy to the agent under study (even though this was clearly in the SOP), and that the physician was *not* initialing and dating *all* lab slips required for entry before the patient was dosed, and the emergency tray was lacking two drugs required to be present in the SOP. Needless to say, the specific derelictions came as a surprise to the personnel responsible. However, the QA intervention immediately effected the correction of the problem.

Sometimes QA auditors can suggest possible solutions to problems or inefficiencies. For example, a QA auditor found that several watches on different participants' wrists were being used to time medication administration and drawing of blood samples. On the day of observation, these three watches varied by as much as 15 minutes. No SOP existed for watch and clock synchronization and no one had thought it important. The QA observer suggested that the clocks be synchronized promptly and that the four blood samples taken at incorrect times be labeled with the time at which they were actually drawn. An SOP was subsequently written and a single wall clock purchased for use with all subsequent studies.

Quality and the entire operation become better with effective QA. Fraud prevention is much easier because QA assures that many specific checks and balances are undertaken in the form of sign-in books, logs, and research charts.

CRITERIA FOR A SUCCESSFUL QA, PI, AND ADMINISTRATIVE RELATIONSHIP

QA points up problems, the majority of which can be corrected simply by the notification of their existence. Almost all employees want to do their jobs well, and when QA points out a shortfall it is usually corrected promptly. Sometimes QA points out problems that do not have immediate solutions, such as recurrent errors, patients getting into a study without a sickle cell test, failure to get laboratory tests back in a timely fashion, or long waits for specialty physicians. These must then be addressed systematically by the PI or the administration.

It is urgent that the findings of QA reach the people who can determine what must be corrected. A good QA points out many things that are minor, undesirable items (e.g., room very uncomfortable on a very cold outside day because heat could not be turned up any higher, the area for phlebotomy is cluttered, or subjects' complaints that the food is inadequate in amount). Sometimes problems are pointed out that cannot be corrected easily. For example, there are not sufficient toilets and showers to accommodate the 40 patients who are studied at one time. It may be agreed that a problem with the lavatory facilities exists, but a planned move to a larger facility in 60 days precludes any short-term solution.

Other items affect ethics, safety, or credibility and must be addressed almost instantly. For example, Mr. A.N., phlebotomist, was observed to take blood according to the protocol but did not attach the identifying label until after six to ten blood samples were obtained. Although the blood samples were in order in the rack, it was clear when the labels were being attached that there was some confusion as to which blood went with which label. Patient 13 was observed to take the tablet given by the nurse and palm it between his fingers while pretending to swallow it. Later the pill was recovered from his pocket. These deficiencies require a review of the procedures and prompt correction. Thus, the phlebotomist should be reminded that every sample must be labeled when taken (SOP already exists). The nurse must observe that the pill is swallowed by inspecting the subject's mouth or actually delivering the pill into the mouth if necessary.

It is the clear responsibility of the PI to review each QA report and to check things that deal with the important parts of the operation. Then he, with his staff, must institute the necessary corrections.

FURTHER READING

Skillicorn, S.A., *Quality and accountability: A new era in American hospitals*, Editorial Consultants, San Francisco, 1980.

Spath, P., *Cost effective quality assurance*, Brown-Spath and Associates, Portland, 1984.

CHAPTER 29

FDA Inspections

Scheduling the Interview   •   The Interview Process   •   CRF and Administrative Record Inspection   •   Exit Interview   •   Types of Findings

The FDA conducts inspections of sponsors, investigators, and IRBs as part of its Bioresearch Monitoring Program. Its inspections of sponsors encompass manufacturing, laboratory testing, and clinical trials, while its inspections of IRBs and investigators are limited to research activities. This monitoring program represents an effort to coordinate the regulatory compliance responsibilities of the many FDA bureaus (Drugs, Biologics, and Devices) that oversee research activities.[1] The FDA views its inspections of investigators and IRBs as vitally important in determining the extent to which the research community is complying with current regulations and ethical standards governing research on human subjects. While this chapter will address itself to the FDA inspection process as it relates to clinical investigators, the reader, nevertheless, should be aware that inspections of IRBs do occur routinely and are carried out by the same FDA field personnel who audit clinical investigators in a particular geographical region. Thus, these IRB inspections, which necessarily involve the records of investigators' submissions to the board, can often provide valuable clues regarding the research practices of particular institutions and may suggest the need to initiate inspections of specific investigators. The Bioresearch Monitoring Program has a twofold purpose: (1) to assure that current regulations applicable to sponsors, investigators, and IRBs are being followed (Table 46) and (2) to assure that the data submitted in support of an application to market a new drug is supported by adequate and accurate clinical records (Table 47). This chapter will outline why certain investigators come to be selected to undergo inspections and how the agency goes about determining whether the regulations have, in fact, been followed in conducting a clinical investigation.

    The agency was granted the authority to inspect clinical investiga-

TABLE 46. FDA Inspector's Audit of Investigators

Review of the sponsor's visit(s)
IRB process
  Dates of approval and start of research
  Changes in protocol
  Final reports
Test article accountability
  Procedures for documenting transactions
  Inventory records
  Site of storage
Protocol and consent processes
Records regarding subjects
  Establish eligibility
  Establish consent
  Establish participation
  Adverse events and reporting
  Retention

---

tors in the 1962 Kefauver-Harris amendments to the Food, Drug, and Cosmetic Act. Under this legislation, the FDA can refuse to accept study results containing data to which the agency has been denied access for inspection purposes. Also, the agency can prohibit investigators from conducting regulated research or prosecute if an inspection reveals fraud or flagrantly substandard performance. FDA inspections of investigators are of two types: (1) routine inspections of randomly selected sites that have participated in submissions currently under review at the agency, and (2) "for-cause" investigations of sites at which serious regulatory or ethical deficiencies are suspected. As a regulatory rather than a funding agency, such as the NIH, the FDA is unique in conducting inspections of investigators that can be used as a

TABLE 47. FDA Inspector's Audit of Data

Subjects
  Confirm eligibility and adherence to protocol
  Reporting on dropouts and reactions
Test article
  Do raw documents confirm administration?
  Other
Lab tests—site and quality of performance
Documentation
  All reports
  Monitor visits
  Work load of investigator
  Reports of adverse experiences

---

basis for criminal prosecution if fraudulent practices are discovered. Alternatively, a study conducted according to the agency's standards inspires great confidence in the data on which the FDA must base its decision to approve a new drug or indication.

In addition to IRB records, ready sources of information regarding an investigator's research practices are available from the sponsor for the FDA. FDA 1572/3 forms, many actual case report forms, and sponsors' summaries of each investigator's performance on a study are included in the IND and NDA filings made on new drugs. This database can be used to identify physicians who are conducting multiple studies in the same disease state and to review their enrollment practices, particularly the recycling of patients into several studies. Review of case records and summaries also allows the FDA to identify sites whose data appear too "clean" or whose recruitment successes seem unrealistic.[2] This close scrutiny of research records and an investigator's work load reflects the agency's recognition of the many pressures that may lead investigators to falsify data or compromise enrollment practices to satisfy recruitment goals.

"For-cause" investigations occur following reports of serious violations found in a routine inspection or may follow an investigator/sponsor-initiated report to the FDA of problems encountered. A report of suspicious practices received from an investigator's patients, sponsors, colleagues, or employees may instigate an inquiry. A for-cause investigation is initiated primarily to determine whether any documents relating to the informed consent process or confirming the subjects' actual existence or participation or full qualification may have been falsified. Although other offenses may be cited in such an audit, the failure to solicit subjects' informed consent and any fabrication of research records are considered fundamental ethical violations that warrant disqualification of the research data. For the most part, a for-cause investigation is limited to the specific area under suspicion.

While the prospect of having one's research activities subjected to such close scrutiny may prove intimidating to a new investigator, the majority of inspections reveal very few violations requiring regulatory action. In the Shapiro and Charrow article,[2] its authors found that fully 88.5% of the routine FDA inspections conducted from June 1977 to September 1983 revealed either no deficiencies or only minor irregularities. Nevertheless, agency personnel tend to view an inspection as an enforcement activity and may approach the audit with the expectation that irregularities will be found. The main purpose of this chapter is to acquaint the investigator and his staff with the components of an FDA inspection, placing emphasis on how to ensure that the audit proceeds as smoothly as possible. A positive audit experience serves a valuable purpose of familiarizing the research team with the high standards and objectivity with which the agency reviews documentation supporting a clinical trial.

SCHEDULING THE INTERVIEW

The FDA inspector will contact an investigator several days in advance to schedule an appointment. The inspection will be scheduled to review a specific study, which will be identified in advance. The audit routinely will not be extended to other studies unless questions or problems arise. While it is not advisable to postpone an audit for more than several days, the investigator may insist that sufficient notice be provided so the necessary records can be assembled and key personnel and any other commitments rescheduled to allow adequate time for the interview. The inspection can be expected to last anywhere from a few days to two weeks, depending upon the size of the study and the quality of the research records. Although the agency does have the authority to inspect an investigator at any time during the study, routine inspections occur most commonly after a study has been concluded. In fact, since many inspections may occur up to two years after a study's conclusion, sufficient care should be taken to assemble the records and verify that they are well organized for the audit. Before beginning the inspection, the FDA representative should present an FD 482 form, which constitutes the notice of inspection, and an identification badge. An inspector who does not display this identification should not be admitted into the facility.

The decision to conduct a for-cause inspection is made at a supervisory level within the FDA, and the investigator should be notified of it at the time that the audit is scheduled. This notice gives the investigator time to make provision for legal counsel to be present if he wishes to do so.

THE INTERVIEW PROCESS

The initial interview with the inspector is designed to elicit information on how the study was conducted and the extent to which the sponsor was involved with the research team during the study. The FDA is concerned with the sponsor's role in supervising the study since the proposed FDA sponsor/monitor regulations emphasize the sponsor's responsibilities to select qualified investigators and properly inform them of their regulatory responsibilities. Additionally, the FDA is heavily dependent on sponsors to communicate data on serious adverse events promptly to the agency. A well-established sponsor–investigator relationship is essential to the successful fulfillment of these very vital functions.

This preliminary discussion of the study procedures gives the inspector a perspective from which to review clinical and administrative records. In particular, the inspector will wish to learn how prospective subjects were identified, selected, and followed for safety and compliance, as well as procedures for administering study medication. Also, the inspector will inquire about the investigator's work load to ascertain whether he had the time available to devote to the study. Following an inspection of the facilities, the bulk of information pertaining to the study will be gathered from a review of the study's clinical, IRB, and drug accountability records. At this point, a list of the names and roles of the study staff with their handwritten initials and dates of employment will facilitate the audit.

For-cause inspections will require a preliminary interview if no previous audit has been conducted so the agency can learn the essentials of how the study was carried out. The results of this initial audit will be used later, if the need arises, to determine the necessity of interviewing subjects, employees, or other affiliated investigators to evaluate suspicions of fraud.

The PI is expected to be knowledgeable about all major aspects of the study and should be able to answer all questions on critical regulatory and scientific practices such as subject selection, safety reporting, and informed consent. If feasible, the PI should review the study before the inspection with the personnel involved to highlight any issues requiring clarification. The inspector does not have the authority to question employees so they need not be made available unless the investigator wishes to do so. Any employee who is likely to become involved in the inspection should be given some instruction prior to the audit. Experienced industry and FDA representatives have recommended that an employee being questioned in an inspection "respond only to the question asked, respond only with the answer that is responsive to that question, and respond only in the area for which that employee has direct and immediate responsibility. An employee [also] shouldn't be afraid to tell the inspector that he or she doesn't know the answer to the question" that was posed if that is the case.[3] Employees need not be apprehensive about the audit process. However, they should recognize that it is a serious activity, which can serve as a basis, albeit rarely, for instituting legal proceedings. Questions should be answered only when an employee feels confident that he has sufficient knowledge of the circumstances surrounding an event to make an informed response.

CRF AND ADMINISTRATIVE RECORD INSPECTION

The major portion of the FDA inspection involves a review of raw data, supporting information presented on the CRF and documentation of the team's compliance with the IRB regulations. The items covered in FDA audits are summarized in Tables 46 and 47. The article on scientific misconduct in clinical research by Shapiro and Charrow offers valuable insight on the types of noncompliance found most often in routine inspections. Of the subgroup of 415 investigators (out of the 964 who made up the study) audited from July 1981 to September 1983, deficiencies were found in the following areas: (1) informed consent document (61%), (2) inadequate drug accountability (31%), (3) protocol nonadherence (27%), (4) inaccurate records (22%), (5) unavailable records (4%), and (6) miscellaneous deficiencies (22%). Within this subgroup, 9% of the investigators were found to have committed serious violations requiring a written statement of correction. For-cause investigations were launched on 4% of the clinical investigators who were audited. In comparing these statistics with those summarizing inspections occurring from July 1977 to June 1981, a significantly greater number of deficiencies were found in the former group in four out of six categories.[4] This trend coincides with the implementation of the IRB regulations, which not only established new standards for informed consent documents but also heightened awareness of research practices and, hence, raised expectations regarding the quality of clinical data.

Unless misconduct is suspected, the record review should encompass only those files needed to confirm compliance with the regulations. Internal personnel records, quality assurance audit reports, and financial agreements with the sponsor are not routinely subject to inspection. Although it is not required, the question of whether to make records such as quality assurance reports or other clinically related documents available to an inspector is a difficult one. Providing documentation of all aspects of the research process does allow the inspector to gain a better understanding of the process by which data have been acquired. That insight is useful in distinguishing between investigators who may be guilty of misconduct and those who have made a genuine effort to comply with the spirit of the regulations. However, investigators who make their internal records available to sponsors should recognize that they are giving up an important legal right to confidentiality of documents generated solely to facilitate the internal functioning of the research activity. The investigator who does make these records available must be prepared to defend any actions he took or failed to take regarding possible protocol violations noted in such documents. If he is prepared to do so, releasing internal records may provide a valuable basis for discussing with the inspector the research procedures that were followed in the study. The chapters on data management discuss at length how a team's written records should be prepared to reflect the process by which research decisions were made and errors rectified. Those chapters should help an investigator to determine whether important internal records have been prepared with the care necessary to be of value in the inspection. The authors have found the inspectors quite willing to be shown supporting methods of data documentation. If a key document could not be located, data gathered by the standard method on a different case have often been accepted as documentation that appropriate data-management procedures were in place.

Records or documents that are subject to inspection but are reported as misplaced may arouse suspicion that some information relevant to the study is not being revealed. Although it is understandable that mishaps may occur in processing large volumes of clinical and regulatory paper work, this problem can be avoided with careful preparation. The ideal time to undertake a complete review of the study files is not just prior to the announced inspection but rather just as the study is concluding. A staff member familiar with the study, or even a representative of the sponsor, can be engaged to conduct a mock audit of the records to determine that all files are complete and in order. Copies of laboratory reports, IRB approval letters, or other documents that cannot be located must then be obtained from the responsible department. The investigator's manual of the Bristol Myers Company prepared by Mariana G. Wilke[5] contains an excellent detailed checklist useful in preparing for an inspection. Tables 46 and 47 are abstracted from this source.

In a routine inspection, agency personnel may review and take copies of subjects' files from which identifying facts (such as names and hospital numbers) have been deleted. While it is advisable to be as cooperative as possible in supplying the agency with information needed to conduct the audit, it is also the team's responsibility to limit dissemination of identifying subject information strictly to circumstances in which its release is truly necessary. Additionally, detailed records should be maintained of whatever photocopied documents are provided to the agency. Ordering a second copy of all the released records that can be maintained in the investigator's file is perhaps the most accurate method of securing such documentation. Audits being conducted for cause give the agency the authority to take copies of records containing information identifying subjects if the FDA has reason to believe that the subjects do not exist or that informed consent was not obtained.

EXIT INTERVIEW

At the conclusion of the inspection, the inspector will meet with the investigator and employees to present his findings. If he has observed any practices that may constitute violations, he will record these on an FD 483 form, which is presented to the PI at the conclusion of the audit. The ensuing discussion gives the investigator the opportunity to clarify any misinterpretations or other errors that the inspector may have made in reviewing the data. This interview also allows the investigator to point out any improvements that have been made in his research efforts in subsequent studies. Although agency personnel are instructed not to adopt the role of consultant in recommending corrective actions certain to satisfy the FDA, they do have valuable insight into the research process, which they may be willing to share for educational purposes. The FDA inspection inevitably results in the team's developing better methods of rectifying specific problems that have been mentioned in the audit. If an FD 483 form is issued, the original document will be left with the investigator. Since inspection reports are subject to the Freedom of Information Act and can be obtained by any sponsor, it is advisable for the investigator to issue a written response to each item in question recorded on the form. This response should be directed to the FDA district manager in whose geographical region the site falls. This address can be obtained from the inspector. Each item cited on the form should be mentioned in the investigator's response, indicating whether the deficiency has been corrected or whether the investigator disagrees with the inspector's assessment. This response, together with the inspector's more detailed report, will be reviewed at a supervisory level within the FDA and a determination made of any further agency action required. As was mentioned earlier, the great majority of FDA inspections reveal no deficiencies requiring regulatory action.

TYPES OF FINDINGS

The results of FDA audits are evaluated and classified as follows: "(1) free of deficiencies and, therefore, entirely satisfactory, (2) generally acceptable but with deficiencies requiring modifications, (3) containing serious deficiencies that require a detailed response in writing from the investigator indicating whether and, if so, how the problem has been corrected, or (4) containing serious deficiencies that merit a further, detailed audit 'for cause.' "[6] The subsequent for-cause investigations determine whether an investigator will be restricted from conducting some types of research involving regulated products or will be disqualified altogether from participating in research on new drugs. Investigators found guilty of fraud or serious misconduct may be prosecuted through the Department of Justice.

The FDA inspection process is an important component of drug regulation that reinforces the importance of adhering to established research techniques in conducting research on human subjects. While investigators may encounter agency personnel of diverse attitudes and levels of experience, they can be certain that the critical aspects of protocol execution, namely, subject recruitment and selection, safety monitoring, and drug administration procedures, will be closely scrutinized in any inspection. They will also discover that an assessment of the investigator's compliance with the regulations will be made exclusively on the written records of the study. Statements of intentions or procedures will be accorded little legitimacy if the written records reveal that those practices were consistently violated. The investigator who is anxious to expedite the audit process will be successful only if he carefully monitors research record keeping while the study is actually being conducted. The investigator must also recognize that although the sponsor can be recruited to conduct reviews of data and assist in organizing records for an inspection, the ultimate responsibility for the integrity of the study rests with the research team. While the investigator should avail himself of the sponsor's resources and expertise, he should, nevertheless, be prepared to be held accountable for the completeness and accuracy of all records subject to inspection.

REFERENCES

1. Nightengale, S.L., The Food and Drug Administration's role in the protection of human subjects, *IRB* **5**:6–9 (January/February), 1983.
2. Shapiro, M.E., and Charrow, R.P., Scientific misconduct in investigational drug trials, *N. Engl. J. Med.* **312**:731–736, 1985.
3. Ross, N., FDA inspections: The limits of authority, *Pharmaceut. Technol.* March:64–70, 1984.
4. Shapiro, M.E., and Charrow, R.P., Scientific misconduct in investigational drug trials, *N. Engl. J. Med.* **312**:731–736, 1985.
5. Wilke, M.G., *Investigator's Manual: Good Clinical Practice in the Conduct of Drug Studies*, Bristol Myers Company, New York, June 1982.
6. Shapiro, M.E., and Charrow, R.P., Scientific misconduct in investigational drug trials, *N. Engl. J. Med.* **312**:731–736, 1985.

SECTION IX
Appendixes

APPENDIX A
Glossary

This list includes abbreviations, definitions of terms with special meaning, and some jargon.

Abbreviated new drug application (ANDA). A submission to the FDA proposing to introduce a generic version of a commercially available product. The generic manufacturer is required to provide data on bioequivalency and manufacturing plans but is not required to conduct clinical trials to establish safety and effectiveness. The data developed by the firm that introduced the patented product are considered adequate to confirm the generic product's safety and efficacy profile.

Adverse drug reaction (ADR). Any new occurrence during the use of an agent or for a reasonable time thereafter that is considered related to the drug.

Adverse on-therapy experience (AOTE). The term used in the pharmaceutical industry to refer to adverse clinical or laboratory events occurring during a drug trial. The term is used most often when the abnormality referred to is of unknown etiology.

Alanine aminotransferase (ALT). Also referred to as the SGPT, this is a laboratory test commonly used to assess liver function.

Ames test. A test of mutagenicity conducted on drugs. The ability of the test agent to alter gene structure is tested using bacteria that reproduce rapidly. The agent and the major metabolic products produced by rodents are tested in this system. The answer is available in a few weeks.

Annual review. The IRB's yearly review of a research project in which the board considers whether the research should be allowed to continue for another approval period. Under FDA regulation, IRB review of ongoing projects must be conducted at least annually.

Aspartate aminotransferase (AST). Also referred to as the SGOT, this is a laboratory test commonly used to assess liver function.

Biologics. A product such as a virus, blood product, or toxin that is produced in living cells or animals. Biologics being used for the diagnosis and treatment of human disease are subject to FDA regulation.

Bioresearch Monitoring Program. The program under which FDA inspects investigators, IRBs, and sponsors conducting research involving regulated drugs, devices, and biologics.

Blind. Refers to the method by which the identity of the test or control agent in a study is concealed from the subject and the investigator. Maintaining the blind requires that all conditions preventing the investigator or the subject from knowing the identity of a subject's test drug be maintained throughout the study.

Case report form (CRF).   Form developed by a sponsor or an investigator on which all data are transmitted to the sponsor and subsequently to the FDA. Computer-compatible forms are being used increasingly.

Clinical research associate (CRA).   The term used in the industry to designate the person who administratively supervises clinical investigators, always performing some of this supervision in the field. A similar person working with the investigator as his employee is designated study coordinator or study technician.

Code of federal regulations (CFR).   A publication of all permanent rules of the executive branch and agencies of the federal government. The code contains 50 titles that cover general areas subject to federal regulation. Title 21 contains the FDA and DEA regulations; Title 45 contains those of the DHHS.

Collaborator.   The personnel listed on the FDA 1572/3 forms as being involved in administering study medication to subjects. These individuals are considered associates of the principal investigator and function under his direction.

Compassionate use.   The continuation of a subject on an investigational agent because a unique therapeutic effect was identified for the subject during the trial. Such use is allowed under a special protocol developed with the sponsor.

Compliance.   All measurable aspects of adherence to a protocol. May refer to the ingestion of medication, keeping of visits, or avoidance of prohibited medications or alcohol.

Conditional approval.   Designation often used by the IRB indicating that approval is granted providing a condition is met. Usually this is a change in the wording of the protocol, the deletion of a portion, or the addition of a safety feature.

Contract firm.   An independent organization that conducts research activities such as clinical or laboratory testing or designs research programs for the pharmaceutical industry. Ordinarily contract firms are for-profit enterprises that perform these services on a specific project for a fee.

Control(s).   The subject or group of subjects receiving the standard therapy being compared with the test agent in a clinical trial.

Control drug.   The standard therapy or placebo against which study medication will be compared in a drug trial.

Controlled substance.   Refers to any addicting or behavior-modifying agents regulated by the DEA.

Cross-over design.   A study design in which each subject acts as his own control. Subjects are assigned to receive the test and control medications in some order determined by the randomization sequence. Subjects and investigators are blinded to which medication is being administered, and there is usually a washout period between phases.

Declaration of Helsinki.   One of the significant documents in the field of human experimentation defining the rights of the participant and the obligations of the investigator.

Department of Health and Human Services (DHHS).   That branch of the federal government containing both the FDA and the NIH.

Department of Health, Education, and Welfare (DHEW).   An earlier designation for the division of the federal government containing the FDA and the NIH. The DHHS essentially replaced this agency in 1980.

Device. A manufactured device being used for medical purposes that is attached to or implanted in the body. Devices are subject to FDA regulation.

Double-blind. A type of study design in which neither the research team nor the test subject knows whether he is receiving the test medication or a control. Study supplies are coded and packaged specially to ensure that the control drug resembles the study medication as closely as possible in taste, color, and shape.

Dropped. The formal discontinuation of a patient from a protocol. The term does not indicate the basis for withdrawal or imply poor performance on the part of any participant or investigator.

Drug Enforcement Administration (DEA). The agency that regulates the use of controlled substances and has some jurisdiction over their use in research.

Emergency use. This term is applied to an emergency situation when an investigator wishes to administer an investigational medication to a patient when the protocol involved has not been approved by the IRB or the patient does not meet the protocol requirements. The emergency use of the medication is permitted in life-threatening circumstances in which commercially available treatment alternatives have failed or do not exist.

Enrollment. The final process of entering the subject into a protocol, signifying that the subject and the PI are fully satisfied that this is an appropriate action. Both have agreed to become collaborators in the conduct of the research.

Exclusion criteria. The list of characteristics specified in the protocol that prohibit a patient from entering a study. They may include medical restrictions, such as laboratory abnormalities, or behavioral characteristics, such as unwillingness to sign an informed consent form. These, combined with the inclusion criteria, define the population under study.

FDA 1572/3 forms. Forms filed by the investigator with the sponsor, who in turn forwards them to the FDA, indicating that the requirements of drug investigation are understood by the PI and the qualifications to conduct the study are met. All other professionals who participate in the investigation are listed and all locations at which the study will be conducted are specified. The FDA 1572 form is submitted for Phase II investigations and the FDA 1573 form is submitted for Phase III and IV investigations.

FDA 1639 form. Form filed by the investigator via the sponsor summarizing an adverse drug reaction that has been observed in the study.

FDA 482 form. Form given to the PI by an FDA inspector notifying him of the inspection.

FDA 483 form. The form issued to a PI by an FDA inspector notifying him of any regulatory violations the inspector has observed during the audit.

Final report. A summary of the study results that an investigator must present to the IRB within three months of a study's conclusion.

Food and Drug Administration (FDA). Refers to the agency, its regulations, and all representative employees. FDA employees who audit clinical investigators in the field are designated inspectors.

For-cause investigation. The type of inspection the FDA conducts on an investigator when the agency suspects fabrication of data or violation of informed consent regulations.

Health maintenance organization (HMO). A nonprofit or business organization that delivers health care to a specific population on a prepaid plan. Increasingly, HMOs are conducting drug and device evaluations.

Human research committee. Synonym for IRB.

Human rights committee. Synonym for IRB.

Inclusion criteria. Essential features that the patient must possess to be included in a study.

Indication. A disease or condition for which a drug has been approved by the FDA. Approved indications are listed in the *Physician's Desk Reference* and may be included in any promotional materials prepared on the product.

Informed consent. The process in which the investigator and the patient engage in dialogue regarding the risks and benefits of a research project and the patient's rights as a prospective subject. This process is documented when the subject signs the informed consent form and agrees to participate.

Institutional review board (IRB). Sometimes referred to as a peer review committee, this board is composed of clinicians, scientists in related fields, laymen, and experts in ethics charged with overseeing safety and making risk–benefit judgments of all research on human subjects.

Intercurrent illness. A term used infrequently in the pharmaceutical industry to refer to adverse clinical or laboratory events that occur while a patient is on study but are clearly related to some underlying disease.

Investigational new drug exemption (IND). An application in which a sponsor requests permission to conduct clinical testing on a new investigational product or new use of an available product. INDs may be filed by either pharmaceutical firms or individual investigators. The submission consists of a page or two and must be acted upon by the FDA within 30 days. IND submission forms may be obtained from the FDA.

Investigator's brochure or manual. A compilation of the animal and clinical data on a new drug that is provided to an investigator to allow him to make an informed decision about the safety of an agent and its anticipated side effects. This brochure is also provided to the IRB for review. Also referred to as an Investigational Use Circular.

Kefauver–Harris amendment. Congressional act issued in 1962 that requires state-of-the-art comparison trials to show drug efficacy. This is the law that led to the requirement of blinded controlled trials in clinical evaluation.

Labeling. The description of a drug and summaries of its proposed usage, safety, and effectiveness in specific diseases. The labeling of a new drug must be approved by the FDA at the time that the NDA is reviewed. Sponsors are not allowed to deviate from the approved labeling in any promotional claims made to physicians and patients.

LD_{50}. The dose of a drug that is lethal to 50% of the animal test population. An important concept in evaluation of toxicity of a drug in animal testing.

Legally authorized representative. As defined by state law, the individual who is authorized to act on behalf of the research subject in the event that the latter is not of legal age or competent to consent to participation in a research project.

Logs. A general term applied to chronological written records of study-related transactions. Examples are logs of blood specimens sent to the lab, appointment books summarizing patients' visits, or logs documenting honoraria provided to patients.

Medical monitor. The physician at the sponsoring pharmaceutical firm who has medical authority for a given drug investigation. This physician usually has the most current information on side effects observed with the medication and has the authority to discontinue a patient from study, break codes, or authorize expenditures for additional diagnostic testing of observed toxicity. The telephone numbers of the medical monitor are usually prominently displayed in the protocol.

National Commission for the Protection of Human Subjects of Biomedical and Behavioral Research. A special commission that was assembled in 1974 to make recommendations to the Department of Health and Human Services regarding the regulation of clinical investigation. This commission contributed greatly to the 1981 regulations governing IRBs.

National Institutes of Health (NIH). The branch of the DHHS that contains the National Cancer Institute, the National Institutes of Allergies and Infectious Diseases (NIAID), and other institutes funding and conducting studies in fields of interest to the public health. The NIH issues general research policy on behalf of all of its agencies.

New drug application (NDA). The application that the sponsor files with the FDA requesting permission to market a new drug for the treatment or diagnosis of specific illnesses. This application contains extensive documentation. The application contains safety information from extensive animal toxicological studies, manufacturing information, and the results of pharmacology and clinical trials in humans.

Nuremberg Code. The code of ethics governing human experimentation that was issued following the trials of Nazi war criminals in Nuremberg. This document remains one of the important codes in the field of clinical investigation.

Office for Protection from Research Risks (OPRR). A branch of the NIH charged with sponsoring studies and investigation of subjects' involvement in clinical trials. The OPRR has been involved in the development of the IRB regulations and those governing special populations.

Open-label. A type of study design in which the agent being given to the subjects is known to both the investigator and the subjects. No placebo is used.

Orphan drug. A drug that is recognized as valuable but having limited market potential. Sponsors have few incentives to undertake the R&D programs needed to bring these drugs to market and generally make them available under research protocols to investigators wishing to obtain them for their patients. Separate regulations have been developed over the past few years to reduce the burdens of regulatory submission for this special class of drugs.

Over-the-counter drugs (OTC). Drugs that can be purchased without a prescription.

Parallel. A type of study design in which two or more groups of subjects are assigned to receive either test or control medication for their entire period of study and are followed on the same protocol.

Peer review. Synonym for the IRB review process.

Physician's Desk Reference (PDR). A proprietary advertisement given free to all practicing physicians that contains approved labeling information on prescription drug products. A separate publication is available on over-the-counter products. Each entry on a product contains information on the indications for usage of the drug, warnings and contraindications, and toxicity data. Photographs of products are included and lists are provided of the dosage strengths and forms in which they are provided.

Phase. Drug investigation is conducted in four phases that reflect the level of knowledge about the agent being studied. Phase I trials are the earliest human trials, usually of pharmacology and dose range. Phase II are the earliest trials conducted in a diseased population. Phase II investigations are performed to determine a drug's safety and efficacy in the target population and to assess whether the dose selected for study is appropriate to treat the disease. Phase III trials are the large safety and efficacy studies conducted in the diseased population. Phase IV studies are the postmarketing surveillance trials conducted to monitor for new toxicity. Phase IV trials may also include studies of the drug's use in new indications. The term phase also may refer to a segment of a cross-over study, e.g., "In the first phase, subjects will receive drug A. In the second, they will receive drug B."

Pioneer drug firm. A drug firm that develops new compounds for testing in animals and all four phases of clinical investigation. In contrast, generic drug manufacturers conduct no R&D on new entities but rather limit their activities to the manufacturing of generic equivalents to brand-name medications.

Principal investigator (PI). The chief medical administrator of a clinical trial, responsible for both the quality of protocol execution and compliance with all FDA regulations and record-keeping requirements. The PI is usually a physician or Doctor of Pharmacy qualified to undertake clinical investigation and administer investigational drugs to subjects. A PI must be named at each institution conducting a particular protocol. That individual must sign the FDA 1572/3 form agreeing to take overall responsibility for the study within that institution. More than one PI may be named at an institution if the responsibility for the study will be shared by a few qualified physicians. In such arrangements, the participants are referred to as coprincipal investigators.

Postmarketing surveillance. Research or surveys conducted after a drug has been approved for marketing to identify any rare adverse reactions that may not have emerged while the drug was being used in the research setting. Postmarketing surveillance may involve protocols to collect data on toxicities of particular concern to the manufacturer or the FDA. Surveillance also includes telephone hot-lines to collect data on spontaneous reporting of adverse experiences by physicians using a drug in practice.

Protocol. The detailed description of all of the activities of the investigation. The exact inclusion and exclusion criteria for patient selection, the tests to be performed, the medications to be administered, and the design of the study are included.

Public Health Service. The branch of the DHHS that contains the Centers for Disease Control, the NIH, and the FDA.

Quality assurance. A program conducted within the research group for self-evaluation of its performance.

Recycling. The practice of utilizing the same patient over and over again in various protocols to facilitate recruitment.

Referring physician.   A physician providing routine medical care to a patient who participates in bringing the patient into a research protocol.

Regulatory documents.   All of the forms that are required for the conduct of drug or device research, including those submitted to the sponsor for the FDA, those required by local regulation, and those submitted to the IRB.

Research and development (R&D).   The division of a pharmaceutical firm involved in developing new compounds.

Risk–benefit assessment.   The process by which the relative risks and benefits of participating in a clinical trial are identified and compared. The risk–benefit assessment is the cornerstone of the IRB process and is also discussed in the context of informed consent in which prospective subjects evaluate the merits and disadvantages associated with a particular project.

Side effects.   Synonym for adverse reactions.

Single-blind.   A type of study design in which the subject is not informed as to whether he is receiving the test agent or a placebo but the investigator does know.

Special population.   A group of prospective subjects, such as the elderly, prisoners, or children, who are considered deserving of special protection to preserve their rights. Special precautions are often taken to mitigate their impaired decision-making capacity, the pressures of incarceration, or their legal status as minors.

Stable of subjects.   A group of subjects to whom the PI provides all medical services gratis to facilitate recruitment.

Standard operating procedure (SOP).   A written procedure for staff members outlining the steps in which an activity is to be carried out and the decision-making authority for certain actions. These are the standards by which a research team should aspire to have its performance judged.

Study coordinator.   The assistant to the PI in the conduct of the study.

Supplemental new drug application (SNDA).   Sponsors file an SNDA with the FDA to request approval for new indications, manufacturing changes, or labeling changes for a prescription product that is already on the market.

Variance.   A permitted deviation from the protocol. This permission is granted in discussion with the medical monitor and should be documented in writing.

Verbal approval.   Verbal permission to undertake an experimental intervention for which there is no time to secure written authorization. IRBs and sponsors may be asked to offer verbal approval for specific procedures, depending on the nature of the emergency. Verbal permissions should always be explained in a written note in the research record, listing the authority who gave approval and any exception involved. Ideally, this approval should be confirmed in writing as soon as possible after it is given.

Vulnerable subject.   A subject who, because of his economic status, race, or social position, is considered especially vulnerable to coercion to participate in a research project. The special populations described above fall into this category and are considered deserving of special protection to preserve their rights.

Waxman–Hatch Act.   A 1984 act of Congress that extended the patent life for exclusivity in marketing a drug by approximately the same number of years that the regulatory process consumed (three or four years). The act also defined the bioequivalence of some generic products and eliminated many barriers to the introduction of new generic products into the market.

Window. The interval during which a scheduled visit must occur to be in compliance with the protocol. Allowable visit windows are ordinarily listed in a protocol to establish the maximum deviation from the visit schedule that will not compromise the statistical validity of the study.

Adverse Reaction Report

DEPARTMENT OF HEALTH AND HUMAN SERVICES
PUBLIC HEALTH SERVICE
FOOD AND DRUG ADMINISTRATION (HFN-730)
ROCKVILLE, MD 20857

ADVERSE REACTION REPORT
(Drugs and Biologics)

Form Approved: OMB No. 0910-0230.

FDA
CONTROL NO.

ACCESSION
NO.

I.	REACTION INFORMATION						

1. PATIENT ID/INITIALS *(In Confidence)*	2. AGE YRS.	3. SEX	4.-6. REACTION ONSET			8.-12. CHECK ALL APPROPRIATE:
			MO.	DA.	YR.	

7. DESCRIBE REACTION(S)

☐ PATIENT DIED

☐ REACTION TREATED WITH Rx DRUG

☐ RESULTED IN, OR PROLONGED, INPATIENT HOSPITALIZATION

☐ RESULTED IN PERMANENT DISABILITY

13. RELEVANT TESTS/LABORATORY DATA

☐ NONE OF THE ABOVE

II.	SUSPECT DRUG(S) INFORMATION

14. SUSPECT DRUG(S) *(Give manufacturer and lot no. for vaccines/biologics)*

20. DID REACTION ABATE AFTER STOPPING DRUG?

15. DAILY DOSE | 16 ROUTE OF ADMINISTRATION

☐ YES   ☐ NO   ☐ NA

17. INDICATION(S) FOR USE

21. DID REACTION REAPPEAR AFTER REINTRODUCTION?

18. DATES OF ADMINISTRATION *(From/To)* | 19 DURATION OF ADMINISTRATION

☐ YES   ☐ NO   ☐ NA

III.	CONCOMITANT DRUGS AND HISTORY

22. CONCOMITANT DRUGS AND DATES OF ADMINISTRATION *(Exclude those used to treat reaction)*

23. OTHER RELEVANT HISTORY *(e.g. diagnoses, allergies, pregnancy with LMP, etc.)*

IV.	ONLY FOR REPORTS SUBMITTED BY MANUFACTURER	V.	INITIAL REPORTER *(In confidence)*

24. NAME AND ADDRESS OF MANUFACTURER *(Include Zip Code)*

26.-26a. NAME AND ADDRESS OF REPORTER *(Include Zip Code)*

24a. IND/NDA. NO. FOR SUSPECT DRUG | 24b. MFR. CONTROL NO.

26b. TELEPHONE NO. *(Include area code)*

24c. DATE RECEIVED BY MANUFACTURER | 24d. REPORT SOURCE *(Check all that apply)*
☐ FOREIGN ☐ STUDY ☐ LITERATURE
☐ HEALTH PROFESSIONAL ☐ CONSUMER

26c. HAVE YOU ALSO REPORTED THIS REACTION TO THE MANUFACTURER?
☐ YES   ☐ NO

25 15 DAY REPORT?
☐ YES   ☐ NO

25a. REPORT TYPE
☐ INITIAL ☐ FOLLOWUP

26d. ARE YOU A HEALTH PROFESSIONAL?
☐ YES   ☐ NO

Submission of a report does not necessarily constitute an admission that the drug caused the adverse reaction.

NOTE: Required of manufacturers by 21 CFR 314.80

FORM FDA 1639 (7 86)   PREVIOUS EDITION MAY BE USED.

INSTRUCTIONS FOR COMPLETING FORM FDA - 1639

GENERAL

- o Use a separate Form FDA - 1639 for each patient.
- o Additional pages may be attached if space provided on the Form FDA - 1639 is inadequate.
- o Non-manufacturers should send forms to the Food and Drug Administration, Division of Epidemiology and Surveillance, HFN-730, 5600 Fishers Lane, Rockville, MD 20857.
- o For questions call: 301 - 443-4580.
- o Patient and initial reporter identification is held in confidence by the FDA and is not subject to release under the Freedom of Information Act.
- o Reports of serious, suspect reactions are encouraged.

SPECIFIC INSTRUCTIONS

I. Reaction Information

Item 2. Age - For children under 5 years of age, also write date of birth (DOB) in Item 1. For congenital malformations, give the age and sex of the infant (even though the mother was exposed).

Item 7. Describe Reaction(s) - Give signs and/or symptoms, diagnoses, course, etc. Underline the single most important descriptive phrase.

II. Suspect Drug Information

Item 14. Suspect Drug - The trade name is preferred. If a generically produced product is involved, the manufacturer should be identified.

Item 15. Dose - For pediatric patients, also give body weights.

Item 20 and 21. NA - is defined as nonapplicable (e.g. when only one dose given or outcome was irreversible).

V. Initial Reporter

Item 26c. Have you also reported this reaction to the manufacturer? Your answer facilitates identification of duplicates in the central adverse reaction file. FDA encourages direct reporting even if a report has been submitted to the manufacturer.

NOTE TO MANUFACTURERS (Refer to 21 CFR 314.80) Detailed instructions are contained in the "Guideline for Postmarketing Reporting of Adverse Drug Reactions."

* U.S.GPO:1986-0-491-338/55173

Statement of Investigator

DEPARTMENT OF HEALTH AND HUMAN SERVICES
PUBLIC HEALTH SERVICE
FOOD AND DRUG ADMINISTRATION

STATEMENT OF INVESTIGATOR

Form approved; OMB No. 0910-0013
Expiration Date   *Still in use

Note: No drug may be shipped or study initiated unless a completed statement has been received *(21 CFR 312.1(a)(12))*.

TO: SUPPLIER OF DRUG *(Name, address, and Zip Code)*

Super Drug Company
100 Alameda Boulevard
Chicago, IL 90009

NAME OF INVESTIGATOR *(Print or Type)*
John D. Jones, M.D.

DATE
April 30, 1986

NAME OF DRUG
Drug XX   Protocol XX-901

Dear Sir:

The undersigned, John D. Jones, M.D. submits this statement as required by section 505(i) of the Federal Food, Drug, and Cosmetic Act and §312.1 of Title 21 of the Code of Federal Regulations as a condition for receiving and conducting clinical investigations with a new drug limited by Federal *(or United States)* law to investigational use.

1. THE FOLLOWING IS A STATEMENT OF MY EDUCATION AND EXPERIENCE.

a. COLLEGES, UNIVERSITIES, AND MEDICAL OR OTHER PROFESSIONAL SCHOOLS ATTENDED, WITH DATES OF ATTENDANCE, DEGREES, AND DATES DEGREES WERE AWARDED

See curriculum vitae

b. POSTGRADUATE MEDICAL OR OTHER PROFESSIONAL TRAINING. GIVE DATES, NAMES OF INSTITUTIONS, AND NATURE OF TRAINING.

See curriculum vitae

c. TEACHING OR RESEARCH EXPERIENCE. GIVE DATES, INSTITUTIONS, AND BRIEF DESCRIPTION OF EXPERIENCE.

See curriculum vitae

d. EXPERIENCE IN MEDICAL PRACTICE OR OTHER PROFESSIONAL EXPERIENCE. GIVE DATES, INSTITUTIONAL AFFILIATIONS, NATURE OF PRACTICE, OR OTHER PROFESSIONAL EXPERIENCE.

See curriculum vitae

e. REPRESENTATIVE LIST OF PERTINENT MEDICAL OR OTHER SCIENTIFIC PUBLICATIONS. GIVE TITLES OF ARTICLES, NAME OF PUBLICATIONS AND VOLUME, PAGE NUMBER, AND DATE.

See curriculum vitae

IF THIS INFORMATION HAS PREVIOUSLY BEEN SUBMITTED TO THE SPONSOR, IT MAY BE REFERRED TO AND ANY ADDITIONS MADE TO BRING IT UP-TO-DATE.

FORM FDA 1573 (10/83)   PREVIOUS EDITIONS ARE OBSOLETE.

2a. The investigator assures that an IRB that complies with the requirements set forth in Part 56 of this chapter will be responsible for the initial and continuing review and approval of the proposed clinical study. The investigator also assures that he/she will report to the IRB all changes in the research activity and all unanticipated problems involving risks to human subjects or others, and that he/she will not make any changes in the research that would increase the risks to human subjects without IRB approval. FDA will regard the signing of the Form FDA 1573 as providing the necessary assurances stated above.

b. A description of any clinical laboratory facilities that will be used. (If this information has been submitted to the sponsor and reported by him on Form FDA 1571, reference to the previous submission will be adequate).

3. *The investigational drug will be used by the undersigned or under his supervision in accordance with the plan of investigation described as follows: (Outline the plan of investigation including approximation of the number of subjects to be treated with the drug and the number to be employed as controls, if any; clinical uses to be investigated; characteristics of subjects by age, sex and condition; the kind of clinical observations and laboratory tests to be undertaken prior to, during, and after administration of the drug; the estimated duration of the investigation; and a description or copies of report forms to be used to maintain an adequate record of the observations and test results obtained. This plan may include reasonable alternates and variations and should be supplemented or amended when any significant change in direction or scope of the investigation is undertaken.)*

4. THE UNDERSIGNED UNDERSTANDS THAT THE FOLLOWING CONDITIONS, GENERALLY APPLICABLE TO NEW DRUGS FOR INVESTIGATIONAL USE, GOVERN HIS RECEIPTS AND USE OF THIS INVESTIGATIONAL DRUG:

a. The sponsor is required to supply the investigator with full information concerning the preclinical investigations that justify clinical trials, together with fully informative material describing any prior investigations and experience and any possible hazards, contraindications, side-effects, and precautions to be taken into account in the course of the investigation.

b. The investigator is required to maintain adequate records of the disposition of all receipts of the drug, including dates, quantities, and use by subjects, and if the investigation is terminated, suspended, discontinued, or completed, to return to the sponsor any unused supply of the drug. If the investigational drug is subject to the Comprehensive Drug Abuse Prevention and Control Act of 1970, adequate precautions must be taken including storage of the investigational drug in a securely locked, substantially constructed cabinet, or other securely locked substantially constructed enclosure, access to which is limited, to prevent theft or diversion of the substance into illegal channels of distribution.

c. The investigator is required to prepare and maintain adequate and accurate case histories designed to record all observations and other data pertinent to the investigation on each individual treated with the drug or employed as a control in the investigation.

d. The investigator is required to furnish his reports to the sponsor of the drug who is responsible for collecting and evaluating the results obtained by various investigators. The sponsor is required to present progress reports to the Food and Drug Administration at appropriate intervals not exceeding 1 year. Any adverse effect that may reasonably be regarded as caused by, or probably caused by, the new drug shall be reported to the sponsor promptly, and if the adverse effect is alarming, it shall be reported immediately. An adequate report of the investigation should be furnished to the sponsor shortly after completion of the investigation.

e. The investigator shall maintain the records of disposition of the drug and the case histories described above for a period of 2 years following the date a new-drug application is approved for the drug; or if the application is not approved, until 2 years after the investigation is discontinued. Upon the request of a scientifically trained and properly authorized employee of the Department, at reasonable times, the investigator will make such records available for inspection and copying. The subjects' names need not be divulged unless the records of particular individuals require a more detailed study of the cases, or unless there is reason to believe that the records do not represent actual cases studied, or do not represent actual results obtained.

f. The investigator certifies that the drug will be administered only to subjects under his personal supervision or under the supervision of the following investigators responsible to him,

John Q. Smith, M.D.

_____

and that the drug will not be supplied to any other investigator or to any clinic for administration to subjects.

g. The investigator certifies that he will inform any subjects including subjects used as controls, or their representatives, that drugs are being used for investigational purposes, and will obtain the consent of the subjects, or their representatives, except where this is not feasible or, in the investigator's professional judgment, is contrary to the best interests of the subjects.

h. The investigator is required to assure the sponsor that for investigations subject to an institutional review requirement under Part 56 of this chapter the studies will not be initiated until the institutional review board has reviewed and approved the study. (The organization and procedure requirements for such a board as set forth in Part 56 should be explained to the investigator by the sponsor.)

Very truly yours,

Name of Investigator X Signature _____   John D. Jones, M.D.

Address 111 Freedom Way, Philadelphia, PA 19119   Telephone (215) 555-8097

Secondary Site: 10 Betsy Ross Lane, Ardmore, PA 19111

(This form should be supplemented or amended from time to time if new subjects are added or if significant changes are made in the plan of investigation.)

APPENDIX D
General Reading

Cox, K.R., *Planning Clinical Experiments*, Charles C Thomas, Springfield, IL, 1968.

Friedman, L.M., Furberg, C.D., and DeMets, D.L., *Fundamentals of Clinical Trials* (2nd ed.), PSG Publishing Company, Littleton, 1985.

Kilpatrick, S.J., *Statistical Principles in Health Care Information*, University Park Press, Baltimore, 1973.

Pocock, S.J., *Clinical Trials: A Practical Approach*, John Wiley & Sons, New York, 1983.

Index